High-Functioning Autism/Asperger Syndrome in Schools

The Guilford Practical Intervention in the Schools Series
Kenneth W. Merrell, Series Editor

This series presents the most reader-friendly resources available in key areas of evidence-based practice in school settings. Practitioners will find trustworthy guides on effective behavioral, mental health, and academic interventions, and assessment and measurement approaches. Covering all aspects of planning, implementing, and evaluating high-quality services for students, books in the series are carefully crafted for everyday utility. Features include ready-to-use reproducibles, lay-flat binding to facilitate photocopying, appealing visual elements, and an oversized format.

Helping Students Overcome Depression and Anxiety, Second Edition: A Practical Guide
Kenneth W. Merrell

Inclusive Assessment and Accountability:
A Guide to Accommodations for Students with Diverse Needs
Sara E. Bolt and Andrew T. Roach

Bullying Prevention and Intervention: Realistic Strategies for Schools
Susan M. Swearer, Dorothy L. Espelage, and Scott A. Napolitano

Conducting School-Based Functional Behavioral Assessments, Second Edition:
A Practitioner's Guide
Mark W. Steege and T. Steuart Watson

Evaluating Educational Interventions:
Single-Case Design for Measuring Response to Intervention
T. Chris Riley-Tillman and Matthew K. Burns

Collaborative Home/School Interventions:
Evidence-Based Solutions for Emotional, Behavioral, and Academic Problems
Gretchen Gimpel Peacock and Brent R. Collett

Social and Emotional Learning in the Classroom:
Promoting Mental Health and Academic Success
Kenneth W. Merrell and Barbara A. Gueldner

Executive Skills in Children and Adolescents, Second Edition:
A Practical Guide to Assessment and Intervention
Peg Dawson and Richard Guare

Responding to Problem Behavior in Schools, Second Edition:
The Behavior Education Program
Deanne A. Crone, Leanne S. Hawken, and Robert H. Horner

High-Functioning Autism/Asperger Syndrome in Schools:
Asessment and Intervention
Frank J. Sansosti, Kelly A. Powell-Smith, and Richard J. Cowan

School Discipline and Self-Discipline:
A Practical Guide to Promoting Prosocial Student Behavior
George G. Bear

Response to Intervention, Second Edition: Principles and Strategies for Effective Practice
Rachel Brown-Chidsey and Mark W. Steege

High-Functioning Autism/Asperger Syndrome in Schools

Assessment and Intervention

FRANK J. SANSOSTI
KELLY A. POWELL-SMITH
RICHARD J. COWAN

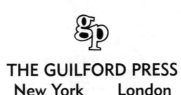

THE GUILFORD PRESS
New York   London

© 2010 The Guilford Press
A Division of Guilford Publications, Inc.
72 Spring Street, New York, NY 10012
www.guilford.com

Printed in Canada

This book is printed on acid-free paper.

Last digit is print number: 9   8   7   6   5   4   3   2   1

Library of Congress Cataloging-in-Publication Data

Sansosti, Frank J.
   High-functioning autism/Asperger syndrome in schools : assessment and intervention / Frank J.
Sansosti, Kelly A. Powell-Smith, Richard J. Cowan.
      p. cm. — (The Guilford practical intervention in the schools series)
   Includes bibliographical references and index.
   ISBN 978-1-60623-670-3 (pbk.: alk. paper)
   1. Autistic children—Education—United States.   2. Autism spectrum disorders   I. Powell-
Smith, Kelly A.   II. Cowan, Richard J.   III. Title.
   LC4718.S26 2010
   371.94—dc22
                                                                            2010007352

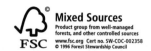

Mixed Sources
Product group from well-managed
forests, and other controlled sources
www.fsc.org Cert no. SW-COC-002358
© 1996 Forest Stewardship Council
FSC

To my wife, Jenine—my successes cannot be understood apart from hers
And to my family, for always believing in my dreams
—F. J. S.

To my husband, Michael, and my children, Hayley and Mitchell,
whose love, understanding, and patience
made finishing this book possible
—K. A. P.-S.

To my parents, Hazel and Gaylen, my sister, Chris,
and other family members, for many years of love and support
—R. J. C.

About the Authors

Frank J. Sansosti, PhD, NCSP, is Assistant Professor in the School Psychology Program at Kent State University. He has extensive experience working with individuals with autism spectrum disorders (ASD) in both school and clinic settings. Prior to his current position, Dr. Sansosti worked as a school psychologist and district-level autism consultant in West Central Florida. While in this role, he provided coaching and technical assistance for early intervention and best-practice approaches for students with ASD in inclusive settings and coordinated efforts between parents, teachers, administrators, and district-level personnel. Dr. Sansosti's primary research and professional interests focus on the development and implementation of behavioral and social skills interventions for young children with ASD, best-practice approaches for the inclusion of students with low-incidence disabilities, and response to intervention. In addition to his research, Dr. Sansosti has been active in conducting professional workshops and presentations for educators working with students with ASD at local, regional, national, and international venues, and he serves as a consultant to multiple school districts.

Kelly A. Powell-Smith, PhD, NCSP, is a senior research scientist with Dynamic Measurement Group, where she conducts research on assessment and intervention related to early childhood language and literacy development. Formerly Associate Professor of School Psychology at the University of South Florida, she spent 12 years training school psychology students in a problem-solving/outcomes-driven approach to service delivery. Dr. Powell-Smith's research interests include using formative assessment data within a problem-solving model for educational decision making, development of early literacy skills, procedures for and outcomes of reintegration, and service delivery to low-incidence populations, including children with Asperger syndrome. She has been a faculty associate of the Florida Center for Reading Research and a consultant with the Eastern Regional Reading First Technical Assistance Center. She has provided formal technical assistance and/or training related to the use of formative assessment and academic interventions in 16 states and in Canada. Over the past 16 years, Dr. Powell-Smith has conducted research related to children with various learning and behavioral difficulties and has led over 150 national, state, and regional workshops and presentations.

Richard J. Cowan, PhD, NCSP, is Associate Professor and Coordinator in the School Psychology Program at Kent State University. Dr. Cowan has been a leader in a number of research projects, publications, presentations, and grants focusing on autism and positive behavior supports. His primary line of inquiry focuses on the development, implementation, and evaluation of academic and behavioral programs for children with ASD. Specifically, he is interested in further investigating the efficacy and utility of various levels of programming (i.e., a range from analogue to naturalistic approaches) to meet the pervasive needs of students with ASD. His research and clinical interests also encompass the implementation and evaluation of positive behavior supports across the universal, targeted, and intensive levels of intervention. In addition to remaining an active researcher and clinician, Dr. Cowan has conducted multiple inservices and workshops at the local, regional, and national levels for a variety of educators and related services personnel.

Preface

There may be no greater challenge facing public educators today than planning for the education of the growing number of students with autism spectrum disorders (ASD). Increased advocacy by parents, lobbyists, professional groups, and celebrities has focused national attention on ASD, with both positive and negative consequences. Subsequently, this attention has affected public schools, as parents increasingly request and, at times, demand state-of-the-art instruction, highly qualified teachers, and extensive support services. Of particular concern is the exponential growth in requests for school-based services for children identified as having high-functioning autism and Asperger syndrome (HFA/AS). Unfortunately, many schools are ill equipped to handle such demands and instead assemble a potpourri of approaches that more often correspond with the latest fad, special education director, or classroom teacher than with contemporary research and practice. Moreover, many educators who work with children with HFA/AS may have limited training or require ongoing professional development related to best-practice strategies. Given decreasing budgets in contemporary education, resources and/or training opportunities are often limited. As a result, schools and districts may find themselves in frequent conflict with outraged parents or, even worse, face due process hearings for failing to meet the academic, behavioral, and social needs of students with HFA/AS.

There is no doubt that the national attention has put pressure on public schools to develop comprehensive programming for students with HFA/AS. However, the picture need not be interpreted as grim. Several decades of research and subsequent practice have identified a variety of effective techniques and strategies that result in lasting student change. Through collaboration, careful planning, and systematic data collection, schools can build systems of supports that not only teach students with HFA/AS skills that enhance academic, behavioral, and social outcomes but also result in positive, productive relationships with families.

This book provides answers and practical solutions to the common questions and concerns posed to us by countless educators, administrators, and student support personnel who work with children and youth with ASD. Specifically, this book provides straightforward "how-to" information to assist in the development of prevention and intervention efforts to meet the academic, behavioral, and social needs of students with HFA/AS. Information shared within this book is based on our practical as well as theoretical and research knowledge about individuals with ASD. Throughout the book are numerous examples, forms, and other reproducible materials to assist educators in daily practice.

Contents

1. Introduction: What Is High-Functioning Autism/Asperger Syndrome?   1

Diagnostic Definitions/Issues   2
Contemporary Conceptualization of HFA/AS   3
Developmental Course   4
  Preschool Years   4
  Elementary School   5
  Middle/High School   7
  Long-Term Outcomes   9
Prevalence   9
  Epidemiology   9
  Educational Placement and Service Delivery Trends   10
Looking Ahead   11

2. Areas of Impairment   13
with REBECCA L. FRITSCHIE

Overview   14
Core Areas of Impairment   14
  Social Interactions   15
  Behavioral Rigidity and Circumscribed Interests   17
  Language and Communication Abilities   19
Associated Areas of Impairment   20
  Responses to Sensory Stimuli   20
  Academic Performance Difficulties   21
  Sleep Disturbances   23
  Motor Abilities   24
  Anxiety and Depression   24
Theoretical Frameworks for Understanding Areas of Impairment   25
  Theory of Mind   25
  Executive Functioning   27
  Central Coherence   28
Conclusion   29

3. Consultation and Collaboration Efforts   **31**

Overview   31
The Ecological Model of School-Based Services   32
The Roles of Parents and Other Key Stakeholders   34
   Parents as Primary Stakeholders   34
   Educators and Student Support Services Personnel as Key Stakeholders   35
   Other Health Professionals and Community-Based Providers as Key Stakeholders   36
Collaborative Problem Solving as a Foundation for Effective Practice   37
Conjoint Behavioral Consultation   40
   Conjoint Needs Identification   41
   Conjoint Needs Analysis   41
   Plan Implementation   42
   Conjoint Plan Evaluation   42
CBC Case Study: Alex   43
Conclusion   45

4. Conducting a Comprehensive Assessment   **46**

Overview   46
Traditional School-Based Assessment   46
Assessing Intellectual Functioning   48
   Issues in Intellectual Assessment   48
   Considerations in Selecting a Cognitive Measure   50
   Measures of Intellectual Functioning   51
Assessing Academic Skills   51
   Traditional Academic Measures   51
   Curriculum-Based Assessment   54
Assessing Adaptive Behavior   61
Assessing Diagnostic Characteristics of HFA/AS   62
Assessing Behavioral Skills   64
   Functional Behavioral Assessment   64
Assessing Social Skills   71
   Interviews   72
   Observations   72
   Rating Scales   74
Assessing Emotional Difficulties   77
Conclusion   78

5. Improving Academic Skills   **80**

Overview   80
General Strategies   81
   Task Presentation   81
   Teacher Communication   82
   Priming   84
   Assignments   84
   Homework and Study Skills   85
Specific Strategies   87
   Reading Support   87
   Writing Support   95
   Math Support   97
Conclusion   101

6. Providing Behavioral Supports   **102**

Overview   102
Effective Behavioral Support   103
Preventative Approaches   104
  Environmental Modifications   104
  Choice and Preference   106
  Visual Supports   106
Direct Intervention Strategies   113
  Teaching Replacement Behaviors   113
  Providing Contingent Positive Reinforcement   114
  Contingency Agreements and Behavioral Contracts   118
  Token Economies   120
  Self-Management   122
Conclusion   125

7. Enhancing Social Skills   **126**

Overview   126
Programming for Social Skills in Schools   127
Schoolwide (Primary) Approaches   128
  Schoolwide Positive Behavior Support   128
  Character Education   130
  Large-Group Social Skills Instruction   131
Small-Group (Secondary) Approaches   133
  Social Skills Groups   133
  Peer-Mediated Approaches   137
Individualized Approaches   143
  Social Stories™   143
  Video Modeling   145
  Power Cards   148
The Future of Social Skills Interventions   149
Conclusion   151

8. Using the Individualized Education Program as a Vehicle   **153**
for Problem-Solving Service Delivery
with JENINE M. SANSOSTI

Overview   153
IEP as Problem-Solving Vehicle   155
Step 1: Problem Identification—Describing Present Levels of Performance   157
  General Considerations   158
  Specific Considerations   160
Step 2: Problem Analysis—Clarifying Areas of Educational Need   162
Step 3: Intervention/Instructional Planning—Goals, Services, and Placement   163
  Goals and Objectives   164
  Service Delivery   169
  Educational Placement   172
  Transition Planning   175
Step 4: Progress Monitoring—Evaluating IEP Outcomes   176
Tools for Enhancing the Quality and Functionality of IEPs   178
Conclusion   180

9. Collecting Data, Evaluating Outcomes, and Ensuring Success   **181**
with JULIE E. GOLDYN

Overview   181
The Importance of Data Collection (Why Collect Data?)   182
Data Collection Process   183
   Step 1: Identify a Target Behavior   183
   Step 2: Define the Target Behavior   183
   Step 3: Determine How to Collect Data   184
   Step 4: Develop an Action Plan   195
How Much Data Should Be Collected?   198
   Baseline Data Considerations   198
   Intervention Phase   198
Factors That Influence Data Collection   199
Graphing Data   200
Methods for Evaluating Data   201
   Visual Analysis   201
Ensuring Success: Maintenance and Generalization   205
   Programming for Maintenance   205
   Programming for Generalization   205
Conclusion   207

Appendix. Reproducible Forms   **209**

References   **231**

Index   **251**

CHAPTER 1

Introduction

What Is High-Functioning Autism/Asperger Syndrome?

STUDENT SNAPSHOT: Marco

Marco is a third-grade student who just began school at Harding Elementary School. During his first 2 weeks of school, his teacher, Mrs. Barton, described him as polite and extremely intelligent. Specifically, Mrs. Barton indicated that Marco spoke very eloquently, had excellent reading skills, and appeared to possess great knowledge of the solar system. As Mrs. Barton interacted more with Marco, she noticed characteristics that were not typical of other students in her classroom. For example, she noticed that Marco had difficulty holding a conversation with other students and teachers despite his extensive vocabulary. Mrs. Barton also said that Marco often exited conversations if they were not about a subject that interested him. On occasion, Marco would stop talking in the middle of a lengthy conversation, usually midsentence. At times, he could be coaxed to finish what he was saying, but more often, he refused and became annoyed, telling everyone to "Shut up!" and "Leave me alone!" as he rapidly tapped his feet on the floor. Most recently, Marco had begun approaching students to ask odd and, at times, personal questions such as "Do you wiggle?" or "Do you pick your nose?" without explanation. Not surprisingly, these interactions often embarrassed or, at times, offended his classmates. Sadly, Marco failed to recognize their discomfort and repeatedly asked the same question until he received an answer. If an individual refused to answer or took too long to respond, Marco would hit him or her and then later cry and say that he did not mean it. Puzzled by these behaviors, Mrs. Barton pondered whether Marco may have an autism spectrum disorder.

DIAGNOSTIC DEFINITIONS/ISSUES

Traditionally, the term *autism* was used to describe children who demonstrated deficits in social development and communication and a range of repetitive behaviors or restricted interests (American Psychiatric Association [APA], 2000). However, since the late 1970s, the categorization of children with autism has been recognized as a spectrum of disorders, currently referred to as *autism spectrum disorders* (ASD) or the autism spectrum. The term *ASD* is used to describe a group of neurodevelopmental disorders characterized by (1) deficits in understanding and using social skills; (2) limited communication; and (3) restricted interests or repetitive behaviors (APA, 2000). The degree of impairment among children with ASD is highly variable, and characteristics of the disability may present themselves in various combinations, from very severe to very mild. At the very severe end of the spectrum are those individuals with autism, sometimes referred to as classic, or Kanner's, autism. These children may be nonverbal, intellectually disabled, and easily recognizable by displays of repetitive behaviors such as hand flapping or rocking (Happé, 1999). At the other end of the spectrum are those children with similar characteristics of autism but who display low average to above average cognitive abilities and normal language abilities, at least superficially. These "less impaired" children may demonstrate odd social mannerisms, a long-winded, pedantic, communication style, and rare or unique special interests (e.g., deep-fry cookers, trains, vacuums, tractors, engines). Such children at the less severe end of the spectrum are commonly referred to as having high-functioning autism or Asperger syndrome (HFA/AS).

> **The degree of impairment among children with ASD is highly variable, and characteristics of the disability may present themselves in various combinations, from very severe to very mild.**

At the present time, there are no diagnostic guidelines for HFA; the term most commonly is used as a clinical descriptor to differentiate individuals with classic autism. By convention, if a child meets the diagnostic characteristics for autism according to the *Diagnostic and Statistical Manual of Mental Disorders* (DSM-IV-TR; APA, 2000) but displays cognitive ability in the low average to above average range, he or she is said to have HFA. Although AS was identified in the literature at about the same time as classic autism, it only recently has been recognized by professionals as a separate disorder (AS first appeared in the DSM-IV in 1994). The current diagnostic criteria for AS include the presence of significant impairment in social interactions and displays of restricted behaviors and/or interests. These impairments are similar to, but usually milder than, those seen in autism. Despite the presence of social and behavioral difficulties, individuals with AS demonstrate no significant delays in the development of language or cognitive abilities.

At present, the DSM-IV-TR represents autism and AS as two distinct conditions with different sets of diagnostic criteria. However, questions remain as to whether HFA and AS represent two distinct conditions or whether they differ only in symptom severity (Volkmar & Klin, 2000; Prior, 2003). During the past decade, a plethora of research has been devoted to examining such a distinction between HFA and AS. The majority of these studies have been conducted to examine the disparity in neurocognitive functioning (e.g., executive functioning domains), language abilities, motor skills, and desire for social relationships between children with HFA and AS (e.g., Ozonoff, South, & Miller, 2000; Tonge, Brereton, Gray, & Einfeld, 1999). Overall, this research has failed to differentiate the two (Wing, 2000). Instead, it appears that many individuals with HFA and AS share the same dysfunction, and the only distinguishable element may be that individuals with AS display greater levels of stress and anxiety (Thede & Coolidge, 2007). Although such research delineating the unique profiles of functioning is important, a discussion of the similarities or differences between HFA and AS is beyond the scope of this book. In this book HFA and AS are combined because it is still undetermined whether their treatment requirements differ. Thus, for the purposes of assessment, prevention, and intervention, understanding the needs of children with HFA/AS is more important than attending to a specific diagnostic label (Kunce & Mesibov, 1998).

CONTEMPORARY CONCEPTUALIZATION OF HFA/AS

HFA/AS is currently understood as a developmental disorder characterized by children who (1) have significant difficulties in social interactions and relationships, (2) display a lack of empathy that is usually milder than that seen in classic autism, and (3) engage in unusual patterns of interest and unique stereotyped behaviors, especially the tendency to overly focus on certain topics of interest (Klin & Volkmar, 1999; Myles, 2005; Thede & Coolidge, 2007). Aside from these diagnostic characterizations, children with HFA/AS generally display average to above average cognitive abilities and sometimes demonstrate superior intellectual skills. Moreover, children with HFA/AS often develop good structural language skills. That is, individuals with HFA/AS may speak in syntactically and grammatically correct structures. In this sense, the content and form of language appear to be intact. However, it is the use of language for communicative purposes (pragmatics) that is significantly impaired (Landa, 2000) and, at times, inappropriate (Sansosti & Powell-Smith, 2006). In sum, HFA/AS is characterized by deficits in social interactions and a restricted range of behaviors and/or interests, yet it is not associated with clinically significant delays in cognitive or language development.

> HFA/AS is characterized by deficits in social interactions and a restricted range of behaviors and/or interests, yet it is not associated with clinically significant delays in cognitive or language development.

From the information provided thus far, it appears that HFA/AS represents the mildest end of the autism spectrum. However, HFA/AS cannot be regarded as a mild disorder because of the severity of the social skill and behavioral limitations (Attwood, 2007), related affective problems such as depression and anxiety (e.g., Berney, 2004; Ghaziuddin, Ghaziuddin, & Greden, 2002), and the heavy burden that is placed on the individual, the family, and the broader community (Frith, 2003). Individuals with HFA/AS often perceive their environment as nebulous, consisting of random, unpredictable, even threatening conditions that one individual with AS called "analogous to a Jackson Pollock painting." When faced with unpredictability, children and youth with HFA/AS, who desire sameness to the greatest degree possible, become easily stressed and emotionally vulnerable (Aspy & Grossman, 2007). As such, children with HFA/AS are at an increased risk for tantrums and aggressive outbursts (Myles & Southwick, 2005), as well as depression and suicide (Ghaziuddin et al., 2002; Kim, Szatmari, Bryson, Streiner, & Wilson, 2000; Lynn, 2007). From this perspective it is important that educators are cautious when thinking of HFA/AS as only a mild form of the larger autism spectrum.

DEVELOPMENTAL COURSE

Preschool Years

At the preschool level, children with HFA/AS may appear to get along well with teachers and other adults. In fact, it may not be unusual for the child to engage in basic social behaviors such as greeting someone or asking someone's name. However, these children have extreme difficulty understanding the social world in which they interact, and they often will demonstrate deficits in sustaining and maintaining relationships with other children and engaging in reciprocal social exchanges. It may not be uncommon for these children to prefer to be on the periphery of activities, acting more as observers than participants. The tendency to remain in the social periphery may be attributed to the fact that children with HFA/AS have difficulty understanding the world around them and become easily upset when they are in novel or unpredictable social situations. If social situations remain unpredictable and confusing, these children may engage in tantrums and other inappropriate behaviors, such as excessive crying, screaming, and, at times, aggression.

> The social rejection that preschool-age children experience may contribute to their desire to remain on the outside edge of group-based games or activities and to instances of inappropriate behaviors when they try to interact in a vague social world.

In order to control their world, preschool-age (and older) children with HFA/AS likely will display a desire to adhere to specific routines and rituals. When a preschool-age child with HFA/AS does engage with peers, the focus of his or her social interactions likely will revolve around his or her circumscribed, and oftentimes obsessive, area of interest (e.g., dinosaurs, tractors, deep-fry cookers, vacuums, engines). Such a high level of knowledge at such an early age may appear as precociousness to the adult observer, but many of these children likely will experience social rejection by their same-age peers. The social rejection that preschool-age children experience may contribute to their desire to remain on the outside edge of group-based games or activities and to instances of inappropriate behaviors when they try to interact in a vague social world.

Many of the aforementioned characteristics do not appear to deviate much from what is seen in children within the autism spectrum. However, the child with HFA/AS is more likely to show some social interest in other children than is the child with classic autism. In fact, Volkmar and Klin (2000) indicate that individuals with HFA/AS "experience social isolation, but are not withdrawn or devoid of social interest" (p. 59). Thus children with HFA/AS (even preschool age) may show an interest in having friends, a finding that contrasts with the pattern found in individuals with classic autism. An interest in the social world combined with an elevated use of language and basic conversational ability may lead early childhood educators to believe that the child does not present as being obviously "different" from other, more typically developing children (Safran, 2001). Rather, educators may view the child as eccentric. Because these children may not stand out as being different enough from their peers, primary care providers and early childhood educators may be reluctant to advocate for a comprehensive assessment. While 95% of parents of preschool-age children with HFA/AS indicate that their children demonstrate a variety of social and behavioral challenges, only 28% of children actually receive a diagnosis by the end of this period (Barnhill et al., 2000; Church, Alisanski, & Amanullah, 2000).

In spite of parents' concerns, many early childhood educators perceive the early social and behavioral difficulties as "at risk" behaviors not directly associated with the autism spectrum (Griswold, Barnhill, Myles, Hagiwara, & Simpson, 2002). This perception may be due to the child's seeming intellectual strength combined with a desire and ability to communicate about topics of interest to adults and peers. In fact, many young children with HFA/AS may appear to understand more than they do (Myles & Simpson, 2001). Such a false impression may delay the delivery of interventions and create a sense of mistrust between parents and educators regarding the needs of the child. Therefore, it is imperative for educators not only to listen carefully to parents' concerns but also to focus on the qualitative social differences of children suspected of HFA/AS. Key elements for educators to be aware of during the preschool years include (1) a tendency to avoid spontaneous social interactions; (2) impairments in the pragmatic use of social communication; (3) perseverance on particular objects or subjects, with a tendency to want to talk only about such interests; (4) difficulty in regulating social-emotional responses; and (5) an appearance of being in one's own world (Bauer, 1996).

Elementary School

As children with HFA/AS enter kindergarten, educators may begin to identify behavioral concerns (e.g., hyperactivity, inattention, aggression, resistance to change) but more often express concern over "immature" social skills and peer interactions (Bauer, 1996). Although children with HFA/AS typically will perform well academically, especially in areas of rote reading and calculation skills, their misunderstanding of the social world, inappropriate behaviors, and "obsessive" interests often will interfere with the classroom setting. When these concerns are severe enough, referrals for special education and related services may be suggested, but generally most elementary-age children with HFA/

> Although children with HFA/AS typically will perform well academically, especially in areas of rote reading and calculation skills, their misunderstanding of the social world, inappropriate behaviors, and "obsessive" interests often will interfere with the classroom setting.

AS remain in the mainstream setting. In fact, only 64% of children are formally diagnosed with HFA/AS by the time they reach 11 years of age (Church et al., 2000).

Within this age group, both parents and educators often report a host of serious developmental concerns. In particular, social skills emerge as a key area of difficulty. In a review of elementary-age children's cumulative records, Church, Alisanski, and Amanullah (2000) reported that none of the 39 children in their sample were perceived by educators to engage in reciprocal relationships with other children, although some were able to form superficial relationships (e.g., usually to share information on topics of interest). Another key finding was that elementary-age children did not demonstrate the ability to take the perspective of others. Specifically, these children frequently misread social cues (e.g., body language, gestures, facial expression) and often acted inappropriately (e.g., blurting out socially inappropriate comments and not understanding the impact of those comments on others) when in the presence of same-age peers. For many elementary-age children with HFA/AS, difficulties with social skills include (1) a lack of awareness of basic, seemingly obvious social rules, (2) a lack of common sense, (3) misinterpretation of social cues and nonverbal messages, and (4) displays of a wide variety of socially unacceptable habits and behaviors (Gagnon & Myles, 1999). When a child does engage socially, language within these social situations likely will be used more often to discuss the child's topic of interest rather than to share in a reciprocal conversation. As was the case during preschool years, misunderstanding and misinterpreting the social world remains a constant challenge.

In addition to the variety of social difficulties, a host of behavioral problems begin to emerge. This is not to say that *all* children with HFA/AS will display problematic behaviors in classrooms or other environments in schools (e.g., playground), but they are not uncommon. In fact, some children with HFA/AS may be overly reactive, whereas others are more withdrawn. Contrary to some commonly held perceptions, problematic behaviors and tantrums that children with HFA/AS may display are not a result of malicious intent. Tantrums and other behavioral meltdowns typically occur as a result of lack of understanding, high stress, distractibility, poor organizational skills, and lack of control over the environment (Myles & Southwick, 2005). Thus any behavioral problems that are observed within structured and unstructured academic settings are likely attributed to the child's inability to function in a world that he or she perceives as unpredictable.

Children with HFA/AS also begin to demonstrate difficulty with problem solving during the elementary school years. Although a student with HFA/AS may demonstrate superior knowledge and problem-solving ability regarding a selected topic of interest, he or she may have difficulty applying these same abilities to traditional learning tasks. Many students with HFA/AS select only one strategy to solve a variety of problems (academic, behavioral, and social) and use it consistently without regard for the situation or outcome (Myles & Southwick, 2005). For example, an elementary-age student who has learned the important spelling rule of "I before E, except after C" may adhere to this strategy rigidly, incorrectly spelling words such as *freight*, *vein*, and *weigh*. The student would likely insist that his or her spelling of these words was appropriate. As a result of continued failures, the student likely feels confused and angry. Continued confusion or anger often leads to behavioral reactions—displayed as emotional outbursts, inappropriate behaviors, and/or tantrums.

Middle/High School

Social and behavioral problems will continue to pervade the lives of children with HFA/AS as they move through middle and high school environments. Often, these difficulties increase, leading a child with HFA/AS to become more isolated or ashamed of his or her eccentric interests. Subsequently, children with HFA/AS are often misunderstood and, at times, left out, teased, and persecuted (Bauer, 1996). Their inability to make friends and "fit in" may result in further behavioral meltdowns and withdrawal, often resulting in some degree of depression. In fact, comorbidity of HFA/AS and depression becomes very common in late childhood and adolescence (Ghaziuddin et al., 2002), which may be due to the individual's awareness of personal inadequacy in social interactions and repeated failures in forming and/or maintaining relationships (Klin, McPartland, & Volkmar, 2005). This awareness is quite different from children with classic autism, who are seemingly unaware of their social deficits. Too often, individuals with HFA/AS are painfully aware that they are different from their peers (Myles, 2005). Pressure to conform is great, and tolerance for differences is at a minimum during this stage of development, and it is likely that children with HFA/AS will demonstrate more behavioral inflexibility and suffer greater emotional vulnerability. Typical behaviors may include increased irritability, withdrawal from social interactions, oversensitivity and excessive behavioral reactions to failure, criticism, and rejection, and an increase in ritualistic behavior.

For middle and high school-age individuals with HFA/AS, social skills deficits continue to be the major area of difficulty. For example, of 18 students in their sample (13 children followed through middle school and 5 individuals followed through high school), Church and colleagues (2000) described these children as having an "inability to read the social cues of their peers, awkward body posture, awkward use of gestures, annoying habits such as making noises or drumming desks, highly variable eye contact, and odd body language" (p. 17). Not only are deficits in social skills apparent, but also the individual may stand out socially among his or her peer group. The fact that individuals with HFA/AS begin to stand out more socially at this developmental stage may be due largely to their level of social-emotional maturity. For example, most typically developing 15-year-olds will be concerned with how they appear to others and often overlook violations of rules by their peers for fear of being labeled a "tattletale," "big mouth," or "rat." This is in direct contrast with an individual with HFA/AS who may be the same chronological age but is functioning emotionally at an 8-year-old level. An individual functioning emotionally as an 8-year-old will be overly concerned with following rules to the letter (and may have difficulty understanding exceptions to the rules). Such behavior is likely to be condemned by peers or, worse, to lead to excessive teasing and/or bullying.

Similar to elementary students, individuals with HFA/AS in middle and high school environments continue to display a host of behavioral difficulties. Because middle and high school environments are replete with change, many individuals with HFA/AS will find it difficult to remain calm and successfully transition from one activity to another. For example, moving to a different classroom between periods may be perceived as threatening due to the highly variable nature of behaviors that occur in school hallways. It may not

> **Because middle and high school environments are replete with change, many individuals with HFA/AS will find it difficult to remain calm and successfully transition from one activity to another.**

be uncommon for a student to begin escalating behavior prior to the end of a period in order to leave class early and avoid what cannot be predicted. In addition, assemblies and other non-scheduled activities may cause misunderstanding for the student and lead to excessive questioning and/or behavioral meltdowns. For example, one student in a middle school was consistently aggressive when assemblies were announced by the principal during morning announcements. The student's behavior quickly escalated and consisted of throwing his book bag, cursing at the teacher and class, and refusing to participate in any "stupid" activity instead of going to history class (his favorite class). In this example, the student demonstrated limited ability to regulate emotions and behaviors, a pattern typical throughout this age range. Overall, individuals are likely to demonstrate limited ability maintaining self-control.

Individuals with HFA/AS in middle and high school likely will continue to demonstrate limited problem-solving skills. However, the heightened level of abstraction may increase the frequency and intensity of successive behavioral reactions by the student. Academically, problem solving becomes more difficult in middle and high school because more abstract concepts are involved (e.g., word problems, advanced comprehension, geometry). This increased abstraction often requires additional levels of problem solving that individuals with HFA/AS may not understand or even know exist. As a consequence, academic subjects that require flexibility in reasoning may cause a great deal of confusion for the student and could lead to an emotional outburst. Socially, the same is true. Students with HFA/AS may not understand that there are few universal and inflexible social rules (Myles & Southwick, 2005). Sometimes they may attempt to follow a learned social behavior consistently because it provides structure to an otherwise confusing world, even though minor nuances of that behavior are required within specific contexts. For example, a middle school student may not understand that although it may appear to be appropriate to curse in the presence of peers, cousins, or with individuals when instant messaging online, the same behavior is likely to draw a much different response from a teacher, principal, or other person of authority. Further complicating this notion of social problem solving is the fact that personal relationships now focus on complex emotions and, at times, intimacy. High school students with HFA/AS may see their peers holding hands and engaging in other public displays of affection (e.g., kissing, hugging) and think that they too can engage in such behaviors. Imagine the confusion and controversy that may occur when a high school student with HFA/AS approaches a member of the opposite sex without understanding that intimate behaviors are not universally displayed. Such social skill errors often are interpreted by educational personnel as sexual overtures when that may not have been the intent; often these behaviors result in immediate disciplinary actions with little understanding of the student's behavior. Overall, individuals with HFA/AS in middle and high school environments likely will have difficulty regulating emotions, resolving conflicts, and demonstrating behavior that matches nuance-specific social situations.

Long-Term Outcomes

To date, very little information exists regarding the long-term outcomes of individuals with HFA/AS. However, reviews of anecdotal reports, case studies, personal accounts, and longitudinal studies may shed some light on the long-term outlook for individuals with HFA/AS. Obviously, limited social understanding, misinterpretation of social cues, and an inability to understand others' perspectives will make it tremendously difficult for adolescents and adults to develop long-standing interpersonal relationships. In addition, issues regarding employment and comorbid health issues remain as critical areas of concern (Barnhill, 2007).

> **Obviously, limited social understanding, misinterpretation of social cues, and an inability to understand others' perspectives will make it tremendously difficult for adolescents and adults to develop long-standing interpersonal relationships.**

The employment prospects for individuals with HFA/AS remain bleak. Because of his or her elevated cognitive abilities, combined with the propensity to have areas of special interest (e.g., computer science, geology, horticulture), an individual with HFA/AS may demonstrate exceptional abilities and/or great expertise in a particular area. Because of these strengths, it may be assumed that individuals with HFA/AS would be able to attend college or technical school to receive specialized training and be successful, productive members of society. However, only 12% of individuals with HFA/AS are employed full time (Barnard, Harvey, Prior, & Potter, 2001). It is likely that, although the individual may demonstrate the technical skills necessary for a particular profession, poor social communication skills, general social skills deficits, and rigid behavioral styles may lead to difficulty obtaining a job (e.g., interviewing for a position), as well as maintaining employment (e.g., thinking quickly in response to questions or problems; Barnhill, 2007; Hurlbutt & Chalmers, 2004). Although the characteristics of HFA/AS may be masked by technical acuity, over time and especially in unpredictable situations, the façade of normality cannot sustain (Frith, 2004).

Individuals with HFA/AS also exhibit difficulties with comorbid mental health needs such as depression and anxiety. Whereas the most common coexisting condition in children with HFA/AS has been identified as attention-deficit/hyperactivity disorder (ADHD), in adolescents and adults it is depression (Ghaziuddin et al., 2002) and anxiety disorders (Berney, 2004; Thede & Coolidge, 2007). To date, it is not known whether depression and anxiety in older individuals with HFA/AS is the result of continued social difficulties and exclusion or the consequence of biological and/or genetic factors. Regardless of the causal link, individuals with HFA/AS are at greater risk for suicidal behaviors and completed suicides (Wing, 2000).

PREVALENCE

Epidemiology

Within the past two decades, it appears that the number of children identified as having ASD has increased substantially. Traditionally, ASD was considered a low-incidence disability, occurring in only 4–6 per 10,000 (or 1 in approximately 1,600) live births (Lotter, 1967). However, the most current estimates from the Centers for Disease Control and Prevention (CDC, 2007) estimate that ASD (including HFA/AS) occurs in 1 in every 150 births, making it the fastest growing developmental disability in the United States. Few studies have investigated the specific occurrence of HFA/AS. However, Hyman, Rodier, and Davidson (2001) suggest that the prevalence of higher functioning ASD may be as high as 63 per 10,000 (1 in 160) births. Other age-specific prevalence rates of HFA/AS have been estimated as ranging from 8.4 per 10,000 (1 in 1,190) in preschool children (Chakrabarti & Fombonne, 2001) to 71 per 10,000 (1 in 140) in children ages 7–16 (Ehlers & Gillberg, 1993). Overall, it does appear that the rates of ASD have increased, although specific numbers related to higher functioning individuals remain highly variable.

In recent years, the astronomical increase in the number of children with ASD has been cause for significant concern. In fact, the "growing epidemic" of autism, sensationalized throughout various forms of lay media (e.g., *Newsweek*, *Time*, *The Today Show*, *Dateline*, *20/20*, *Oprah*), has raised public concern, as well as promulgated various presumptions as to causal factors, such as viruses contained within immunizations (Wakefield, 1999) or mercury from the thimerosal preservative used specifically within the measles, mumps, and rubella (MMR) vaccine (Geir & Geir, 2004). To date, numerous studies have found no causal link between immunizations and increased prevalence of ASD (e.g., Fombonne & Chakrabarti, 2001; Honda, Shimizu, & Rutter, 2005; Smeeth et al., 2004). Despite ever-increasing studies that have refuted such claims, more and more parents do not have their children vaccinated.

Educational Placement and Service Delivery Trends

Given epidemiological increases, it logically follows that state departments of education also have reported significant increases in the number of students with ASD receiving special education. The Individuals with Disabilities Education Act (IDEA) requires each state's Department of Education (DOE) and the U.S. Department of Education (USDOE) to record specific childhood disabilities, including autism, for each school year. In 1991, the autism disability category was added as a reporting requirement for the first time. However, it was not until 1992 that data on the prevalence of special education services specific to children with ASD were available from states. From 1992 to 2006, the total number of children served under the autism category of the IDEA grew from 15,580 to 224,594, an increase of 1,342% (Fighting Autism, 2008). During this same time, the number of students served in all other disability categories increased by only 31%. From the available information, it is likely that all states have witnessed significant impacts in the number of students with ASD.

Unfortunately, no information exists regarding the current percentage of students receiving services specifically for HFA/AS. Estimates of children receiving special education services are based solely on the number of services provided under the IDEA category of autism, which may or may not include children with HFA/AS. It is possible that the significant increase in the number of children receiving special education services under the

IDEA category of autism is a gross underestimate of the actual frequency of services necessary to support the education of students with HFA/AS and classic autism. This is due to the fact that some children with classic autism and most children with HFA/AS are not included in IDEA counts because they attend private schools, are home schooled, or do not meet a state's eligibility criteria for the autism disability category. For

> **It is possible that the significant increase in the number of children receiving special education services under the IDEA category of autism is a gross underestimate of the actual frequency of services necessary to support the education of students with HFA/AS and classic autism.**

example, Bertrand et al. (2001) found that 66% of children with classic autism and only 50% of children with higher functioning ASD had autism listed as their special education designation for services in the state of New Jersey. In a more recent study conducted in Atlanta, of those children with ASD, only 41% were receiving services under the autism category of IDEA (Yeargin-Allsopp et al., 2003). This underreporting may be due to the fact that states have different eligibility criteria for the autism disability category and that children with HFA/AS may not qualify for such services. Because of their elevated cognitive and language abilities, children with HFA/AS may receive services under another IDEA category such as other health impaired, specific learning disability, or emotional disturbance, if they qualify for any services at all. Regardless of which category is chosen, the potential exists that children with HFA/AS represent a large underserved student population (Safran, 2008).

Aside from the issue of the exact number of students served, placement in general education settings has become a dominant service delivery issue for individuals with HFA/AS (Simpson & Myles, 1998). Data from the Office of Special Education Programs (OSEP; 2004) suggests that children with ASD (statistics specifically related to HFA/AS currently are not available) are increasingly served in inclusive settings. Specifically, participation of students with ASD in the general education curriculum (more than 80% of the day) increased at a faster pace than that of all disability categories combined. Whereas only 4.8% of students with ASD were included in 1990–1991, nearly 29.1% were in general education for 80% or more of their day in 2003–2004, representing a growth rate of 24.3%. Increases in inclusion of students with ASD from 1991 to 2004 outpaced those of other low-incidence disabilities such as mental handicaps (8% growth) and emotional disturbance (17.4% growth) and were comparable to those of high-incidence disabilities, such as specific learning disability (26.4% growth). Moreover, educators commonly comment on the increasing numbers of students with characteristics of HFA/AS within general education classrooms (Myles, 2005). With this in mind, developing and implementing effective programming for children with HFA/AS becomes a challenge for educators.

LOOKING AHEAD

The remaining chapters of this book provide more detailed information regarding HFA/AS and supply the reader with practical solutions to assist in the development of prevention and intervention efforts to meet the academic, behavioral, and social needs of students with HFA/AS. Chapter 2 includes detailed information related to areas of impairment that individuals with HFA/AS display. Chapter 3 covers information related to providing collaborative consultation via multiple stakeholders for assisting in the development of effective supports and interventions for students with HFA/AS. Chapter 4, considered the foundation of this book, discusses assessing the domain-specific features of HFA/AS within an ecological context. Chapters 5, 6, and 7 provide detailed and specific information regarding academic, behavioral, and social-emotional interventions, respectively. Chapter 8 discusses the importance of creating an effective individualized education plan (IEP) that is objective and measurable for a student with HFA/AS. Finally, Chapter 9 discusses the importance of using data to make important educational decisions and offers strategies for practitioners to employ to monitor progress of prevention and/or intervention efforts. It is hoped that readers will come away from this book with the understanding, knowledge, and skills necessary to promote positive outcomes for students with HFA/AS in a variety of educational settings.

CHAPTER 2

Areas of Impairment

with REBECCA L. FRITSCHIE

STUDENT SNAPSHOT: Dino

Dino is a middle school student with AS. Academically, he is performing at grade level and above, yet his social, behavioral, and emotional skills are limited. He has extreme difficulty making and keeping friends and engages in many socially inappropriate behaviors. For example, Dino has told racist jokes, "mooned" his classmates, and/or made personal comments that are hurtful to others, such as "Your shoes are really ugly!" His interest in continuously variable transmissions borders on obsession, and he incessantly attempts to engage others in conversations about them. In the hallway between class periods, Dino verbally calls out rule infractions that students have committed and states what appropriate behaviors should be occurring. Because of this, his classmates often say he is "weird" and "retarded" as he walks on by. When Dino is excited or nervous, he becomes fidgety, begins to scream, and, at times, throws his book bag at others. As a result, Dino has been suspended several times. Lately, Dino has been complaining that nobody likes him and he would be better off dead. These statements are followed by a period of social withdrawal that lasts for days at a time.

Rebecca L. Fritschie, MEd, is an EdS student in the school psychology program at Kent State University. Currently, Ms. Fritschie is completing her yearlong internship in school psychology in Pennsylvania. Throughout her graduate training, Ms. Fritschie has been active in assisting with research focusing on personality traits, intelligence, and ASD. Her professional interests include working with children with ASD and their families, promoting positive school climate, and enhancing home–school collaboration.

OVERVIEW

Children and adolescents with HFA/AS typically demonstrate impaired functioning in several core areas of development. These areas of impairment include (1) difficulties with social interactions and relationships, (2) repetitive or restricted behaviors, interests, and/or activities, and (3) abnormalities in specific aspects of communication, although no clinically significant delays in language acquisition are usually displayed in individuals with AS (APA, 2000). In addition, children with HFA/AS typically do not show evidence of clinically significant delays in cognitive development. Typically they exhibit a developmentally appropriate expression of curiosity about their environment (i.e., active exploration of surroundings) and the ability to acquire age-appropriate self-help and adaptive behavior skills, except for those that are needed in social situations (Ozonoff, Dawson, & McPartland, 2002). For example, although children and adolescents with HFA/AS are often able to take care of their basic needs, such as eating, dressing, grooming, and toileting, they have a limited skill set in terms of interacting with others, sharing conversations, and maintaining interpersonal relationships.

In addition to the core impairments that are needed to make a formal diagnosis using the DSM-IV-TR (APA, 2000), individuals with HFA/AS also may exhibit a variety of associated difficulties. These difficulties can include (1) atypical responses to sensory stimuli (e.g., Attwood, 2007; Bromley, Hare, Davison, & Emerson, 2004), (2) academic performance problems (e.g., Sansosti & Powell-Smith, 2006; Myles & Simpson, 2003; Ozonoff et al., 2002), (3) sleep disturbances (e.g., Allik, Larsson, & Smedje, 2006; Polimeni, Richdale, & Francis, 2005; Paavonen et al., 2002), (4) motor difficulties (e.g., Attwood, 2007; Freitag, Kleser, Schneider, & von Gontard, 2007; Manjiviona & Prior, 1995), and (5) disorders of anxiety and/or depression (e.g., Tonge et al., 1999; Kim et al., 2000; Macintosh & Dissanayake, 2006b).

No two individuals with HFA/AS will display all of the characteristic areas of impairment and/or associated features of these disorders. Thus it is important to recognize each individual's unique differences when working within educational settings.

Certainly, as with many other disorders, the characteristics of HFA/AS are highly variable and range in severity. Furthermore, no two individuals with HFA/AS will display all of the characteristic areas of impairment and/or associated features of these disorders. Thus it is important to recognize each individual's unique differences when working within educational settings.

CORE AREAS OF IMPAIRMENT

Similar to individuals with classic autism, students with HFA/AS demonstrate significant difficulties in social interactions, behavioral rigidity, and communication. Although similar, displays of behaviors across these three domains may be less severe or, at times, more peculiar in students with HFA/AS. Table 2.1 provides common teacher observations of students with HFA/AS. Descriptions and examples of the three core areas of impairment are provided next.

TABLE 2.1. Common Teacher Observations of Students with HFA/AS

Social skills/interactions

1. Difficulty interacting with others, despite demonstrating a desire for friends
2. Difficulty initiating and/or maintaining any social relationship
3. Difficulty following social rules/norms
4. Difficulty understanding facial expressions, gestures, and/or voice tone
5. Limited social and/or emotional reciprocity
6. Limited engagement in social activities
7. Difficulty understanding another's perspective
8. Occasional engagement in inappropriate social exchanges

Behavioral rigidity/interests

1. Engagement in rigid motor mannerisms (e.g., hand flapping, pacing)
2. Insistence on adherence to routines and/or rituals
3. Greater interest in parts of objects than in objects themselves
4. Demonstration of substantial factual knowledge of a relatively narrow topic of interest (e.g., roller coasters, weather patterns)
5. Focus of the majority of social interactions on identified topic of interest

Language/communication

1. No apparent delay in the development of language or ability to communicate
2. Difficulty initiating and/or maintaining a conversation
3. Tendency to dominate conversations, talking excessively about a topic of interest
4. Difficulty taking turns during a conversation
5. Failure to respond consistently to comments or questions from others
6. Use of very formal language when speaking socially
7. Demonstration of odd prosody when engaging with others
8. Interpretation of jokes, sarcasm, and/or idioms literally

Social Interactions

As in classic autism, children and adolescents with HFA/AS demonstrate significant difficulties in their ability to interact with both peers and adults. Compared with individuals with classic autism, children and youth with HFA/AS have a tendency to display greater interest in having friends (Bacon, Fein, Morris, Waterhouse, & Allen, 1998; Klin, McPartland, & Volkmar, 2005), as well as an increased capacity for social-emotional expressiveness and responsiveness (Macintosh & Dissanayake, 2006a). Despite their desire to seek friendships and share emotions, individuals with HFA/AS exhibit numerous impairments in their ability to initiate and maintain social relationships. Most often, the

> The difficulties that children with HFA/AS exhibit when interacting socially are the result of an inability to understand and appropriately respond to social information ..., as well as adhere to seemingly obvious social rules and values.

difficulties that children with HFA/AS exhibit when interacting socially are the result of an inability to understand and appropriately respond to social information (Dawson, Meltzoff,

Osterling, Rinaldi, & Brown, 1998), as well as adhere to seemingly obvious social rules and values (Myles, 2005).

In general, children and adolescents with HFA/AS have a general weakness in understanding nonverbal cues such as facial expressions, gestures, and tone of voice. Such a weakness makes it difficult for individuals with HFA/AS to decipher the thoughts, feelings, intentions, and perspectives of others. This means that children and adolescents with HFA/AS likely will have difficulty interpreting when another child is upset, happy, or uninterested in playing a game or talking about a particular subject. Furthermore, it is unlikely that an individual with HFA/AS will engage in expected nonverbal behaviors when communicating. That is, he or she may demonstrate poor eye contact (or have a stiff, staring gaze), display awkward or clumsy body posture and limited or inappropriate facial expressions, and/or fail to use gestures while interacting and communicating with others (APA, 2000; Gillberg, 2002).

Individuals with HFA/AS also express limited social and emotional reciprocity. Often unresponsive to auditory cues (e.g., their names being called, requests from a peer or teacher), some individuals may appear to be unaware of the people and circumstances that surround them. In fact, it is not uncommon for educators to describe children and adolescents with HFA/AS as being in their "own little world" (Ozonoff et al., 2002). These individuals may prefer to engage in solitary activities or take part in activities only from the periphery, rather than actively participating in games or group activities with others (APA, 2000; Ozonoff et al., 2002). In fact, Bauminger, Shulman, and Agam (2003) noted that individuals with HFA/AS play with other children less often and for a shorter period of time in comparison with their typically developing peers. Moreover, they may not share feelings of enjoyment about interests, activities, or accomplishments.

An important aspect of social and emotional reciprocity that children and adolescents with HFA/AS demonstrate impairment in is the ability to consider others' perspectives and to appreciate the fact that other individuals think, feel, and view the world differently than they do, a concept commonly referred to as *mindblindness* (Baron-Cohen & Swettenham, 1997; Ozonoff et al., 2002). Unlike individuals with classic autism, the level of mindblindness displayed by children and youth with HFA/AS is mainly manifested in a one-sided social approach to others whereby they overly pursue a topic of interest (e.g., Hoover vacuum cleaners, dinosaurs) regardless of the other individual's interest or reaction (APA, 2000). For example, a child or adolescent may continue to talk about Disneyland or the latest Spider-man movie while seemingly ignoring the listener's signs of boredom (e.g., rolling of the eyes, looking away) or attempts to leave. This failure may appear as disregard for others' feelings and may come across as insensitive. However, this is not the child's intention. Instead, individuals with HFA/AS have a poor capacity to recognize, relate to, and understand the feelings of others, making it difficult for them to understand why others do not share their same level of passion.

Taken together, individuals with HFA/AS frequently demonstrate unawareness of how to engage and respond socially. As a result, they likely will violate many social conventions and engage in a large amount of socially inappropriate behavior(s) at one time or another. For example, children and adolescents with HFA/AS may infringe upon another's personal space (e.g., touching a peer's shirt that has a picture the child really likes) and may be unable to refrain from asking extremely personal questions (e.g., "Why are your parents divorced?") or to keep thoughts and/or opinions to themselves (e.g., blurting out "you have really ugly shoes"). In addition, these individuals are often described as responding to others using a blunt, seemingly tactless manner (Ozonoff et al., 2002; Gillberg, 2002), as well as being confused as to why their behavior(s) may affect others as they do. A lack of understanding of the social world, combined with socially inappropriate behavior(s), often results in numerous social errors.

Despite the social errors they make, many children and adolescents with HFA/AS desire and frequently attempt to actively seek friendships. However, they lack the skills to acquire and maintain such relationships. Very often, desires for companionship are suppressed due to a history of failed social encounters and negative response from peers (Bauminger et al., 2003). Continued rejections and/or history of negative interactions with others may cause individuals with HFA/AS to remove themselves from social situations. In turn, this causes them to become victims of a downward spiral, whereby they never learn how to interact appropriately with others and, subsequently, fail to develop friendships that are developmentally appropriate for their age (Ozonoff et al., 2002; APA, 2000). In fact, children and adolescents with HFA/AS often display social maturity that is at one-third to two-thirds their age level (Myles, 2005). For example, a 16-year-old female with HFA/AS may enjoy playing with Barbie dolls and insist on carrying a Barbie backpack to school, even though this interest is not typical for adolescents.

Behavioral Rigidity and Circumscribed Interests

As in classic autism, children and adolescents with HFA/AS frequently display behaviors, interests, and activities that are not only restricted and repetitive in nature but also are abnormally intense or focused (Attwood, 2007; APA, 2000). These patterns of behavior, interests, and activities can be separated into two distinct groups: "lower level" and "higher level" behaviors (Turner, 1999). Lower level behaviors are characterized by stereotyped motor movements or atypical, involuntary actions (e.g., hand flapping, object spinning). Conversely, more advanced, higher level behaviors involve insistence on following elaborate routines and focusing on circumscribed interests (e.g., arranging toys by order of color, eating only five Pringles at lunchtime). Wing and Gould (1979) suggest that although children and youth with HFA/AS do display lower level behaviors, they are more likely to engage in higher level behaviors.

With regard to lower level behaviors, individuals with HFA/AS may engage in rigid motor mannerisms, although usually not to the same degree or intensity as do individuals with classic autism. These behaviors may include spinning, finger flapping, clapping, hand flapping or twisting, pacing, stereotyped walking, and/or complex whole-body movements, among others (South, Ozonoff, & McMahon, 2005; APA, 2000). Oftentimes these repetitive movements, frequently referred to as "self-stimulatory" or "self-stimming" behaviors, denote expressions of excitement, happiness, frustration, and/or agitation (Attwood, 2007). For practitioners, educators, and parents it is important to understand that these behavioral difficulties are not performed intentionally. Rather, they are due to difficulty in identifying and describing one's emotions (Fitzgerald & Bellgrove, 2006), as well as the individual's sense of loss of control or inability to predict outcomes (Myles & Southwick, 2005). That is, lower level behaviors likely occur during highly stressful periods that are difficult to interpret or that evoke anxiety and/or confusion. Therefore, it is the role of practitioners, educators, and parents alike to determine the functions of these behaviors in order to best intervene and prevent them.

When examining higher level behaviors, children and adolescents with HFA/AS often display an inflexible adherence to seemingly nonfunctional routines or rituals, desiring sameness, and requiring environmental predictability (APA, 2000; Gillberg, 2002). This is especially true at younger ages. For example, children may line up their toys or crayons in rows or patterns; watch the same video continuously; insist on the same sequence of events during everyday activities, such as food preferences; play the same game on the recess playground; or engage in other compulsive behaviors (South et al., 2005). Change, surprise, chaos, and uncertainty are not easily tolerated, and the lack of predictability or sameness causes feelings of stress and/or anxiety for the child (Attwood, 2007). Children and adolescents with HFA/AS prefer things to be the same and function best when they can predict what is going to occur within the environment. By engaging in routines or ritualistic behaviors, individuals with HFA/AS attempt to control their environment. To this end, it is important to provide children and adolescents with HFA/AS with a predictable and structured environment across all ages.

During all aspects of development, children and adolescents with HFA/AS are often preoccupied with parts of objects rather than the whole object itself (APA, 2000). They are unable to see the big picture because they are overly focused on small details, such as colors, shapes, marks, or patterns of an object. Rather than using these objects in the ways intended, children and adolescents with HFA/AS may use them in atypical ways. For example, a child or adolescent may continuously roll a pencil between his or her hands or open and close the door of a classroom repeatedly. Individuals with HFA/AS also may be particularly interested in the sensory qualities of objects, such as how they smell or feel, and therefore they can be observed at times incessantly sniffing or rubbing things. They seem to show preference for objects that move (e.g., ceiling fans, the spinning wheels of a toy truck) and may even demonstrate a bizarre attachment to specific objects (e.g., a ball of lint, an empty box; Ozonoff et al., 2002).

Perhaps the most common feature of rigid behavior displayed by individuals with HFA/AS is their obsessive and, at times, all-absorbing interests. These children and adolescents may collect volumes of detailed, factual information and trivia related to a relatively narrow topic.

Perhaps the most common feature of rigid behavior displayed by individuals with HFA/AS is their obsessive and, at times, all-absorbing interests. These children and adolescents may collect volumes of detailed, factual information and trivia related to a relatively narrow topic (e.g., roller coasters, NASCAR racing). At times, circumscribed interests may appear to be developmentally appropriate for the child's or adolescent's age (e.g. dinosaurs, weather patterns). At other times, such interests may appear to be quite unusual (e.g., train engine numbers, telephone pole insulators). In addition, it is not uncommon for interests to change once the child collects all of the information available regarding a specific topic. Regardless of the topic of interest or the frequency by which it may change, individuals with HFA/AS tend to focus most of their social advances and conversations on their specific topic of interest (Ozonoff et al., 2002) and talk about it to the point at which they annoy others. For example, an elementary-age student, Angelo, was fascinated with "pyramid juice," an elixir that ancient pharaohs drank to improve their vitality. Angelo talked incessantly about pyramid juice and often became upset when other students would change the subject to a discussion of soccer. Uninterested in soccer, Angelo would quickly attempt to change the conversation back to pyramid juice. Such behavior was quickly rebuffed, and Angelo's peers walked away from him to talk about soccer.

Language and Communication Abilities

For children and adolescents with AS, no clinically significant delays in the development of language are observed, as these individuals are generally using single words by the age of 2 and communicative phrases, such as "more milk" and "go bye-bye," by the age of 3 (APA, 2000). Additionally, individuals with AS may develop an unusually rich and sophisticated vocabulary at a very young age and have been referred to as "little professors" due to their advanced language skills and formal speaking style (Myles & Simpson, 2003; Ozonoff et al., 2002). Conversely, individuals with HFA initially may be delayed in attaining language, although eventually they are able to speak at a level that is close to what is expected for their age. Despite these subtle differences in the two disorders, both children and adolescents with HFA/AS often display abnormalities in certain aspects of communication, specifically their conversation skills (Ozonoff et al., 2002).

First, children and adolescents with HFA/AS have difficulties holding conversations with others and frequently demonstrate impairment in their ability to initiate, maintain, and end verbal exchanges. When they do converse with parents, teachers, or peers, these individuals have a tendency to dominate the conversation, talking excessively about topics that interest them (e.g., trains, vacuum cleaners, engines, dinosaurs). During such monologues, individuals with HFA/AS likely will exhibit poor pragmatic use of language, using metaphors that are meaningful only to them while conveying little communicative intent during a conversation. Additionally, individuals with HFA/AS may fail to take turns in a conversation or to respond to the comments of others (social reciprocity). For example, attempts by the listener to elaborate on the speech's content or logic or to shift to related topics are often unsuccessful due to the individual's verbosity. At times, children and adolescents with HFA/AS may engage in conversation that may come across as incoherent, with abrupt transitions and a conclusion or point that may never be made (Ozonoff et al., 2002; Klin, Sparrow, Volkmar, Cicchetti, & Rourke, 1995).

Second, the manner in which children and adolescents with HFA/AS speak also may be uncharacteristic when compared with typically developing individuals of the same age. More often than not, individuals with HFA/AS are overly formal and pedantic (i.e., too concerned with correct rules and details of grammar) in their style of speaking. Although this is not necessarily incorrect or inappropriate, it may deter others, especially peers, from wanting to interact with them. For example, when asked by a teacher whom he played with at recess, Tyler, a third-grade student with HFA, declared, "Charles is with whom I played with on the playground during recess." Although grammatically correct, such a statement is likely to fall outside the norms of simple conversations that 8- or 9-year-olds typically have.

In addition to using overly formal speech, individuals with HFA/AS may exhibit unusual prosody of speech. Speech prosody includes intonation, pitch, rate, loudness, and rhythm, some or all of which may be affected. Individuals with HFA/AS have been observed to speak in either very high or very low monotone voices, with little change in intonation or pitch. In addition, they may talk extremely loudly, or so softly that they can barely be understood. Moreover, some individuals with HFA/AS may speak at an extremely slow pace or so quickly that their words become jumbled together. Overall, individuals with HFA/AS exhibit a host of difficulties with regard to understanding and using prosody, and they may be unaware of how different they sound from others (Ozonoff et al., 2002; Klin et al., 1995).

Finally, many children and adolescents with HFA/AS take the literal interpretation of what is said to them and often use language literally themselves. These individuals frequently are unable to understand abstract concepts and nonliteral, figurative language, such as metaphors, humor, irony, sarcasm, and teasing. For example, a child with HFA/AS might interpret a sarcastic expression such as, "well, isn't that nice?" as meaning it really is nice. Likewise, it is unlikely that an individual with HFA/AS would be able to identify the double meaning and communicative purpose of the headline "Red Tape Holds Up New Bridge." Although they typically are able to understand the cognitive basis of humor, they may not enjoy it due to lack of understanding of its intent (Ozonoff et al., 2002; Klin et al., 1995; Gillberg, 2002). For example, a middle school child with AS was extremely confused and engaged in aggressive behavior when he did not understand the intent of an April Fool's Day prank started by his peers. It is likely that such difficulties with communication result from an individual's failure to understand and utilize conventional rules of conversation (APA, 2000) and from his or her tendency to organize the world of people and things into discrete labels according to more concrete, factual perceptions of their environment (Myles & Simpson, 2003).

ASSOCIATED AREAS OF IMPAIRMENT

Responses to Sensory Stimuli

Like individuals with classic autism, children and adolescents with HFA/AS often respond unusually to sensory stimuli, such as sound, light, touch, texture, taste, smell, pain, and temperature, reacting in either hypersensitive (i.e., oversensitive) or hyposensitive (i.e., under-sensitive) ways. For example, some individuals with HFA/AS may have a high threshold for withstanding painful bumps or bruises, yet they may be extremely sensitive to clothing touching their skin (e.g., the tag on the back of their shirt) or people touching them (e.g., giving them a hug or kiss). The most common oversensitivity for these individuals is specific sounds (Attwood, 2007; Bromley et al., 2004). Many children and adolescents with HFA/AS have a propensity to be overly startled by sudden noises. Moreover, they may perceive sounds of a certain pitch to be unbearable or notice very faint sounds that others might not hear, such as a siren in the distance. Additionally, many children and adolescents with HFA/AS may withdraw from certain stimuli due to overloading of the senses. For example, an elementary school child, Timmy, routinely covered his ears in order to try to block out the "intolerable" sound of a school fire alarm sounding during a drill.

In contrast, children and adolescents with HFA/AS also may demonstrate a lack of sensitivity to various stimuli. This typically occurs when responding to particular sounds, such as their names being called; they also may be unusually able to endure pain and tolerate cold weather. In fact, some sensory stimuli may even evoke pleasure, such as cool air coming from an air conditioner or the smell of a parent or teacher's perfume. Generally, children and adolescents with HFA/AS appear to be confused by and fail to understand why others do not have the same level of sensitivity to stimuli that they themselves do. In addition, the way in which children and adolescents with HFA/AS respond to different sensory stimuli, whether fearful or not, can frequently cause problems in daily living situations, such as at home or in school (Attwood, 2007).

Academic Performance Difficulties

Although children and adolescents with HFA/AS typically do not demonstrate clinically significant delays in cognitive development, they often experience difficulties in academic functioning and are overwhelmed by most academic tasks (Sansosti & Powell-Smith, 2006). It has even been suggested that many of these students also demonstrate learning profiles that are similar to that of children with specific learning disabilities (Klin & Volkmar, 2000). Unfortunately, these problems usually do not become apparent until after the first few years of formal schooling, when instructional material becomes

> **Although children and adolescents with HFA/AS typically do not demonstrate clinically significant delays in cognitive development, they often experience difficulties in academic functioning and are overwhelmed by most academic tasks (Sansosti & Powell-Smith, 2006).**

more abstract and children are required to interpret, integrate, and generalize information (Ozonoff et al., 2002). It may appear to educators, practitioners, and parents that children and adolescents with HFA/AS know and/or understand more than they actually do because of their "professor-like" speech and advanced vocabulary, which may mask their academic deficits (Myles, 2005). However, preoccupation with special interests, inattention, limited problem solving and planning, and organizational challenges often make it difficult for individuals with HFA/AS to benefit from education without appropriate support and accommodations (Church et al., 2000). Figure 2.1 provides a brief checklist of the most common academic difficulties students with HFA/AS display.

Very often, children and adolescents with HFA/AS appear to be inattentive and easily distracted during both structured and unstructured academic activities. These individuals are often perceived to be daydreaming (i.e., wandering around the room, staring into space) and unaware of the environment around them. When they do attend to tasks, attention is likely to be fleeting (Myles & Southwick, 2005). For instance, educators often remark that a student with HFA/AS may start to follow directions for a task but quickly lose focus. As a result, educators may perceive that students with HFA/AS are purposefully inattentive, and they may find themselves constantly having to redirect these students and to restate directions for them (Sansosti & Powell-Smith, 2006). High levels of inattention likely are due to distractions in the environment, such as noises (e.g., the ticking of a clock), objects (e.g., bulletin boards, instructional manipulatives), and overstimulation of the senses (e.g., flickering of fluorescent lights). Individuals with HFA/AS also may be driven to distraction due to high levels of confusion and stress.

1. Student is inattentive		
a. during structured activities	☐ Yes	☐ No
b. during unstructured activities	☐ Yes	☐ No
2. Student is attentive but attention lasts:	☐ A few minutes	☐ A few seconds
3. Inattentiveness appears to be the function of:	☐ classroom distraction	
	☐ people and/or peers	
	☐ confusion and/or stress	
	☐ overstimulation	
	☐ objects (inside or outside classroom)	
4. Student demonstrates good reading accuracy:	☐ Yes	☐ No
but has poor text comprehension:	☐ Yes	☐ No
5. Student exhibits poor problem-solving skills:	☐ Yes	☐ No
6. Student organizational skills are limited:	☐ Yes	☐ No
Poor organization consists of:	☐ misplaced academic supplies	
	☐ unpreparedness	
	☐ messy desk/backpack/locker	
7. Student fails to turn work in on time:	☐ Yes	☐ No
8. Student turns work in, but it is incomplete:	☐ Yes	☐ No
9. Student frequently is forgetful:	☐ Yes	☐ No
10. Student handwriting is messy:	☐ Yes	☐ No

FIGURE 2.1. Checklist of common academic difficulties of students with HFA/AS.

Aside from inattention, children and adolescents with HFA/AS exhibit poor, inflexible problem-solving skills. They lack the ability to generalize and to apply knowledge and skills across multiple environments and situations. Instead, these individuals use the same rigid problem-solving method for all academic tasks (e.g., reading, writing, mathematical calculations), even when this strategy has proved to be ineffective for them in the past. For example, an elementary-age student who has learned the spelling rule of "I before E, except after C" may adhere to this strategy rigidly, incorrectly spelling words such as *freight* and *weigh*. Poor problem solving also may present itself in reading tasks. Children and adolescents with HFA/AS often have difficulty differentiating fact from fiction, extracting meaning from text, and discriminating relevant from irrelevant information. Consequently, these deficits lead to poor comprehension (Myles, 2005).

In addition, individuals with HFA/AS may have difficulties with organizing, planning, and prioritizing. For example, they have a tendency to misplace academic supplies (e.g., writing utensils, notebooks), fail to plan ahead regarding what materials are necessary in order to complete at-home assignments, and incorrectly allocate time and energy to their work. Likewise, they may have very messy desks, work stations, backpacks, or lockers, and finding anything in these areas becomes a daunting and challenging task (for both the student and the teacher). As a result, these individuals are often unable to complete academic assignments on time or fail to turn them in at all (Sansosti & Powell-Smith, 2006). Poor organization goes beyond the placement of academic materials and supplies. Many individuals with HFA/AS also demonstrate poor organization of thoughts, as well as actions. For example, a middle school student, Joe, often (almost daily) forgot the combination of his locker. When his teachers provided Joe with a card with his locker combination on it, he often forgot it at home. When they wrote the combination of his locker on his backpack, he frequently forgot it was there. When Joe was able to get into his locker, he often forgot what he needed. Subsequently, these behaviors often led Joe to be late for class and not to have the correct materials. This pattern of forgetfulness and lack of planning is common and creates a challenge for educators when teaching organizational skills.

Sleep Disturbances

Research has suggested that sleep disturbances are common among children and adolescents with HFA/AS (e.g., Allik et al., 2006; Polimeni et al., 2005; Paavonen et al., 2002). It appears that these individuals may have greater frequencies of and more types of sleep problems than children and adolescents with classic autism. For example, Polimeni et al. (2005) indicated that individuals with HFA/AS were more sluggish and disoriented and had slower reactions and speech after waking than did both typically developing individuals and children and adolescents with classic autism. In addition, parent reports of sleep disturbances of individuals with HFA/AS regularly include difficulties in falling asleep, frequent and longer lasting nighttime awakenings, earlier morning awakenings, shorter overall sleep duration, and lower sleep quality (e.g., Allik et al., 2006; Polimeni et al., 2005; Paavonen et al., 2002; Patzold, Richdale, & Tonge, 1998). Unfortunately, issues of disordered sleep can have a significant negative impact on the daytime functioning of these individuals, including elevated behavioral outbursts, daytime drowsiness, and learning problems (Paavonen et al., 2002; Patzold et al., 1998).

Motor Abilities

Children and adolescents with HFA/AS are frequently described by teachers as having gross-motor-skill impairments. These impairments include a lack of coordination and balance, as well as difficulties in the timing and execution of motor tasks. As a result, educators may state that a child or adolescent with HFA/AS is clumsy, awkward, or has a bouncy gait while walking or running (Attwood, 2007, Freitag et al., 2007; Manjiviona & Prior, 1995). One teacher of an elementary-age student, Eli, frequently commented that Eli often bumped into objects and "had a tendency to trip over his own two feet." Not surprisingly, these gross-motor impairments make it extremely difficult for individuals with HFA/AS to participate successfully with other peers in physical education classes or on the playground. This inability to perform developmentally and age-appropriate gross-motor tasks has been associated with increased peer rejection and teasing (Attwood, 2007) and social withdrawal (Freitag et al., 2007).

In addition, children with HFA/AS may demonstrate delays in fine-motor tasks such as drawing pictures, cutting on lines, and, specifically, handwriting (Manjiviona & Prior, 1995). Very often, difficulties occur in acquiring skills that require motor dexterity and hand–eye coordination. Such activities may include cutting, opening a jar, using utensils, tying one's shoelaces, and learning how to ride a bicycle (Attwood, 2007). Children and adolescents with HFA/AS also may demonstrate difficulty copying information from books, papers, the board, or other formats displaying information (e.g., overhead projections). Perhaps the most significant fine-motor difficulties experienced by individuals with HFA/AS relate to writing. During early elementary grades, children with HFA/AS may not be able to copy letters correctly. By mid- to late elementary grades, they likely will labor over the simplest of writing tasks, concentrating the majority of their efforts on letter formation (Moore, 2002). As a result, many individuals with HFA/AS are described by educators as having very messy and oftentimes illegible writing samples. Moreover, educators may express concern that the students fail to pay attention to the directions and are not completing writing assignments. Difficulties in the area of writing are especially problematic because assessment of proficiency is often measured by written performance (Myles & Adreon, 2001).

Anxiety and Depression

In the past decade, more research and clinical information has been shared to suggest that many children and adolescents with HFA/AS may be more susceptible to anxiety and other affective mood problems (e.g., Tonge et al., 1999; Kim et al., 2000). In fact, both teachers and parents have reported that individuals with HFA/AS have substantially more problems with internalizing symptoms as compared with their typically developing peers (Macintosh & Dissanayake, 2006b). Anxieties may begin to emerge at early ages due to: (1) preoccupation with possible violations of routines and rituals, (2) being placed in situations without clear schedules or expectations, or (3) anticipation of failed social encounters. Over time, such anxieties may evolve into more depressive symptoms. This typically occurs during adolescence, when individuals with HFA/AS begin to develop a greater insight into their differences from others and experience a growing desire to have friendships (Kim et al., 2000).

For instance, Hedley and Young (2006) indicated that individuals with HFA/AS who perceived themselves as being more dissimilar to others reported higher depressive symptoms. In general, feelings of victimization and chronic frustration from repeated failure to engage others socially may contribute to the development of both depression and anxiety disorders in children and adolescents with HFA/AS (Bauminger et al., 2003).

> **Feelings of victimization and chronic frustration from repeated failure to engage others socially may contribute to the development of both depression and anxiety disorders in children and adolescents with HFA/AS (Bauminger et al., 2003).**

Unfortunately, an increased prevalence of anxiety and depression has been reported among children and adolescents with HFA/AS (e.g., Berney, 2004; Ghaziuddin et al., 2002; Kim et al., 2000; Lynn, 2007). It has been suggested that such problems directly interfere with these individuals' ability to enter into and to sustain mutually enjoyable relationships with their peers (Tonge et al., 1999). As a result, it is important for practitioners, educators, and parents to be aware of the way in which these disorders may possibly present themselves in children and adolescents with HFA/AS. Characteristics of these conditions may include a worsening in behavior, inattention, social withdrawal, overreliance on obsessions and compulsions, hyperactivity, aggressive or oppositional behavior, agitation, and/or changes in eating and sleeping (Kim et al., 2000).

THEORETICAL FRAMEWORKS FOR UNDERSTANDING AREAS OF IMPAIRMENT

In an attempt to further explain many of the common characteristics that children and adolescents with autism spectrum disorders demonstrate, researchers have developed and focused on three main theoretical perspectives: theory of mind, executive functioning, and central coherence. These theoretical frameworks, which are often said to overlap, help to articulate the possible underlying causes of the impairments associated with both classic autism and HFA/AS. These theories provide parents, educators, and practitioners with a better understanding of the difficulties experienced by children and adolescents with these disorders. Fortunately, this enhanced understanding also helps to facilitate the development of more individualized and effective interventions for individuals with HFA/AS.

Theory of Mind

The term "theory of mind" (ToM) has been used to describe the ability to infer and appreciate the mental states (e.g., beliefs, interests, desires, perceptions, intentions, feelings) of others and to apply this understanding to explain and/or predict individuals' behavior. Whereas most typically developing children are able to "mentalize" (Frith, 2003), or presume the mental states of peers and adults by the age of 4 (Wimmer & Perner, 1983), children and adolescents with HFA/AS are impaired in this ability, a concept referred to as "mindblindness." Individuals on the autism spectrum are not automatically programmed to think about mental states and instead seem to have a preference for information about the physical/observable, rather than the psychological, world (Baron-Cohen, 2002; Frith, 2003). In addition, these individuals frequently show lack of interest in

> Whereas typically developing children are able to "mentalize" (Frith, 2003), or presume the mental states of peers and adults by the age of 4 (Wimmer & Perner, 1983), children and adolescents with HFA/AS are impaired in this ability, a concept referred to as "mindblindness."

the human face and fail to focus on facial features that reveal emotions, such as the eyes (Pelphrey et al., 2002); many of them also lack joint attention (i.e., the tendency to attend to something that another person is looking at) and are unable to share in another individual's interest and gain insight into his or her feelings (Frith, 2003). As a result, children and adolescents with HFA/AS often are unable to understand that individuals think, feel, and view the world differently than they do. For that reason, they have difficulty distinguishing their own thoughts and feelings from those of others.

Unfortunately, ToM skills and the ability to recognize and think about others' thoughts and feelings are of central importance for social interaction, understanding, and communication (Frith, 2003). Therefore, the concept of mindblindness is believed to explain a wide range of the social deficits displayed by individuals with HFA/AS. For example, due to a disturbance in ToM, children and adolescents may have difficulty in following the conventions of topic maintenance when speaking, in understanding the communicative intent of others (Landa, 2000), and/or in reading an individual's level of interest, emotional expression, and nonverbal cues during interaction. Individuals with HFA/AS also may express impairment in both using and understanding nonliteral language, such as jokes, irony, sarcasm, and idioms (e.g., to "kick the bucket," to "knock someone's socks off"; Klin, Jones, Schultz, Volkmar, & Cohen, 2002; Landa, 2000). Furthermore, because ToM deficits cause impairment in an individual's ability to explain and predict the behavior of others, it is difficult for children and adolescents with HFA/AS to distinguish the accidental from the intentional nature of others' behaviors. For instance, a child may believe that his classmate bumped into him intentionally, even though the hallway was overly crowded and the individual could not avoid the contact. Lastly, the inability of some individuals with HFA/AS to recognize words that are associated with mental states (e.g., *upset*, *confused*) or to use words to describe their own feelings also may correlate with a lack of ToM skills (Baron-Cohen & Swettenham, 1997).

In general, the concept of mindblindness seems to prevent children and adolescents with HFA/AS from being able to understand how their own behaviors (e.g., talking excessively about the weather or engaging in specific snacktime routines) may affect the thoughts and feelings of others (Sansosti & Powell-Smith, 2006). Although many children and adolescents with HFA/AS can be taught to consciously use ToM skills in low-demand, one-on-one situations, these individuals have difficulty utilizing these same strategies in more high-demand social situations (e.g., in a novel classroom with many unfamiliar people; Hill & Frith, 2003). Consequently, it is essential that ToM interventions, like all systematic interventions, are practiced in real-world settings and are generalizable.

Executive Functioning

Executive functions consist of a broad group of cognitive strategies, which include working memory (i.e., recalling and manipulating information), planning, mental flexibility, task initiation and performance monitoring, self-regulation, behavior inhibition, and attention skills. These mental processes are involved in and are critical for controlling inappropriate, impulsive behavior, overriding automatic behavior, maintaining an appropriate and flexible problem-solving approach, switching between several activities, and prioritizing during a given time frame, among other cognitive tasks. In all individuals, the prefrontal cortex of one's brain, also known as the frontal lobe, is responsible for controlling executive functioning (Goldberg, 2001). Unfortunately, it appears that individuals with autism spectrum disorders undergo a period of accelerated brain growth during the first 2–4 years of life (Redcay & Courchesne, 2005), resulting in poor neural connections within the brain (Courchesne & Pierce, 2005). Whereas in typically developing children, faulty connections are eliminated or pruned, in individuals with both classic autism and HFA/AS pruning does not occur, causing brain size to increase (Redcay & Courchesne, 2005). Overgrowth in the brain's prefrontal cortex is thought to account for the deficits in executive functioning exhibited by these individuals. Thus executive dysfunction is believed to result in the behaviors commonly demonstrated by children and adolescents with HFA/AS, as well as those with classic autism.

In general, children and adolescents with HFA/AS typically perform poorly on problem-solving tasks that require planning skills (Bennetto, Pennington, & Rogers, 1996; Ozonoff & Jenson, 1999), working memory, set shifting (i.e., the ability to move back and forth between tasks; Bennetto et al., 1996; Hughes, Russell, & Robbins, 1994), and inhibiting a natural response (Geurts, Verté, Oosterlaan, Roeyers, & Sergeant, 2004). More specifically, due to deficits in mental flexibility, children and adolescents with HFA/AS frequently display restricted interests, engage in repetitive behaviors, and are resistant to change. They often fail to learn from their mistakes and continue to use ineffective problem-solving strategies while simultaneously refusing to consider the recommendations of peers, parents, and/or teachers. At times, it is even difficult for these individuals to generate new thoughts or to use different words or phrases (Turner, 1997). For many children and adolescents with HFA/AS, a lack of mental flexibility may also explain why they have fixed ideas regarding the functional use of objects (Attwood, 2007). For example, a child with HFA/AS might insist that a kitchen pot be used only for cooking purposes and not as a drum to create sounds.

> **Due to deficits in mental flexibility, children and adolescents with HFA/AS frequently display restricted interests, engage in repetitive behaviors, and are resistant to change. They often fail to learn from their mistakes and continue to use ineffective problem-solving strategies.**

Characteristically, children and adolescents with HFA/AS also may be impaired in their ability to self-regulate and to inhibit their own behaviors. For instance, these individuals often are unable to control and appropriately express their emotions (Hill & Frith, 2003), thereby frequently throwing temper tantrums and having meltdowns. In addition, they may continue to engage in "self-stimming" behaviors (e.g., hand flapping), even after being asked to stop, or they may fail to refrain from uttering inappropriate remarks, such as "That's an ugly dress." Furthermore, as displayed by individuals with HFA/AS, the lack of social reciprocity (i.e., the natural back-and-forth of conversations) and their difficulty in starting and maintaining conversations with others can be attributed to poor performance monitoring and task initiation (Bennetto et al., 1996). Likewise, deficits in these mental processes (i.e., performance monitoring and task initiation), as well as in planning skills, may explain why children and adolescents with HFA/AS are typically impaired in their ability to manage their time, prioritize, stay organized (Hill & Frith, 2003), disengage and shift attention when needed, and recall information they had previously been attending to (Attwood, 2007)—all of which may adversely affect the success of these individuals both within the classroom and in the community.

Overall, not all children and adolescents with HFA/AS have executive-function deficits, and many of the mental processes related to executive functioning cannot be directly linked to the behaviors exhibited by these individuals. Additionally, it is important for parents, teachers, and practitioners to understand that executive dysfunction is not exclusive to children and adolescents on the spectrum but also can be seen in individuals with obsessive–compulsive disorder, attention-deficit/hyperactivity disorder, and Tourette syndrome (Hill & Frith, 2003).

Central Coherence

The term *central coherence* is used to describe the general tendency of individuals to integrate, or simultaneously process, incoming pieces of information into meaningful wholes. Happé (1999) suggests that this information processing style (i.e., central coherence) lies on a continuum from strong to weak. Those individuals with a strong central coherence, who include most typically developing individuals, are able to recognize and understand the gist of information and events yet fail to attend to or memorize details. Conversely, individuals with a weak central coherence, such as children and adolescents with autism spectrum disorders, tend to sequentially process information by focusing on the fine details or parts

> **Individuals with a weak central coherence, such as children and adolescents with autism spectrum disorders, tend to sequentially process information by focusing on the fine details or parts of a stimulus, causing them to overlook the global picture (Frith, 2003).**

of a stimulus, causing them to overlook the global picture (Frith, 2003). More recently, Murray, Lesser, and Lawson (2005) have referred to this concept as *monotropism*, whereby individuals on the spectrum exhibit an unusual strategy for allocating attention, focusing on one thing at a time and, consequently, piecing the world together fact by fact.

In general, due to this cognitive style, children and adolescents with HFA/AS are often able to demonstrate proficiency on tasks that require them to memorize specific facts and details (e.g., identifying familiar faces based on recognition of certain facial features) and/ or to focus on the individual elements of a stimulus rather than the whole (e.g., finding hidden objects incorporated into a larger picture; Baron-Cohen & Swettenham, 1997). This enhanced ability to discriminate details also may explain why individuals with HFA/AS frequently have superior rote memory (i.e., the ability to learn by repetition) and/or display an encyclopedic knowledge in specific areas of interest (e.g., roller coasters, NASCAR racing; Hill & Frith, 2003). Unfortunately, though, these children and adolescents appear to be unable to discriminate relevant from irrelevant information, as they have the tendency to fixate on minor, as opposed to major, stimuli. Due to a weak central coherence, this incoming information often remains segmented; therefore, the knowledge of individuals with HFA/AS is of limited utility (Myles & Simpson, 2003).

As a result of this processing style, children and adolescents with HFA/AS are often impaired in their ability to draw conclusions and to interpret information based on context, a skill that is important in both social and academic settings. A weak central coherence may explain why an individual with HFA/AS who has the appropriate ToM skills continues to struggle socially in real-world settings (Happé, 1997). For example, even though this child or adolescent may be able to correctly read social cues, this does not mean that he or she understands where and when to apply these skills (Frith, 2003), resulting in difficulties during interactions with peers and adults. Furthermore, academically, children and adolescents with HFA/AS typically demonstrate poor reading comprehension, as they may remember the details of a story (e.g., the names of all the characters or what one character said to another) yet be unable to state the main idea or theme of a story, highlight the story's relevant information, and/or compare and contrast concepts within the story (Attwood, 2007). Similarly, these individuals fail to take into account the context clues of sentences, causing them to be unable to determine the meanings or pronunciations of words, such as homographs (e.g., *tear* and *read*), which are spelled one way yet have two meanings and are pronounced differently based on these meanings (Hill & Frith, 2003). Overall, parents, educators, and practitioners need to be aware of the strengths and weaknesses associated with having a weak central coherence and use this information to their advantage when designing and implementing social and academic interventions for individuals with HFA/ AS.

CONCLUSION

As was discussed throughout this chapter, children and adolescents with HFA/AS demonstrate both core and related deficits in major areas of development. These impairments, which include difficulties with socialization, concentration on repetitive behaviors and restricted interests, abnormalities in communication, unusual responses to sensory stimuli, academic difficulties, sleep disorders, motor problems, and anxiety and/or mood disorders, can have significantly negative impacts on the general functioning of these individuals. Understanding the characteristics of HFA/AS and the theories underlying these difficulties (i.e., ToM, executive functioning, and central coherence) is essential to the development of effective interventions for these students. Overall, it is imperative for parents, educators, and practitioners to be aware of each child or adolescent's strengths and weaknesses in order to provide the supportive and stimulating environments that these individuals require to excel within their own limitations.

CHAPTER 3

Consultation and
Collaboration Efforts

OVERVIEW

The education of students with HFA/AS is perhaps one of the greatest challenges facing educators and families to date (Cowan & Allen, 2007). Debate regarding the best methods for teaching students with HFA/AS, the specific skills to be taught, and the most appropriate settings for education abounds. In addition, parents and educators may embrace differing perspectives regarding the role of education for students who perform within average limits academically but demonstrate behavioral and/or social skills difficulties. Regardless of individual viewpoints, families and educators will need to interact routinely to best support the educational needs of a student with HFA/AS. In fact, it is not uncommon for a team of educators such as general and special education teachers, school psychologists, speech and language pathologists, and occupational therapists, to name a few, to cooperate regularly with one another, with the student, and with the student's family. Moreover, educational teams at times may need to interact with other health professionals (e.g., psychiatrists, physicians, private therapists) outside of the school setting. As such, it often is necessary to employ a collaborative, transdisciplinary approach when working with students with HFA/AS and their families so that multiple sources of information can be obtained and shared.

In this chapter, we discuss how collaborative consultation can serve as a foundation to the education and support of students with HFA/AS. Such a foundation is predicated on Bronfenbrenner's (1979, 1986) ecological theory that highlights the importance of a transdisciplinary approach to educational programming. Due to the complex nature of assisting students with HFA/AS, a discussion regarding the roles of families and other key stakeholders is highlighted, followed by a review of the problem-solving consultation model. The conjoint behavioral consultation (CBC; Sheridan & Kratochwill, 2008; Sheridan, Kratochwill, & Bergan, 1996) model is described in detail as a model to encourage collaborative, transdisciplinary problem solving across settings. Such topics are addressed within the context of understanding the roles of school-based practitioners in the provision of services for students with HFA/AS.

THE ECOLOGICAL MODEL OF SCHOOL-BASED SERVICES

School-based practitioners have long recognized the importance of assuming an ecological approach to the education and treatment of children with special needs (Gutkin & Curtis, 1999; Sheridan, Kratochwill, & Bergan, 1996).

> **School-based practitioners have long recognized the importance of assuming an ecological approach to the education and treatment of children with special needs.**

Sheridan and colleagues point out that there are several advantages to using ecological theory to drive services for children with special needs: (1) it extends beyond the traditional, setting-specific behavioral approach to understanding behavior; (2) it extends beyond traditional systems theory by focusing on the interrelations among *and* between various systems that influence child development; and (3) it helps practitioners interpret behavior through a comprehensive lens that is compatible with most approaches to educational problem solving (Sheridan & Kratochwill, 2008; Sheridan, Kratochwill, & Bergan, 1996).

Bronfenbrenner's (1979, 1986) ecological theory model recognizes that children operate within and across multiple related environments. That is, the ecological model assumes that children exist as a part of a complex social system wherein development occurs as a "mutual accommodation" between the individual child and the multiple environments in which he or she operates (Bronfenbrenner, 1986).

> **Bronfenbrenner's (1979, 1986) ecological theory model recognizes that children operate within and across multiple related environments.**

Bronfenbrenner's ecological approach to understanding human behavior and development assumes that children are affected by at least five interrelated systems: the microsystem, the mesosystem, the exosystem, the macrosystem, and the chronosystem (see Figure 3.1). Whereas the *microsystem* is concerned with the relationship between the individual child and his or her immediate environment (e.g., the child either at home or at school), the *mesosystem* considers the relationship and connections between two primary environments (e.g., the influence of interactions between the home and school settings). The *exosystem* considers the influence of settings that the child does not directly occupy yet that still affect the child's learning and development (e.g., the workplace of a parent or the home of a teacher). The *macrosystem* level focuses on the influence of cultural, governmental, and global factors on child development (e.g., how a long-lasting war might influence the quality of a child's education). Finally, the *chronosystem* highlights the influence of the micro-, meso-, exo-, and macrosystems on the learning and development of a child over time (i.e., across the lifespan).

School-based practitioners are likely most concerned with mesosystemic influences on the development of a child (Christenson & Sheridan, 2001). Although educators, school psychologists, and related services personnel might focus their energy on microsystems

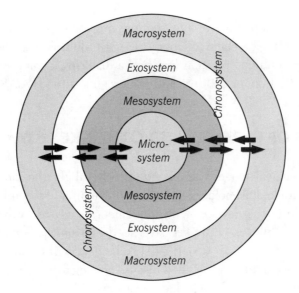

FIGURE 3.1. Bronfenbrenner's ecological model.

level influences on behavior and development, a mesosystemic approach allows them to better understand the child's behavior through the consideration of multiple related environments and their impact on the development of academic and behavioral skills. For example, if a child with HFA/AS is demonstrating an elevated level of noncompliance and off-task behavior in the classroom, it may be helpful for the team to investigate whether an event occurring in the home environment (e.g., difficulty sleeping) may be influencing the child's behavior in the school setting. In behavioral terms, this type of influence is referred to as a *setting event*—that is, a temporally or contextually removed stimulus that may bear a functional relationship to the behavior (Wahler & Fox, 1981). Thinking beyond immediate antecedents and consequences when addressing a behavior may have profound implications for how educational teams approach assessment and intervention (Cowan & Sheridan, 2009). It is important to note that, in this example, the parent acts as a common factor across settings and providers. It is advisable for school-based practitioners to both (1) understand the pivotal role parents play in the education and treatment of their child and (2) acknowledge the unique skills and child-specific knowledge parents possess as members of the educational team (Christenson & Sheridan, 2001; Sheridan, Cowan, & Eagle, 2001).

An ecological approach to the education and treatment of children with special needs reminds school-based practitioners of the importance of seeking comprehensive data to inform their practice. A multidimensional assessment approach (McConaughy & Ritter, 2002) involves gathering multisource data (i.e., data from several key stakeholders, including parents, teachers, and medical personnel) through multiple means (e.g., utilizing ratings scales, interviews, direct observations, records review) across a variety of settings (e.g., home, school, community treatment organization) in an effort to gain a comprehensive understanding of a student's strengths and needs. The development of a thorough picture of the student regarding both academic performance and behavioral skills allows the student's educational team to develop effective interventions or, when appropriate, an individualized education program (IEP). Through collaborating with multiple stakeholders, student support personnel are in a unique position to assist in fostering a comprehensive approach to assessment and intervention for children and adolescents with HFA/AS.

THE ROLES OF PARENTS AND OTHER KEY STAKEHOLDERS

A review of the ecological model was intended to highlight the paramount importance of working with multiple stakeholders to both (1) develop a broad understanding of each student and (2) guide in the development, implementation, and evaluation of individualized programming for children with pervasive needs. Given the complexity of HFA/AS, a variety of stakeholders will be involved. Following are detailed discussions regarding the roles and importance of including various stakeholders in the provision of support services for students with HFA/AS.

> **Given the complexity of HFA/AS, a variety of stakeholders will be involved.**

Parents as Primary Stakeholders

Although the education and treatment of children with HFA/AS often requires several key stakeholders (e.g., parents, teachers, student support services personnel, medical professionals, community-based providers), it is helpful when multidisciplinary team leaders recognize that parents assume a pivotal role in their children's education and treatment. Common roles for the parents include acting as coaches (i.e., encouraging the use of skills in applied settings), cotherapists, interpreters of behavior and language, providers of information about the children's educational and developmental history, and coordinators of service (Siegel, 2003). Within the context of participating in the planning, coordination, and coimplementation of educational, behavioral, and medical programming for children with HFA/AS, parents acquire an incredibly broad knowledge base and skill set. Given their in-depth experiences and history of their children's development, parents often possess a wealth of knowledge regarding their children's behavior. As such, parents should be actively engaged throughout the evaluation and intervention processes. Of all participants in educational teams, parents are the most likely to possess an understanding of how their children develop within the context of Bronfenbrenner's (1986) concept of the *chronosystem*, which focuses on how various systems influence a child's education and development throughout the formative years. This is a unique and critical viewpoint often missing from most contemporary multidisciplinary team meetings.

> **Given their in-depth experiences and history of their children's development, parents often possess a wealth of knowledge regarding their children's behavior.**

A rationale for the active engagement and participation of parents reaches beyond the face validity of including their relative expertise. Parents have long been involved in educational programming to enhance the academic, behavioral, and social successes of both children deemed at risk for academic failure and children identified with special needs in the school setting (Comer, 1984; Epstein et al., 2002; Christenson & Sheridan, 2001; Sheridan, Kratochwill, & Bergan, 1996). Furthermore, research indicates that parental involvement in education has been associated with increased student achievement, improved school attendance, enhanced study skills, increased roles of homework completion and accuracy, and fewer discipline concerns for a variety of learners (Epstein et al., 2002; Sheridan, Kratochwill, & Bergan, 1996; Cowan, Swearer, & Sheridan, 2004). Indeed, parent involvement may be one of the most critical elements associated with successful outcomes for children with HFA/AS.

Educators and Student Support Services Personnel as Key Stakeholders

Within the context of a relative expertise approach to the education and treatment of children with HFA/AS, teachers maintain a critical role in the process. Whereas general educators possess a solid understanding of typical child development, of universal approaches to the education of children, and of the development and implementation of curricular materials, special educators possess an understanding of differentiated instruction, of curricular modifications, of the development of IEP, and of how to address the needs of a variety of learners. When engaging in collaborative problem solving, including both general and special educators in the process may be most beneficial to the child with HFA/AS because he or she most likely will receive instruction in a general education classroom with additional supports and/or modifications (Myles, 2005). Educational teams composed of general educators, special educators, autism specialists/consultants, and paraprofessionals alike can serve as a solid foundation from which to develop individualized educational programming through the use of a variety of accommodations as delivered through a continuum of placement.

Another invaluable group of educational professionals, commonly referred to as student support services personnel, include school psychologists, speech pathologists, occupational therapists, and school/guidance counselors. In addition to their knowledge and skills related to assessment, prevention, intervention at multiple levels, and crisis response, school psychologists frequently serve as consultants, wherein they offer their expertise in both content (i.e., knowledge about adaptive and disruptive behaviors of students with HFA/AS) and process (i.e., knowledge and understanding of the problem-solving process; Gutkin, 1996). Although other school-based personnel (e.g., school counselors, social workers, special educators, special education coordinators) can serve as consultants in collaborative consultation, school psychologists have long been recognized as leaders in this domain (Gutkin & Curtis, 1990, 1999).

Speech pathologists offer yet another area of expertise as related to programming for children with HFA/AS. Armed with their knowledge about communication and language development, speech pathologists often serve as both language assessment experts and interventionists. There are many aspects of communication that may interfere with a student's academic or social-communicative successes, including receptive language, expressive language, social-communicative functions of language, and pragmatic speech. With regard to receptive language, children with HFA/AS may have difficulty with idioms (e.g., "The early bird gets the worm") and understanding humor in applied contexts (Attwood, 2007; Klin et al., 1995; Myles & Simpson, 2003; Myles, Trautman, & Schelvan, 2004). With regard to expressive language, children with HFA/AS may speak in a manner that is much too proper for colloquial conversation, setting themselves apart from their typical peers (Ozonoff, et al., 2002). Should any of these communication patterns interfere with the child's learning or social functioning, having a speech pathologist as part of the problem-solving team can be invaluable.

A smaller, yet equally important, group of student services support personnel that may serve as part of a collaborative team include occupational and physical therapists, guidance counselors, and rehabilitation counselors. Occupational and physical therapists should be involved as part of the multidisciplinary team when issues pertaining to the assessment and intervention of fine-motor skills, gross-motor skills, recreational and leisure skills, and when other functional and adaptive motor skills are involved. School guidance counselors and rehabilitation counselors can offer expertise and guidance to assist the student in exploring employment and/or postsecondary education options. A brief overview of the relative expertise and roles of these related services personnel is included here as a reminder of how important it is to consider collaborations among multiple key stakeholders in the education and treatment of children with HFA/AS.

Other Health Professionals and Community-Based Providers as Key Stakeholders

It is estimated that between 25 and 37% of children with ASD have comorbid medical conditions (Barton & Volkmar, 1998). A variety of medical conditions are commonly comorbid with a diagnosis of an ASD, including seizures, gastrointestinal conditions (e.g., celiac disease, constipation, diarrhea), sleep difficulties, eating and nutritional difficulties, poor muscle tone, and altered pain threshold (Satter, 2007). Given the variety and potential severity of complications often associated with such medical conditions, it is critical for parents and educational professionals to collaborate with medical professionals. Such collaborations may bring together pediatric neurologists, developmental pediatricians, psychiatrists, nurses, and social workers to develop a better understanding of how associated conditions may affect behavior and overall wellness across settings. In addition to adding unique viewpoints to the assessment process, these professionals may assist in developing a variety of medical interventions (e.g., psychopharmacological intervention) to enhance educational programming for students with HFA/AS. Although not a cure, medical intervention such

> It is estimated that between 25 and 37% of children with ASD have comorbid medical conditions (Barton & Volkmar, 1998).... Given the variety and potential severity of complications often associated with such medical conditions, it is critical for parents and educational professionals to collaborate with medical professionals.

as prescription medication may assist in treating symptoms that impair educational and social functioning (e.g., aggressive behavior, self-injurious behaviors, depressed or elevated moods, poor attention, obsessions, compulsions, sleep problems; Bodfish, 2004). In fact, it would not be uncommon for an educational team to assist in determining the effectiveness of a medication regimen. Such a collaborative partnership represents but one of many possible scenarios involving parents, educators, and medical professionals.

Aside from the aforementioned medical conditions, many children and, in particular, adolescents with HFA/AS possess comorbid mental health conditions such as anxiety and depression (Tonge et al., 1999; Kim et al., 2000). Therefore, a close collaborative relationship should be forged, when necessary, with a variety of mental health professionals, including pediatric psychologists, child clinical psychologists, and social workers. Community-based mental health professionals often participate in the provision of comprehensive services for children with HFA/AS. Because it is not uncommon for children with HFA/AS to have higher levels of cognitive ability than children with classic autism, these individuals are often better equipped to participate in behavioral and cognitive-behavioral therapy with community-based mental health providers. For example, a parent might seek the services of a pediatric psychologist for an adolescent with AS demonstrating social anxiety. Although this condition clearly may have a direct impact on the child's educational performance, the student's parent may opt to seek consultation outside of the school to assist in more intensive, symptom-specific treatment. In this scenario, both educators and clinic-based therapists may be involved in the treatment of social anxiety in this adolescent with AS. Specifically, whereas a community-based psychologist may help the child learn specific social skills and coping strategies through direct instruction, modeling, guided practice, and parent consultation, school-based practitioners are well positioned to provide an environment enriched with multiple embedded opportunities for the child to practice a variety of emerging skills. This would require ongoing communication and collaboration among key stakeholders across settings, which is often fostered by having a parent acting as a liaison.

COLLABORATIVE PROBLEM SOLVING AS A FOUNDATION FOR EFFECTIVE PRACTICE

As indicated previously, it may be in the best interest of children with HFA/AS and their families if they are engaged in a transdisciplinary approach to the provision of services. Consultation is an indirect model of service delivery that has been well documented as a conduit for supports for students with academic, behavioral, and social needs (Gutkin & Curtis, 1990, 1999). In addition, consultation has been conceptualized as a powerful means of establishing relationships among key stakeholders (Christenson & Sheridan, 2001; Sheridan, Eagle, Cowan, & Mickelson, 2001). There are two primary goals of consultation: remediation and prevention (Gutkin, 1996). Within the context of remediation, consultation provides a role for school psychologists and other professionals to assist parents,

> **Within the context of remediation, consultation provides a role for school psychologists and other professionals to assist parents, teachers, and other service providers in decreasing disruptive behaviors and/or developing adaptive behaviors and social skills.**

teachers, and other service providers in decreasing disruptive behaviors and/or developing adaptive behaviors and social skills. With regard to prevention, Gutkin (1996) argues that consultants can provide consultees with two distinct types of information: (1) "content" information, as derived from the educational and psychological bases of knowledge about the specific disruptive and/or adaptive behaviors and (2) "process" information that pertains to the process of problem solving. That is, engaging in consultation affords consultees the opportunity to learn information about both the specific need or concern (i.e., content knowledge) and the process of problem solving (i.e., process knowledge), which may result in independent prevention and remediation in the future. Consultation also has been conceptualized as having implications for a multi-tiered approach to preventive intervention (i.e., universal, targeted, and intensive-level applications; Cowan & Sheridan, 2009; Kratochwill, 2008).

Several models of consultation have been considered in the provision of school-based services to students with special needs, including behavioral consultation (BC; Bergan & Kratochwill, 1990; Kratochwill & Bergan, 1990), CBC (Sheridan & Kratochwill, 2008; Sheridan, Kratochwill, & Bergan, 1996), ecobehavioral consultation (Gutkin, 1993), instructional consultation (Rosenfield, 1992), mental health consultation (MHC; Caplan, 1970), and organizational consultation (Maher, Illback, & Zins, 1984). Whereas a variety of consultation models have influenced school-based services for children demonstrating academic, behavioral, and/or social needs (Gutkin & Curtis, 1990, 1999), it could be argued that BC and CBC have received the greatest amount of attention and empirical support in the fields of education and psychology (Bramlett & Murphy, 1998; Kratochwill, 2008; Sheridan, Welch, & Orme, 1996).

Both BC and CBC are grounded in perhaps one of the best documented approaches to offering collaborative student support, the five-step problem-solving consultation model

> **Both BC and CBC are grounded in perhaps one of the best documented approaches to offering collaborative student support, the five-step problem-solving consultation model.**

(Kratochwill, 2008; Kratochwill, Elliott, & Callan-Stoiber, 2002). According to Kratochwill and colleagues, a best practices approach to problem solving involves the following sequential steps: (1) establishing relationships, (2) problem identification, (3) problem analysis, (4) plan implementation, and (5) plan evaluation. The first step of the problem-solving model (i.e., establishing relationships) is such a critical component of the collaboration process that it has been described elsewhere as the "zero step" (Swanger-Gagne et al., 2007), suggesting that before the team can proceed through the problem-solving sequence, it is essential that the consultant or facilitator take the time to establish a relationship with other team members (i.e., consultees). Failing to do so may result in minimal trust and engagement by multiple members of the consultation team.

Sheridan and Kratochwill (2008) refer to the first step of BC–CBC as "preconsultation." During preconsultation the consultant often focuses on building relationships with the consultees while at the same time gathering information about the individual student's strengths and needs in an effort to streamline the consultation process.

Within the context of BC–CBC, *problem identification* involves engaging team members in identifying and prioritizing the child's needs, agreeing on the most critical need, developing a behavioral definition for the priority need, selecting a reliable and valid data collection system, and gathering baseline data regarding both the target behavior and the conditions surrounding that behavior. *Problem analysis* involves both baseline data analysis and plan development. Baseline data analysis involves reviewing data in terms of frequency, intensity, and/or duration, as well as developing hypotheses about what might be causing or maintaining the target behavior (i.e., the function of the behavior). Upon consideration of the functional hypotheses, *plan development* includes brainstorming possible solutions, agreeing on a functionally relevant and feasible intervention, and developing the specifics of the intervention (i.e., addressing the *who, what, when,* and *where* questions related to implementing the intervention). Following *plan implementation*, the team meets again to conduct a *plan evaluation*. During this phase of behavioral consultation, the team considers outcome data to determine whether the goal has been met. If the goal is met, the team determines specific mechanisms for maintaining treatment gains and establishing generalization across settings. If the goal is not met, the team determines which of the previous steps may be beneficial for the team to reconsider for the student at that time. Although BC and CBC follow the same general problem-solving sequence, they differ in terms of who is involved in the consultation process. Whereas BC was developed within the context of teacher-based consultation (i.e., consultation between a consultant—often a school psychologist—and a teacher), CBC involves consultees from both the home and school environments (i.e., teachers and parents or caregivers).

CBC (Sheridan & Kratochwill, 2008; Sheridan, Kratochwill, & Bergan, 1996), a derivative of BC (Bergan & Kratochwill, 1990; Kratochwill & Bergan, 1990), expands beyond focusing on the school as a primary setting to include the home system in the collaborative problem-solving process. Originally developed to foster home–school collaboration within the context of applied behavioral consultation, CBC provides a structured approach to problem solving across these two microsystems (Christenson & Sheridan, 2001). Since its inception, CBC has been further developed to include the consideration of other systems, including pediatric psychology and other community-based domains (Cowan et al., 2004; Sheridan & Cowan, 2004). CBC may be defined as a partnership-based, indirect service delivery model wherein caregivers (e.g., parents, grandparents, foster parents), educators, and service providers work collaboratively to address the academic, behavioral, developmental, and/or social needs of students for whom multiple parties bear some responsibility for education and treatment (Sheridan & Kratochwill, 1992; Sheridan et al., 2005). Because CBC recognizes the importance of parents as key stakeholders, as well as the implications of a transdisciplinary approach to collaborative problem solving, it should be considered as a hallmark when working with students with HFA/AS.

CONJOINT BEHAVIORAL CONSULTATION

The CBC model borrows from both behavioral and ecological theories (Sheridan & Kratochwill, 2008; Sheridan, Kratochwill, & Bergan, 1996). From behavioral theory, CBC incorporates components that foster gathering behavioral data on a continuous basis in an effort to inform functional assessments and data-based decision making (Sheridan, Cowan, & Eagle, 2001). In addition, CBC recognizes the importance of implementing empirically validated interventions within the context of interpreting and changing behavior from an applied behavior analysis (ABA) perspective (Cowan & Sheridan, 2009). ABA technology encourages the team to consider how antecedent, sequential, and consequential conditions affect behavior; it also is compatible with the notion of preventive intervention through the use of antecedent manipulation and intensive application of consequence-based intervention.

From ecological theory, CBC incorporates Bronfenbrenner's (1979, 1986) system, in which children and their behaviors operate within and across the following systems or levels: microsystem, mesosystem, exosystem, macrosystem, and chronosystem. CBC focuses primarily on mesosystemic relationships wherein key stakeholders (e.g., parents, educators, service providers) from multiple related settings (e.g., home, school, community-based agencies) work together toward common behavioral and educational outcomes (Sheridan & Cowan, 2004). With its emphasis on home–school collaboration, CBC provides a vehicle through which families are meaningfully involved in ongoing educational programming for children who are at risk for academic failure or who exhibit characteristics associated with specific disabilities (Sheridan, Cowan, & Eagle, 2001). In doing so, CBC acknowledges the unique expertise and knowledge possessed by families and caregivers (Christenson & Sheridan, 2001; Sheridan et al., 2005). In addition to the consideration of mesosystemic interactions between and across the home and school environments, CBC may be used as a vehicle through which individuals from other community-based environments (e.g., day care setting) participate in collaborative problem solving.

> With its emphasis on home–school collaboration, CBC provides a vehicle through which families are meaningfully involved in ongoing educational programming for children who are at risk for academic failure or who exhibit characteristics associated with specific disabilities.

Participants include the consultant (in most cases, the school psychologist) and the consultees (e.g., parents, educators, service providers, other relevant parties). Given that CBC is an indirect service delivery model, it generally does not include the child for whom services are being provided. However, there may be times when active participation by the student is deemed relevant (e.g., selecting reinforcers, having older children participate in the development of self-monitoring forms, etc.) at particular phases (e.g., planning for treatment). In CBC, the consultant guides the team through the following procedural stages that operationalize the model: (1) conjoint needs (problem) identification, (2) conjoint needs (problem) analysis, (3) plan (treatment) implementation, and (4) conjoint plan (treatment) evaluation (Sheridan & Kratochwill, 2008; Sheridan, Kratochwill, & Bergan, 1996). Although the CBC stages are applied in a collaborative, dynamic manner that may be adapted to meet the needs of the child and his or her team (e.g., recycling through any stage to further inform the next), the conjoint needs identification, conjoint needs analysis, and conjoint plan evaluation phases are generally conducted through a structured interview. These interviews help ensure the fidelity of the CBC problem-solving process (see Sheridan & Kratochwill, 2008, for additional details and contemporary scholarship). The protocol by which each of these steps is executed within the context of CBC is highlighted in the following and discussed in greater detail in Chapters 4 and Chapter 10.

Conjoint Needs Identification

During this assessment phase of the process, the CBC team collaboratively participates in the conjoint needs identification interview, which addresses the following objectives: (1) defining the target concern in concrete, observable behavioral terms; (2) identifying tentative surrounding conditions of the behavior (e.g., antecedent and consequential conditions); (3) providing a tentative present level of behavior (i.e., specifications regarding the frequency, intensity, or duration of the behavior); (4) establishing an agreed-upon goal for behavior change; and (5) establishing and implementing a baseline data collection procedure.

Conjoint Needs Analysis

The conjoint needs analysis stage comprises two primary objectives: problem analysis and plan development. During problem analysis, the consultation team considers the antecedent and consequent conditions surrounding the behavior (Sheridan, Kratochwill, & Bergan, 1996) in an effort to hypothesize about what may be causing or maintaining that behavior. Information obtained from functional assessments is then used for appropriate support plan development. During plan development, the hypothesized function of the behavior as derived from baseline data collection should link directly to an intervention. In addition to collaboratively considering the hypotheses regarding what may be causing or maintaining a particular disruptive behavior, the team is encouraged to consider a systematic approach to enhancing the likelihood of the child's demonstration of an adaptive replacement behavior. If the disruptive behavior may be prevented or enhanced through antecedent strategies, the team considers the manipulation of such variables to prevent or increase the student's behavior. In addition to antecedent manipulation, the team considers the use of consequential strategies to enhance the likelihood of a positive, adaptive response while at the same time decreasing the likelihood of disruptive, maladaptive behavior.

> The conjoint needs analysis stage comprises two primary objectives: problem analysis and plan development.

Regardless of whether the target behavior is academic or behavioral in nature, it is imperative that the team select from interventions that have proven effective through rigorous research methods. The standard here is that experimental research has demonstrated that the intervention resulted in statistically significant changes in the child's behav-

> **Regardless of whether the target behavior is academic or behavioral in nature, it is imperative that the team select from interventions that have proven effective through rigorous research methods.**

ior through carefully controlled methodology. Another means of determining treatment effectiveness is derived through multiple replications of trials within the context of well-controlled single-subject research studies (Kratochwill & Stoiber, 2000; Stoiber & Kratochwill, 2000). The literature on effective interventions for students with HFA/ AS is replete with words used to describe interventions for which there exists research to validate their effectiveness. Examples of such terminology include *evidence-based interventions, research-based treatments,* and *efficacious interventions.* The National Autism Center has developed a set of standards outlining effective, research-based educational and behavioral interventions for children with ASD. The National Standards Report has been recognized as a leader in informing parents, educators, and related professionals of the most promising interventions to be used in the education and treatment of children with HFA/AS (see *www.nationalautismcenter.org* for more information and to request the report).

Once the team conjointly identifies the most appropriate intervention, final treatment planning begins. At this point, the team determines the specifics of the intervention, outlines the steps associated with the specified treatment, and assigns roles related to treatment delivery. It is imperative that all CBC team members are involved in this phase and are in agreement as to when, where, and how the intervention will be implemented across settings. It is also important for the team to plan for ongoing data collection to aid in both (1) determining intervention effectiveness and (2) making data-based decisions regarding the alteration or continuation of intervention.

Plan Implementation

There is no structured meeting associated with this phase of CBC. The primary objective of plan implementation is to do what it takes to maximize the likelihood that the intervention will be implemented with fidelity so the plan results in meaningful outcomes for the child (Sheridan, Kratochwill, & Bergan. 1996). At this point, the consultant is advised to remain in close contact with all concerned parties in an effort to monitor their needs, to provide knowledge and skills enhancement as needed, to reward their successes in treatment implementation, and provide guidance should an alteration or change be deemed necessary (Sheridan & Cowan, 2004).

Conjoint Plan Evaluation

During this phase, which may include more than one meeting, the primary objectives include: (1) evaluating the data to determine whether the goals have been met; (2) evaluating the overall effectiveness of the intervention; (3) planning for the continuation, modification, or termination of the intervention; (4) planning for maintenance and generalization of any observed treatment gains; and (5) discussing a means of continued collaboration (Sheridan & Kratochwill, 2008; Sheridan, Kratochwill, & Bergan, 1996). Given the pervasive needs of children with HFA/AS and the complexity of disruptive behaviors, it may be necessary to recycle through the CBC process, as determined through an evaluation of treatment phase data. This might involve returning to a new understanding of the behavior to design and implement a new data collection system.

> **Given the pervasive needs of children with HFA/AS and the complexity of disruptive behaviors, it may be necessary to recycle through the CBC process, as determined through an evaluation of treatment phase data.**

Alternatively, it could involve revisiting the hypotheses related to what might be causing or maintaining the behavior of concern, which in turn may lead to the development of a revised treatment plan. Regardless of the next step(s) in the dynamic CBC process, it is critical that all concerned parties are involved in joint decision making, as this is one of the primary assumptions of the CBC model (Christenson & Sheridan, 2001).

CBC CASE STUDY: ALEX

Alex was an 8-year-old, third-grade male student diagnosed with HFA at age 5. His parents were actively engaged in his educational career, consistently making an effort to collaborate with members of his educational team to maximize Alex's experience at school. Alex's educational team described him as an extremely bright, energetic student who performed well in subject areas of interest to him (i.e., literature, science, and social studies). Ms. Jones, Alex's teacher, indicated that she sincerely believed that Alex benefited both academically and socially from participating in the general education classroom. However, she reported that when it came to mathematics, he was often off task and failed to complete assignments on a regular basis. She reported that this was a concern for both in-class math assignments and related homework. Ms. Jones was concerned that Alex's math grade was beginning to suffer as a result of his noncompletion of assignments. In addition, she was concerned that Alex was missing out on learning and mastering key math concepts that would aid him in higher order math tasks in the future.

Ms. Jones referred Alex to the school psychologist for behavioral consultation due to his failure to complete math assignments on a regular basis. Because Alex's parents were so involved with Alex's education, and in an effort to gain a more comprehensive understanding of Alex's noncompletion of math assignments, the school psychologist opted to utilize a CBC team approach to improving Alex's performance in the area of math. During the conjoint needs identification meeting, it was determined that, although Alex's failure to complete assignments was of major concern, his off-task behavior during this time was not disruptive to others. However, his parents and teacher feared Alex was missing out on critical math content while engaging in off-task behavior (e.g., drawing quietly at his desk, going over to the computer area and playing science games). Ms. Jones reported that when motivated to do so, Alex demonstrated the ability to complete math problems with a higher than average accuracy rate. Alex's parents agreed that Alex had demonstrated the ability to complete most math assignments with accuracy and that clearly a performance deficit was linked to his noncompletion of math assignments. The team agreed to monitor both assignment completion and accuracy for a week using math worksheets as permanent products. This allowed the calculation of percentage of completion and percentage of accuracy as a potential outcome variable. In addition, the team agreed that the school psychologist would observe Alex in the classroom and that his parents would observe him during homework using an interval recording system that captured both on-task and off-task behaviors in relation to the completion of math assignments (i.e., an adapted version of the *Behavioral Observation of Students in Schools [BOSS]*; Shapiro, 2004). Finally, the school psychologist and Alex's parents agreed to track antecedent and consequential conditions surrounding on- and off-task behavior in an effort to gain additional insight as to what may have been causing or maintaining Alex's relatively high level of off-task behavior.

During the conjoint needs analysis meeting, the team conducted a brief functional assessment and developed an intervention plan linked to the resulting hypothesis. Baseline data indicated that in the classroom setting, Alex completed two out five assignments (i.e., 40%), and for those assignments he completed, he achieved an accuracy rate of 84%. At home, baseline data indicated that Alex completed one out of three assignments (i.e., 33%), with an accuracy rate of 82%. In addition, it was observed that Alex was on task for 23% of the observed intervals during independent math seatwork as compared with 68% for the typical classroom male peer. As the team considered these data within the context of a functional behavior assessment, it was determined that Alex frequently was allowed to escape from working on his math assignment through easy access to preferred activities. Ms. Jones made the observation that because Alex was not disruptive while off task, classroom staff often allowed him to engage in a preferred activity with the assumption that the assignment could be completed as homework. In addition, the team observed that Alex was most likely to complete an assignment either when it was a preferred type of math worksheet or when a preferred activity appeared immediately following math on the classroom schedule. Alex's parents reported that Alex often drifted away from the assignment at home, mainly focusing his attention on either computer games or a nearby television/game system. Based on the conclusion that Alex was motivated by escape, his team came up with an intervention plan that allowed Alex to earn escape from math work contingent on the completion of math problems. Specifically, for every two math problems Alex completed, he was allowed to cross out one math problem on the same worksheet using a favorite scented marker (adapted from Doyle, Jenson, Clark, & Gates, 1999). One condition was that his teachers added to the length of the worksheet in an effort to ensure assignments of adequate length. This intervention was designed to be first implemented in the classroom, then in the home setting if the math assignment was sent home to be completed (no additional homework assignments were given). When the assignment was complete, Alex was allowed to select from three teacher- or parent-approved preferred activities for the remainder of that allotted time period in the respective setting.

Following plan implementation, the team met on two occasions to conduct ongoing conjoint plan evaluation. During the 1st week of intervention, Alex's completion rate for the classroom went up to 80%. The one assignment that was sent home was completed. No major changes were made following this initial week of intervention implementation. During the 2nd and 3rd weeks of intervention, Alex's completion rate was 100% in the classroom, thus removing the need for intervention at home. His average accuracy rate across settings was 94% (class average = 92% accuracy) during intervention. During the time period during which Alex was expected to be working on his assignment, it was observed that he was on task 72% of the intervals, as compared with 68% for the typical classroom male peer. All parties were pleased with his improved performance and rated both the consultation process and intervention to be highly acceptable.

CONCLUSION

Given the pervasiveness of the symptoms associated with HFA/AS, it is essential to utilize a comprehensive, transdisciplinary approach such as CBC. The fields of education and psychology have long recognized the potential benefits associated with both ecological and behavioral approaches when developing individualized treatment plans for children either at risk for academic failure or those children identified with specific disabilities (Sheridan, Kratochwill, & Bergan, 1996; Sheridan & Kratochwill, 2008). Furthermore, the consultation literature is rich with examples of positive outcomes associated with the implementation of treatment plans consisting of input from and participation by individuals from more than one setting (e.g., Sheridan, Eagle, Cowan, & Mickelson, 2001). Indeed, scientist–practitioners

> The consultation literature is rich with examples of positive outcomes associated with the implementation of treatment plans consisting of input from and participation by individuals from more than one setting.

have made an impressive contribution to better understanding how to meet the needs of students with special needs. However, given the pervasive needs of students with HFA/AS combined with an ever-increasing need for accountability within the public education system, the need for collaborative systems that are assessment driven and accountable is of primary importance.

CHAPTER 4

Conducting a Comprehensive Assessment

> The overriding purpose of all assessments is to gather information
> to facilitate effective decision making.
> —WITT, ELLIOTT, DALY, GRESHAM, and KRAMER (1998, p. 17)

OVERVIEW

Assessing students with HFA/AS often is a complicated process, to say the least. Frequently, contradiction, uncertainty, and disagreement exist regarding the best tools for assessing the unique and idiosyncratic patterns of academic, behavioral, and social skills characteristics of students with HFA/AS. Moreover, students with HFA/AS do not fit a uniform profile of needs that can be used to formulate a specific assessment approach. Aside from such characteristics, common school-based assessment practices tend to rely solely on traditional standardized, norm-referenced assessment instruments such as IQ tests, academic achievement tests, and behavioral rating scales. These instruments frequently fall short of providing information necessary for intervention development. Therefore, a more comprehensive assessment practice that evaluates a child's total level of functioning, as well as the environments in which that child is expected to function, is needed. Within this chapter, examples of tools and descriptions of strategies are provided to inform practitioners of the best approaches to assessing children with HFA/AS within school-based settings that lead to positive, lifelong outcomes.

TRADITIONAL SCHOOL-BASED ASSESSMENT

Historically, school-based assessments have focused on whether students are eligible for special education services. As such, traditional school-based assessment practices for children and youth with HFA/AS tend to overrely on published standardized, norm-referenced instruments. Within the traditional model, a practitioner (typically a school psychologist) completes an evaluation using instruments that assess a child's intellectual ability, academic achievement levels, behavioral profile, and, at times, adaptive behavior functioning. The information gathered from these instruments is then compiled to describe the child's current level of performance—usually interpreted or described in terms of the severity of the child's deficits in comparison with same-age peers. In most cases, this information is used to suggest or verify that the pattern of weaknesses identified align with a set of diagnostic criteria. Subsequently, the child is determined eligible for one of the special education categories as outlined in the Individuals with Disabilities Education Improvement Act (IDEIA, 2004). Within this traditional framework, assessment is the application of a set of diagnostic criteria to a particular individual.

> **The assessment of children and youth with HFA/AS in schools must be viewed as a process that leads to meaningful interventions intended to improve lifelong functioning rather than the mere act of following a list of procedures for determining eligibility for services.**

Two problems are intrinsic to this traditional assessment approach. First, although this approach to assessment may help some students with HFA/AS access special education services, other students with HFA/AS will not meet special education eligibility requirements and yet will continue to demonstrate a need for school-based supports. In fact, most children and youth with HFA/AS receive the majority of their education within general education classrooms due to their elevated levels of intellectual functioning and academic skills (Myles, 2005). Assessment for the sake of eligibility may be a means to an end, but when a student fails to qualify for special education services it can be the means to a dead end. Second, traditional assessment approaches often emphasize student weaknesses (e.g., "admiring the problem") but fail to identify the root causes (functions) or conditions underlying those weaknesses. Understanding the causal factors of student problems is critical for developing effective interventions in both special education and general education environments. Therefore, the assessment of children and youth with HFA/AS in schools must be viewed as a process that leads to meaningful interventions intended to improve lifelong functioning rather than the mere act of following a list of procedures for determining eligibility for services.

This paradigm shift toward intervention-based assessment requires educators to develop a tool kit of assessment practices that both evaluate the ecological context of student difficulties and determine the causes and/or conditions under which behaviors occur. To be most effective, school-based practitioners should make use of a comprehensive assessment that evaluates the child's total functioning (Goldstein, Naglieri, & Ozonoff, 2009). A comprehensive assessment for a student with HFA/AS will incorporate aspects of both traditional and functional assessment practices that yield detailed information regarding the student's intellectual, behavioral, and social levels of functioning. In the sections that follow, both traditional and functional assessment instruments and strategies are reviewed in reference to this intervention-based paradigm. By viewing assessment tools through an intervention-focused lens, practitioners can evaluate and select instruments that will guide teams toward the development of meaningful solutions.

ASSESSING INTELLECTUAL FUNCTIONING

Issues in Intellectual Assessment

Of the many tools a school-based practitioner can employ to assess the functioning of a student with HFA/AS, tests of intellectual functioning may have the least to offer in terms of direct intervention-development utility. The notion that optimal learning occurs when instruction is matched exactly to the aptitudes (cognitive profiles) of the learner (commonly referred to as aptitude–treatment interaction, or ATI) never has been realized. Moreover, there has been a lack of reliable evidence regarding relationships between subtest profiles obtained on IQ tests and socially important academic and behavioral outcomes of students (Kamphaus, 2001; Watkins, 2000, 2003). In fact, decades of research have failed to demonstrate the practical utility of both ATI and subtest profile analysis approaches and confirmed the need for responsive, intervention-based problem solving when making educational decisions (Deno, 1990; Fuchs & Fuchs, 1986; Gresham & Witt, 1997; Reschly, 2008).

Despite efforts to reform the nature of making special education eligibility decisions by using intervention-based data, many states and local education agencies (LEAs) continue to require the administration of an IQ test when interventions have shown limited success and the child has been referred for a formal psychoeducational evaluation. In this context, practitioners must be aware that obtaining IQ scores represents only a small component of the larger evaluation process and may be most useful for the purpose of developing hypotheses to be examined by further assessment procedures.

The idea that children and youth with HFA/AS frequently obtain unique score profiles when administered a standardized IQ measure has gained considerable popularity. Traditionally, this profile has been characterized by higher verbal than performance skills (Ghaziuddin & Mountain-Kimchi, 2004; Joseph, Tager-Flusberg, & Lord, 2002; Ozonoff, South, & Miller, 2000). Ghaziuddin and Mountain-Kimchi (2004) reported that 50% and 82% of individuals with HFA and AS, respectively, showed higher verbal than nonverbal IQ scores. Although this intellectual profile is common, it does not describe all children with HFA/AS and provides little information for building meaningful interventions. Moreover, such variability in verbal and nonverbal performance may be found in populations of typically developing children (Watkins & Glutting, 2000). Therefore, a discrepancy between verbal and performance skills in a student with HFA/AS cannot be described as unusual, and it should *never* be considered in diagnosis or in educational planning within school-based settings.

> Therefore, a discrepancy between verbal and performance skills in a student with HFA/AS cannot be described as unusual, and it should *never* be considered in diagnosis or in educational planning within school-based settings.

More contemporary understanding of children and youth with HFA/AS has moved the focus away from the differences between verbal and nonverbal skills assessed by most IQ tests to more specific characteristics of cognitive skills in relation to higher order executive functions. Executive functions are a set of intellectual abilities that control and regulate a wide array of behaviors. For example, executive functions permit an individual to initiate and stop actions, to monitor and change behavior as needed, and to plan future behavior when faced with novel tasks and/or situations. Therefore, executive functions are an important component in both academic learning and social understanding because they allow an individual to anticipate outcomes and adapt to changing situations. Many separate skills are subsumed under the category of executive functions; however, researchers (e.g., Courchesne et al., 1994; Liss et al., 2001; Minshew & Goldstein, 2001) have demonstrated that individuals with HFA/AS often exhibit particular cognitive difficulties in relation to attention, flexibility, and working memory.

Attention theorists have demonstrated a delayed response time in the brains of individuals with ASD when they are required to disengage or shift attention from one stimulus to another (Courchesne et al., 1994). Specifically, Courchesne and colleagues (1994) have demonstrated that individuals with ASD continue to attend to stimuli within their environment for 3–5 seconds longer than typically developing children. Difficulty in shifting attention from one focus to another likely translates to a loss of information necessary for engaging in appropriate behaviors or completing comprehension tasks successfully. For example, if a student with HFA/AS is engaged in reading a favorite book during morning routine and a teacher tells the class to put their things away and get their math activity books out, it may take the student with HFA/AS a few more seconds to attend and listen. As a result, the child likely will have difficulty understanding the nature of the directions and potentially not follow them because he or she did not (or could not) attend to the first few seconds.

These attention-shifting delays have been expanded on further and used to describe an overall impaired cognitive style characterized by rigid, inflexible thinking and limited organizational planning (Liss et al., 2001; Ozonoff, Pennington, & Rogers, 1991). As such, individuals with HFA/AS have difficulty with tasks that require managing time, material, and/or space, as well as evaluating ideas, planning a course of action, and communicating details in an organized manner. Furthermore, working-memory theories have posited that individuals with HFA/AS have difficulty both in the ability to maintain information over brief periods of time and to manipulate ideas internally when planning a response. Specifically, research in this domain has demonstrated that individuals with HFA/AS tend to have poor memory for complex visual and verbal information despite having strengths in memory for facts, recollection of patterns or sequences, and word recognition (Minshew & Goldstein, 2001; Steele, Minshew, Luna, & Sweeney, 2007; Williams, Goldstein, & Minshew, 2006).

From a practical perspective, school personnel assessing a student with HFA/AS by use of traditional methods most likely will obtain results characterized by widely discrepant skills across subtests. Specifically, students with HFA/AS likely will perform well in areas requiring sustained attention (e.g., building a design with blocks), basic recognition of facts (e.g., vocabulary, spelling), and simple information processing (e.g., organizing pictures chronologically to complete a story). Furthermore, students with HFA/AS likely will demonstrate weaknesses in shifting attention (e.g., solving logical puzzles containing multiple scientific rules), flexible thinking (e.g., deducing a rule that identifies a set of symbols), and complex information processing (e.g., reading comprehension, written expression tasks), particularly those that require speed or motor skills. Furthermore, students with HFA/AS may demonstrate difficulty on tests or test items that require the use of social skills or social inference. The presence of such cognitive strengths and weaknesses often masks the true intellectual functioning of a student with HFA/AS because his or her obtained IQ score is an average of highly discrepant scores (Klin, Saulnier, Tsatsanis, & Volkmar, 2005). Moreover, the presence of strength within one domain is not indicative of strength in another. For example, Donny, an 11-year-old student with AS, might recognize and read words at the high-school level, but his comprehension of written material may be at the second-grade level. To avoid invalid conclusions when interpreting IQ scores, examiners must be aware of the potential for widely varying skill levels across domains of functioning, as well as the effects of executive functions on student performance.

Considerations in Selecting a Cognitive Measure

Student services personnel, primarily school psychologists, have a number of tools available to them for assessing the intellectual functioning of students with HFA/AS. However, the assessment of specific cognitive skills of students with HFA/AS is laden with both systemic and child-centered issues, as discussed previously. Therefore, several issues should be considered when choosing a cognitive measure. First, the purpose for assessing the intellectual functioning of students with HFA/AS should be considered. Is conducting an IQ test merely a means to an end? Or is it that hypotheses will be identified and utilized to support the development of effective assessment procedures directly linked to appropriate interventions for the student? Clearly, the latter is a more appropriate means and one that, hopefully, leads to a beneficial end. Second, the examiner must have knowledge regarding how executive functioning domains may interfere with test administration and overall performance. Ideally, the examiner will have knowledge of the information highlighted previously, in addition to experience interacting with students with HFA/AS. Such an understanding not only will assist the examiner in selecting an appropriate instrument but also will provide the examiner with information regarding how the symptoms of HFA/AS may have interfered with test performance. Third, the examiner must be aware that some students with HFA/AS may exhibit inappropriate behavior during an evaluation. For example, a student with HFA/AS may engage in such behaviors as slamming his hands on the desk, yelling that he cannot do this anymore, or attempting to kick the examiner halfway through an evaluation. Behavioral difficulties such as these are not malicious. Rather, inappropriate behaviors often are indicators of fatigue, stress, or a loss of control and predictability in the student with HFA/AS. Therefore, examiners need to structure the testing environment in a way that reduces anxiety and increases the student's attention and motivation to complete tasks. For example, a visual checklist may be needed to provide a child with the sequence of events during the evaluation. Providing such a visual support enables the child to understand what is coming next and likely decreases the level of anxiety the child exhibits. Within this written schedule, examiners should provide opportunities for breaks or access to preferred items and activities as a reward for hard work. Breaks are necessary for students with HFA/AS who may exhibit short attention spans or low tolerance for working on abstract tasks on a standardized IQ test and provides them with the motivation to continue. This approach will prove more satisfying to both examiners and examinees.

Measures of Intellectual Functioning

Although a number of IQ tests are available, there are no instruments designed specifically to assess the cognitive profiles of children with HFA/AS, nor any instruments that are considered to be the best. Instead, examiners must select from a number of contemporary instruments that align more closely with the unique and idiosyncratic characteristics of students with HFA/AS. Broadly speaking, measures of intellectual functioning that rely less on the use of complex verbal ability and/or social inference may be more appropriate for assessing students with HFA/AS. Instruments that rely heavily on the need for verbal understanding, such as the Wechsler Intelligence Scale for Children—Fourth Edition (WISC-IV; Wechsler, 2003) and the Stanford–Binet Intelligence Scale—Fifth Edition (SB-5; Roid, 2003), may underestimate the student's true abilities. Selection of the right instrument for each child with HFA/AS helps ensure that an accurate assessment of intellectual functioning is obtained. Ideally, examiners will want to select instruments that provide information on specific, rather than global, constructs that provide useful insights into the child's problem-solving strategies. Table 4.1 briefly summarizes the characteristics of several instruments that may be most appropriate for assessing the cognitive ability of children with HFA/AS (see Flanagan & Harrison, 2005, for detailed information on IQ assessment instruments).

> **Broadly speaking, measures of intellectual functioning that rely less on the use of complex verbal ability and/or social inference may be more appropriate for assessing students with HFA/AS.**

ASSESSING ACADEMIC SKILLS

Traditional Academic Measures

The administration of a traditional published norm-referenced academic achievement measure typically follows a referral for a formal psychoeducational evaluation to determine eligibility for special education. Assessment of academic functioning for students with HFA/AS using traditional, standardized approaches is laden with the same issues and concerns mentioned with regard to IQ testing (i.e., limited utility for identifying interventions, questionable usefulness for students ineligible for special education). Administration of academic achievement measures, in combination with IQ tests or other norm-referenced measures, for the sake of determining eligibility for special education services fails to align with the call for intervention-based assistance when working with students who may be at risk for failure and falls short of aligning interventions appropriately matched to student need. Although it is understood that many states

> **Administration of academic achievement measures, in combination with IQ tests or other norm-referenced measures, for the sake of determining eligibility for special education services fails to align with the call for intervention-based assistance when working with students who may be at risk for failure and falls short of aligning interventions appropriately matched to student need.**

TABLE 4.1. Cognitive Measures for Assessing Individuals with HFA/AS

Measure	Age range (years)	Presentation of instructions	Response modes	Includes time limits?	Practice or teaching items	Benefits	Drawbacks
DAS-II	3–17	Spoken	Speaking, drawing, arranging geometric pieces, marking in response booklet	Yes, on three subtests	Scored teaching items	Permits flexibility in administration; examiners can easily interpret strengths and weaknesses.	Individuals with ASD not included in standardization. May not be suitable for students with language deficits.
KABC-II	3–18	Spoken	Speaking, pointing, completing puzzles, arranging geometric pieces	Yes, on four subtests. Bonus points awarded for speed	Unscored demonstration items; scored teaching items	Individuals with ASD included in standardization. Examiners can examine simultaneous versus sequential processing.	Verbal conceptualization subtests may be difficult for students. May not be suitable for students with language deficits.
Leiter-R	2–20	None; examiner uses pantomimed gestures	Pointing, arranging cards, marking in response booklet	No. Bonus points awarded	Scored teaching items	Useful for students with impaired language skills; includes series of teaching trials.	Individuals with ASD not included in standardization. Gestural instructions may be difficult for examiners to give and for students to understand. Requires strong attention from student.
UNIT	5–17	None; examiner uses pantomimed gestures	Pointing, placing chips on grid, arranging cards, drawing, building block designs	Yes, on one subtest	Unscored demonstration items; scored practice items	Useful for students with impaired language skills; includes series of teaching trials; brief administration time.	Gestural instructions may be difficult for examiners to give and for students to understand. Narrow range of abilities assessed.
WJ-III COG	2–90+	Spoken	Speaking, pointing, marking in response booklet	Yes. On seven subtests (both batteries)	Scored and unscored demonstration items	Allows a practitioner to interpret scores across several levels; may be useful for examining executive functioning.	Individuals with ASD not included in standardization. Lengthy to administer. Listening subtests may be difficult for students.

Note. DAS-II, Differential Ability Scales—Second Edition (Elliot, 2007); KABC-II, Kaufman Assessment Battery for Children—Second Edition (Kaufman & Kaufman, 2004); Leiter-R, Leiter International Performance Scale—Revised (Roid & Miller, 1997); UNIT, Universal Nonverbal Intelligence Test (Bracken & McCullum, 1998); WJ-III, Woodcock–Johnson Tests of Cognitive Abilities—Third Edition (Woodcock et al., 2001).

and LEAs likely will continue to require the administration of traditional published norm-referenced measures as part of a formal psychoeducational evaluation, efforts should be made to use such measures functionally. That is, practitioners may use measures of academic functioning as part of a comprehensive assessment when determining potential eligibility to identify areas of functioning to be included within a student's IEP or to identify broad areas of difficulty that require additional and more purposeful academic assessment(s). In this context, it is imperative that practitioners understand the academic strengths and weaknesses of students with HFA/AS.

Similar to their intellectual skills, the academic skills of students with HFA/AS can be described best as being highly variable. Currently, no single pattern of skills accurately characterizes the academic functioning of students with HFA/AS. Instead, each individual likely will demonstrate a range of highly discrepant scores across a variety of academic tasks. In fact, many anecdotal reports from educators have indicated that individual academic performance ranges from significantly below average to significantly above average. Most common are reports praising the elevated, and oftentimes superior, early word reading skills of a student (or students) with HFA/AS, followed quickly by comments related to the same student's significant difficulty comprehending written material. Studies investigating the academic achievement profiles of individuals with HFA/AS have confirmed what many educators previously have hypothesized. Specifically, Griswold et al. (2002) noted strengths in oral expression and word identification/vocabulary skills combined with weaknesses in written expression on the Wechsler Individual Achievement Test (WIAT; Wechsler, 1992) for a group of students diagnosed with AS. In addition, these authors discovered lower mathematical skills, especially when students with AS were required to solve equations or answer mathematical calculation problems. From the extant literature it appears that the most significant academic difficulties that individuals with HFA/AS experience emerge as demands for abstract reasoning, flexible problem solving, and language-based critical thinking increase (Myles & Simpson, 2003). Therefore, students with HFA/AS likely will demonstrate lower performance on subtests that require application and synthesis of learned information or advanced comprehension or that use complex verbal directions.

As is the case with intellectual functioning, no one instrument is designed to assess the academic profiles of students with HFA/AS. Rather, practitioners must select from an array of instruments that align best with the unique characteristics of each individual with HFA/AS. To make appropriate selections, practitioners must be familiar not only with a student's intellectual and academic strengths but also with how the student's weaknesses in such areas may interfere with test administration and overall performance. Selection of the right instrument for each child with HFA/AS helps ensure that an accurate assessment of academic functioning is obtained.

Two types of traditional norm-referenced academic achievement tests are presented here as part of an overall evaluation for students with HFA/AS. First, academic skills can be measured using broad achievement measures such as the Woodcock–Johnson Tests of Academic Achievement—Third Edition (WJ-III; Woodcock, McGrew, & Mather, 2001), the Kaufman Tests of Educational Achievement—Second Edition (KTEA-II; Kaufman &

Kaufman, 2004), or the Wechsler Individual Achievement Test—Second Edition (WIAT-II; Wechsler, 2001). These instruments measure skills and knowledge across a broad array of reading, writing, and math and may be used as the foundation for identifying general patterns of skills for students. Second, academic proficiency may be measured using narrowband instruments that measure particular skills (e.g., reading fluency, vocabulary). Such instruments may be specific to areas of reading (e.g., Gray Oral Reading Test—Fourth Edition, [GORT-4]; Wiederholt & Bryant, 2001), writing (e.g., Test of Written Language—Fourth Edition [TOWL-4]; Hammill & Larsen, 2009), or math (e.g., Key Math Diagnostic Arithmetic Test—Third Edition [KeyMath-3]; Connolly, 2008). This second type of instrument may be used to assist in identifying specific academic difficulties in particular areas and often can provide greater detail than broad academic achievement tests. Table 4.2 briefly summarizes the characteristics of some traditional norm-referenced instruments that may be used for assessing academic skills in children with HFA/AS. Practitioners are encouraged to examine this table, as well as to investigate other academic measures commercially available.

Aside from the types of instruments available, practitioners must be skilled in advanced interpretation of such instruments. Although scores from these tests can be used, in part, for determining special education eligibility for a student with HFA/AS, these scores alone are of little value when developing effective interventions or IEP goals. Of greater value to teachers who work with and may be responsible for developing and implementing intervention goals for students with HFA/AS are specific interpretations of each subtest or, at times, item scores based on accompanying qualitative information and behavioral observations. School psychologists or other diagnosticians who administer any achievement test (or IQ test for that matter) must assemble data regarding the individualized needs of the student that will provide specific information related to intervention development and identification of appropriate goals.

Curriculum-Based Assessment

Curriculum-based assessment (CBA) is the descriptor broadly applied to testing strategies used for direct and repeated assessment of student performance in the curriculum for the purpose of gaining information useful for educational decision making (Powell-Smith, 1996; Shinn, 2008). According to Deno (1987), CBA uses "direct observation and recording of a student's performance in the local curriculum as a basis for gathering information to make instructional decisions" (p. 41). CBA is not a unitary type of assessment but, rather, represents a collection of assessment models. Historically, four CBA models have been discussed in the literature (cf. Hintze, Christ, & Methe, 2006; Powell-Smith, 1996; Shapiro, 2004; Shinn & Bamonto, 1998; Shinn, Rosenfield, & Knutson, 1989). These four CBA models include: (1) CBA for instructional design (CBA-ID; Gickling & Havertape, 1981; Gickling, Shane, & Croskery, 1989); (2) criterion-referenced CBA (CR-CBA; Blankenship, 1985); (3) curriculum-based evaluation (CBE; Howell, Hosp, & Kurns, 2008; Howell & Nolet, 2000); and (4) curriculum-based measurement (CBM; Deno, 1985; Shinn, 1989, 2008). In addition, the Dynamic Indicators of Basic Early Literacy Skills (DIBELS; Kaminski, Cummings,

TABLE 4.2. Academic Achievement Measures for Assessing Individuals with HFA/AS

Measure	Age range (years)	Presentation of instructions	Response modes	Includes time limits?	Practice or teaching items	Benefits	Drawbacks
GORT-4	3–18	Spoken	Speaking, reading	No. Reading speed is recorded	Unscored practice items	Identifies reading strengths and weaknesses; serves as a device for documenting growth	Discontinuing procedure may lead to premature termination of testing. Some students may have difficulty with comprehension tasks.
KeyMath3	4–21	Spoken	Speaking, pointing	No	Unscored practice items	Covers full spectrum of math concepts and skills; aligns with national math standards; absence of reading and writing tasks	Students with communication delays may find it difficult to follow along and respond.
KTEA-II	4–25	Spoken	Speaking, pointing, writing	Yes	Unscored teaching items	Enhanced reading subtests included; listening and reading	Listening required for some subtests may be difficult for students.
TOWL-4	9–17	Spoken	Speaking, reading, writing	Yes, on one subtest	Unscored practice items	Provides in-depth assessment of writing skills	Subtests that require listening comprehension and prewriting planning may be difficult for some students.
WIAT-II	4–85	Spoken	Speaking, reading, pointing, writing	Yes, on two subtests	Unscored practice items	Assesses inferential comprehension; allows assessment of nonsense word decoding	Levels of reading comprehension may be higher due to use of pictures. Listening required for some subtests may be difficult for students.
WJ-III	2–90+	Spoken	Speaking, reading, pointing, writing	Yes, on four subtests (both batteries)	Scored and unscored demonstration items	Good achievement battery; assesses basic skills, fluency, and application for each academic area	Individuals with ASD not included in standardization; lengthy to administer. Listening required for some subtests may be difficult for students.

Note. GORT-4, Gray Oral Reading Test—Fourth Edition (Wiederholt & Bryant, 2001); KeyMath3, KeyMath—Third Edition (Connolly, 2008); KTEA-II, Kaufman Test of Educational Achievement—Second Edition (Kaufman & Kaufman, 2004); TOWL-4, Test of Written Language—Fourth Edition (Hammill & Larsen, 2009); WIAT-II, Wechsler Individual Achievement Test—Second Edition (Wechsler, 2001); WJ-III, Woodcock–Johnson Tests of Academic Achievement—Third Edition (Woodcock et al., 2001).

Powell-Smith, & Good, 2008; Kaminksi & Good, 1996) are a downward extension of CBM reading (Kaminski & Good, 1998).

Several commonalities exist across the various CBA models. For example, in most cases testing procedures are short in duration. Tasks are designed to be teacher friendly in that they do not eat away instructional time unnecessarily. In addition, CBA is often characterized by frequent and direct measurement of student academic skills. Finally, the data collected typically are linked to instructional planning. According to Shapiro (2004), the common underlying assumption across CBA models is "that one should test what one teaches" (p. 16). However, Shinn and Bamonto (1998) contend that the models do not have much in common when it comes to such issues as the purpose for testing, test development, technical adequacy, and empirical support. Although an in-depth discussion of each of the CBA models is beyond the scope of this chapter, Table 4.3 provides a summary of the primary purpose, framework for use, skill domains assessed, and materials and procedures, as well as resources for further information for the various types of CBA. In addition, the interested reader is referred to Hintze et al. (2006); Powell-Smith (1996); Shinn and Bamonto (1998); and Shinn et al. (1989).

Curriculum-based assessment serves several important purposes in the overall assessment of academic functioning for students with HFA/AS. First, CBA can be used to ameliorate findings from traditional academic achievement tests. In this way, CBA may provide more functional and specific information pertaining to the specific academic difficulties, thereby providing more in-depth data to inform intervention development. Second, because most students with HFA/AS receive their education within general education classrooms or may not qualify for special education, CBA can be used to identify functional academic skill

> **Because most students with HFA/AS receive their education within general education classrooms or may not qualify for special education, CBA can be used to identify functional academic skill deficits and to plan for appropriate interventions.**

deficits and to plan for appropriate interventions. Third, certain types of CBA lend themselves particularly well to goal-setting and progress-monitoring functions, making them useful within a response-to-intervention (RTI) context.

Three CBA types are discussed here in more detail: curriculum-based measurement (CBM), the Dynamic Indicators of Basic Early Literacy Skills (DIBELS), and curriculum-based evaluation (CBE). These three models were chosen because (1) their use is linked to a systematic decision-making framework and (2) they are a focus of contemporary practice and research. First a brief introduction to each of these models is provided. Then the application of these models relative to skills most likely to be of concern for students with HFA/AS is discussed.

Curriculum-Based Measurement

CBM is a set of brief (i.e., 1-minute) standardized measures of basic academic skills (e.g., reading, math, written expression, spelling). These measures were designed to be used as indicators of overall skill within a basic-skills domain. For example, the 1-minute measure of oral reading serves as an *indicator* of overall reading skill. An abundance of research supports the use of CBM as indicators of basic skills useful for screening, goal setting and progress monitoring. Importantly, the use of these measures is tied to a specific decision-making model referred to as the problem-solving model (Deno, 1995, 2002). Although the historical roots of CBM are tied to its use in special education settings (Deno, 1985; Deno & Mirkin, 1980), CBM has been adopted for more widespread use in general education settings since that time (see Shinn, 2008, for a review). Further, although initially CBM materials were drawn from curricula, over time research on this topic concluded that it was not necessary that these tests be constructed using curricular materials (see Fuchs & Deno, 1994; Powell-Smith & Bradley-Klug, 2001, for review).

Although CBM can provide a useful way to index and monitor basic skills of concern for any student, for students with HFA/AS the oral reading fluency (R-CBM), math applications (MA-CBM), and written expression (WE-CBM) measures likely will be of greatest use. R-CBM provides an index of a student's overall reading proficiency, including comprehension. Because R-CBM is a 1-minute measure, it is a very efficient and useful start to rule out reading fluency and decoding as issues that affect student reading comprehension. Nonetheless, if these skills are on track and the student's primary difficulties are with comprehension, further diagnostic assessment will be needed.

MA-CBM provides an index of student skill in completing grade-level mathematics applications problems (Fuchs, Fuchs, & Hamlett, 1995). When administered individually, this 4-minute measure provides an opportunity to directly observe the student's problem-solving efforts. Because students with HFA/AS are more likely to encounter difficulties with applied problems rather than with computation, direct observation of their skills will provide rich data useful for intervention development.

Finally, WE-CBM is conducted by providing the student with an age-appropriate story starter and asking him or her to write for 3 minutes (Powell-Smith & Shinn, 2004). WE-CBM may be useful to track the written expression skills of students with HFA/AS. Whereas these students may perform at high levels when asked to express themselves orally, they often experience challenges with organizing and planning that negatively affect their written expression. Three ways to score WE-CBM include counting total words written, words spelled correctly, or correct writing sequences (Deno, Marston, & Mirkin, 1982; Powell-Smith & Shinn, 2004). The correct-writing-sequences score may be the most important indicator to monitor for students with HFA/AS. This scoring method accounts for semantics and syntax in addition to spelling. The measure also provides an opportunity to observe the student's approach to writing. Given that students with HFA/AS often experience difficulty with the planning and organizational requirements of writing tasks, the opportunity to directly observe students engaged actively in this structured writing task likely will be as valuable as the score itself.

Dynamic Indicators of Basic Early Literacy Skills

DIBELS shares many features and design characteristics with CBM. The measures are standardized, have adequate technical adequacy data for the types of decisions for which

TABLE 4.3. Types of Curriculum-Based Assessment Approaches

Type	Primary purpose(s)	Framework for use	Skill domains	Materials and procedures	Resources for further information
CBA-ID	To determine appropriate student placement in instructional material	No specific procedures or decision rules, but typically used to identify instructional, independent, and frustration levels	May extend to any curricular area	Typically examiner-developed materials and nonstandardized procedures.	• Gickling & Havertape (1981) • Gickling et al. (1989) • Hintze et al. (2006) • Shapiro (2004)
CR-CBA	To determine appropriate instructional content by testing sequential instructional objectives		May extend to any curricular area	Typically examiner-developed materials and nonstandardized procedures.	• Blankenship (1985) • Hintze et al. (2006)
CBE	To provide a structured evaluation and decision-making process focused on curriculum-driven if/then principles, alterable variables, and student outcomes	Step-by-step evaluation inquiry process including: 1. Fact finding and problem validation. 2. Developing assumed causes. 3. Validating assumed causes. 4. Summative decision making. 5. Formative decision making.	Reading (decoding and comprehension), math, written expression, language, social skills	Examiner-developed and readily available materials (i.e., may make use of elements of CBA and CBM); both standardized and nonstandardized procedures are used.	• Howell (2008) • Howell et al. (2008) • Hosp & MacConnell (2008) • Howell & Nolet (2000) • Kelley (2008) • Robinson & Howell (2008)
CBM	To evaluate the effects of instructional programs and interventions via screening and progress monitoring	Problem-solving model including: 1. Problem identification. 2. Problem certification. 3. Exploring solutions. 4. Evaluating solutions. 5. Problem solution.	Basic skills in reading, math, written expression, and spelling	Standard materials available from various sources including: 1. AIMSWeb (*www.aimsweb.com*). 2. EdCheckup (*www.edcheckup.com*). 3. Intervention Central (*www.interventioncentral.org*) Standardized administration and scoring procedures are used.	• Shinn (1989) • Shinn (1998) • Shinn (2008)
DIBELS	Screening to identify students in need of support and progress monitoring to determine effectiveness of instructional support	Outcomes-driven model including: 1. Identifies need for support. 2. Validating need for support. 3. Planning support. 4. Evaluating and modifying support. 5. Reviewing outcomes.	Early literacy skills including: phonemic awareness, alphabetic principle, fluency with connected text, vocabulary, and comprehension	Standard materials available from the following sources: 1. DIBELS Data System (free download; *dibels.uoregon.edu*). 2. Sopris West. 3. Wireless Generation (Palm Pilot version) (*www.wirelessgeneration.com*). Standardized administration and scoring procedures are used.	• Kaminski & Good (1998) • Kaminski, Cummings, Powell-Smith, & Good (2008)

Note. CBA-ID, curriculum-based assessment for instructional design; CR-CBA, criterion-referenced curriculum-based assessment; CBE, curriculum-based evaluation; CBM, curriculum-based measurement; DIBELS, Dynamic Indicators of Basic Early Literacy Skills.

they were designed to be used, have multiple forms for repeated assessment, do not take much time to administer and score, are indicators of critical early literacy skills, and, perhaps most important, are sensitive to small changes in student performance (Kaminski et al., 2008). DIBELS measures include indicators of the following critical early literacy skills: phonemic awareness (e.g., phoneme segmentation fluency; PSF), alphabetic principle/phonics (e.g., nonsense word fluency; NWF), accuracy and fluency with connected text (e.g., oral reading fluency; ORF), comprehension (e.g., ORF plus retell), and oral language/vocabulary (e.g., word use fluency). Each of these measures is designed to be a brief *indicator* of overall skill in the corresponding early literacy skill domain. Thus these measures are not designed to be comprehensive diagnostic assessments of the corresponding skill domain. One characteristic that is unique to DIBELS is the provision of empirically derived benchmarks that indicate the likelihood of the student's meeting the next benchmark. As such, research-based targets are available for goal-setting and progress-monitoring purposes. Finally, DIBELS was designed to be used in the context of a prevention-oriented decision-making model referred to as the outcomes-driven model (see Kaminski et al., 2008, for discussion).

For students with HFA/AS who are experiencing difficulties in the development of their reading skills, an important first step might involve ruling out problems with their automaticity in critical reading subskills (e.g., phonemic awareness). Because DIBELS provides an efficient means of determining whether these skills are on track, it can be used to help make this determination. For example, difficulties with phonological awareness or the development of the alphabetic principle can be determined with the PSF measure and the NWF measure. Each of these measures are 1-minute timed measures and have good technical adequacy for screening and progress-monitoring purposes. In addition, a student's development with oral language and vocabulary may be indexed with the word use fluency (WUF) measure.

What is more likely to be the case for students with HFA/AS is difficulties with reading connected text—in particular, comprehension. Use of measures such as R-CBM and DIBELS ORF may help determine whether decoding or comprehension difficulties (or both) exist. Often students with HFA/AS decode quite well but experience difficulties with comprehension. In part, these challenges may be explained by difficulties experienced with social cognition. "Understanding written text may recruit the same social cognitive processes that underlie oral discourse" (Donahue & Foster, 2004, p. 363). An oral reading fluency measure including a retell component is among the DIBELS measures. Two critical features of this measure set it apart from R-CBM. First, empirically derived benchmarks are provided, as mentioned previously. Second, and most relevant here, DIBELS ORF includes a retell component. Retell serves two important purposes that are particularly relevant to students with HFA/AS. First, retell sends the message to the student that reading is conducted for the purpose of gaining meaning, not for the purpose of being fast at reading. Second, retell allows the examiner to directly index whether a student

> **What is more likely to be the case for students with HFA/AS is difficulties with reading connected text—in particular, comprehension. Use of measures such as R-CBM and DIBELS ORF may help determine whether decoding or comprehension difficulties (or both) exist.**

is tracking meaning. As such, this measure may serve as an important starting place from which to develop hypotheses about reading comprehension difficulties that may be followed up by more in-depth, comprehensive assessment of reading comprehension.

Curriculum-Based Evaluation

CBE is a systematic process of inquiry and decision making that makes use of a variety of CBA strategies. However, at the heart of CBE is the notion of testing out hypotheses about student performance that are tied to alterable variables. Howell, Hosp, and Kurns (2008) describe such hypotheses as a series of "curriculum-driven *if/then* statements" (p. 351) related to the hypothesized or assumed causes of the academic difficulty. The CBE process provides rules about developing these assumed causes, the foremost of which is that they must be related to alterable variables (i.e., something we can change; Howell et al., 2008; Howell & Nolet, 2000). Assessment materials are either gathered or designed to facilitate answering questions and interventions are then aligned based on whether the answers are yes or no. For example, if the question is "Does Victor have difficulty with comprehension of expository text?" then assessments are gathered to help answer this question with respect to why he is having difficulty comprehending these texts. Assumed causes might be that Victor has not been taught grade-level decoding skills to mastery, that he is not yet sufficiently fluent to gain meaning from text, or that Victor is not using metacognitive strategies (i.e., executing a planned approach to reading, monitoring his understanding as he reads, etc.).

The CBE process begins with defining and validating the problem. These goals may be accomplished with CBM and/or DIBELS approaches, as described previously. In addition, other data may be used (e.g., classroom assignments, traditional achievement test data). Following this step, the goal for the student is established. Once assumed causes are generated, then specific-level assessments may be required to examine them in order to develop a comprehensive and appropriately targeted intervention. In the case of Victor, to explore the issue of metacognitive strategies, a think-aloud interview might be used to examine such things as self-monitoring, reflection, discriminating essential details from extraneous information, and problem solving (Howell, 2008). During this interview, Victor may be prompted with such questions as "How could you decide what information in this passage is most important?" In addition, Victor might be asked to show the interviewer how to identify specific text structure elements (e.g., main idea, supporting details, irrelevant information) by highlighting or underlining them while reading.

Instructional programming is developed based on the data obtained from the specific-level assessments. Once a program or intervention is developed, the CBE process indicates that progress-monitoring data are collected to determine intervention effectiveness. In CBE, these progress-monitoring assessments may include CBM or DIBELS, as well as classroom assessments, or specific-level testing procedures used earlier in the process (Howell et al., 2008). Thus, this process affords practitioners a great deal of flexibility when designing assessment protocols for examining intervention effects. Because of the detailed nature with which (1) assumed causes are described, (2) ways to conduct specific-level assessments are listed linked to such causes, and (3) higher order skills within academic domains are addressed (e.g., advanced reading skills), the CBE process is very useful for students with HFA/AS. Particularly noteworthy are the CBE procedures for evaluating reading comprehension, language (including pragmatics), written expression, and math described in Howell and Nolet (2000). Resources for obtaining detailed information about CBE with respect to a variety of academic skill domains, as well as social functioning, are listed in Table 4.3. Intervention ideas for commonly occurring academic difficulties for students with HFA/AS are detailed in Chapter 5.

ASSESSING ADAPTIVE BEHAVIOR

Adaptive behavior is defined as the age-appropriate skills or abilities that enable an individual to live independently and to function aptly in daily life. Examples of adaptive behavior include daily skills such as caring for oneself, dressing, grooming, managing money, cleaning, dealing with conflict, and making and keeping friends. Generally speaking, adaptive behavior includes those skills and abilities necessary to perform both personal and social activities self-sufficiently. Although a host of adaptive behavior problems among individuals with HFA/AS have been reported anecdotally, little research has been conducted in this area to suggest that it is a widespread concern (Klin, Sparrow, Marans, Carter, & Volkmar, 2000). However, recent studies demonstrate that many individuals with HFA/AS exhibit significant delays across myriad adaptive behavior domains despite having average to above-average intelligence and intact communication skills. For example, Myles et al. (2007) demonstrated that individuals with AS obtained low or moderately low levels of adaptive functioning across all measured adaptive behavior domains, including communication. Moreover, in a review of contemporary research, Lee and Park (2007) concluded that the adaptive behaviors of individuals with HFA/AS were at lower levels than would be expected, particularly in the areas of communication, daily living skills, motor skills, and socialization. In short, the adaptive behavioral functioning of students with HFA/AS is often lower than their level of intellectual and/or communicative skills (Klin, Saulnier, Tsatsanis, & Volkmar, 2005). Given this conclusion, many students with HFA/AS likely will struggle to achieve even the simplest of daily tasks.

> Recent studies demonstrate that many individuals with HFA/AS exhibit significant delays across myriad adaptive behavior domains despite having average to above-average intelligence and intact communication skills.

Whereas the assessment of adaptive behaviors is a cornerstone of practice for students with classic autism and more profound cognitive disabilities, such appraisals typically are not incorporated into a school-based evaluation for students with HFA/AS. This assessment is often not undertaken because educators have believed that individuals with HFA/AS do not suffer from significant delays in adaptive behaviors aside from their limited socialization skills. Given the fact that many students with HFA/AS likely will demonstrate delays in independent functioning across much broader domains, assessment of adaptive behavior appears appropriate. Perhaps the most relevant purpose of an adaptive behavior assessment is the identification of potential life skills to be included in the student's IEP and targeted for instruction. When targeting such goals, educators should stress the extent to which instruction will promote age-appropriate independence. A primary consideration in targeting goals is to utilize the "criterion of ultimate functioning" (Brown, Nietupski, & Hamre-Nietupski, 1976), which poses the question "If the student does not learn to do the task, will someone else have to do it for him or her?" When the answer to this question is "yes," planning for and incorporating instruction in the particular adaptive behavior are necessary.

Assessment of adaptive functioning typically involves the use of rating scales completed as part of a structured interview with a parent, a teacher, or another individual who is familiar with the child's daily routines and activities (see Sattler & Hoge, 2006, for detailed information on adaptive behavior assessment instruments). Within school settings, the Scales of Independent Behavior—Revised (SIB-R; Bruininks, Woodcock, Weatherman, & Hill, 1984) and the Vineland Adaptive Behavior Scales—Second Edition (VABS-II; Sparrow, Cicchetti, & Balla, 2005) are the most widely used instruments. Both of these instruments provide detailed information regarding a student's level of functioning in the broad domains of communication, daily living skills, socialization, and motor functioning. When administered in interview format, both the SIB-R and the VABS-II can take up to 60 minutes to complete. Alternate formats (i.e., parent and teacher rating forms, abbreviated administration) can be used with both instruments to reduce the amount of time required to complete the assessment. However, the full interview formats are preferred because they allow an examiner to gain more detailed information about a student's level of functioning. When a full interview format cannot be conducted, and when parent and/or teacher time is an issue, the Adaptive Behavior Assessment System—Second Edition (ABAS-II; Harrison & Oakland, 2003) can be used. The ABAS-II consists of a series of forms that are completed by parents, teachers, and, when appropriate, the individual. Each form assesses an individual's functional skills across 10 domains and can be completed in 15–20 minutes.

ASSESSING DIAGNOSTIC CHARACTERISTICS OF HFA/AS

Obtaining information related to the diagnostic characteristics of HFA/AS often is a small part of the larger assessment process and typically is reserved for those individuals who are being considered for special education eligibility. This form of assessment most often utilizes rating scales designed to measure the severity of impairment within several core areas of development: (1) social interactions and relationships, (2) repetitive or restricted behaviors, interests, and/or activities, and (3) communication and language use (see Table 4.4 for an overview of several common instruments). These scales are designed to quantify the severity of impairment by aligning specific items to behavioral indicators associated with the diagnostic characteristics of autism and AS. From this perspective, these scales emphasize student weaknesses ("admire the problem") and fail to identify the root causes (functions) or conditions underlying those weaknesses. Of the many tools and strategies available to assess the overall functioning of a student with HFA/AS, rating scales may have the least to offer in terms of direct intervention-development utility.

TABLE 4.4. Scales Used to Assess Diagnostic Characteristics of HFA/AS

Measure	Age range (years)	Number of items	Purpose	Benefits	Drawbacks
ASDS	5–18	50	Differentiates individuals with AS from other persons with autism and other behavior disorders	Yields overall and domain standard scores	Questions are answered in yes/no format; questionable standardization sample; substandard psychometric properties
ADI-R	Above 2	93	Assesses the presence and severity of symptoms of ASD across three main areas: language and communication, reciprocal social interactions, stereotyped behaviors and interests	Thorough assessment that is useful for assisting in diagnosis as well as treatment and educational planning	Children with ASD were not included in the standardization sample; takes 1.5 to 2.5 hours to complete; only raw scores are calculated; requires significant training prior to use
GADS	3–22	32	Evaluates individuals with unique behavior problems and discriminates persons with AS from persons with autism or other behavioral disorders	Individuals with ASD included in standardization; examines domains that are characteristic of AS; behaviors rated on a 4-point scale; yields overall and domain standard scores	Items may not be sensitive enough to the variability of functioning in children with HFA/AS; definitions for scores may not be robust enough to capture prolonged difficulties; substandard psychometric properties
GARS-2	3–22	42	Assesses the severity of autism characteristics in three categories: communication, social interaction, and stereotyped behaviors	Individuals with ASD included in standardization; behaviors rated on a 4-point scale; provides operational definitions for each item; yields overall and domain standard scores	Items may not align with the elevated skills of individuals with HFA/AS; may not be sensitive enough to capture withdrawn features of more social individuals
KADI	6–22	32	Distinguishes individuals with AS from those who have other forms of higher functioning autism	Standardized on individuals with higher functioning ASD; useful for distinguishing features of AS from autism	Standardization data based almost exclusively on parent report; no teacher data exist
PDDBI	1–12	124	Assesses levels of both adaptive and maladaptive functioning in domains specific to ASD: communication, social interaction, ritualistic activities, and learning skills	Individuals with ASD included in standardization; age-normed; useful for clinical, educational, and research applications; taps into withdrawal and anxiety-related symptoms; yields a variety of standard scores (*T*-scores)	Both the parent and teacher forms are lengthy; fewer items aligned specifically with higher functioning individuals

Note. ASDS, Asperger Syndrome Diagnostic Scale (Myles, Jones-Bock, & Simpson, 2000); ADI-R, Autism Diagnostic Interview—Revised (Rutter, Le Couteur, & Lord, 2003); GADS, Gilliam Asperger's Disorder Scale (Gilliam, 2001); GARS-2, Gilliam Autism Rating Scale—Second Edition (Gilliam, 2006); KADI, Krug Asperger's Disorder Index (Krug & Arick, 2003); PDDBI, PDD Behavior Inventory (Cohen & Sudhalter, 2005).

63

Although the administration of a diagnostic rating scale may be necessary within school-based assessment, practitioners should focus more of their attention on identifying unique strengths and/or special interests of a child with HFA/AS. It is not uncommon for individuals with HFA/AS to demonstrate significant and, at times, perseverative interests across a wide variety of topics (e.g., bridges, vacuum cleaners, trains). For example, Nathan, a 12-year-old student with HFA, spent several hours a day reading about and discussing dinosaurs. Nathan's extreme fascination with dinosaurs led him to memorize all of the specific facts about the tyrannosaurus, mapusaurus, and other creatures that lived during the Mesozoic era. Although many educators may want to limit the use of special interests, reserving them for use contingent on the demonstration of some targeted behavior (e.g., staying on task), it may be advantageous to use a student's interest across content areas and within lessons. Special interests can be an important asset in developing interventions because they likely will increase motivation for the student to engage in nonpreferred activities. Granted, care will need to be taken to systematically embed special interests into activities.

> Although the administration of a diagnostic rating scale may be necessary within school-based assessment, practitioners should focus more of their attention on identifying unique strengths and/or special interests of a child with HFA/AS.

ASSESSING BEHAVIORAL SKILLS

Functional Behavioral Assessment

One of the most effective approaches to addressing challenging behaviors is functional behavioral assessment (FBA). Like other assessment approaches, FBA is a process for gathering information to answer a set of assessment questions. More specifically, FBA is designed to gather information about events in a person's environment that are contributing to or maintaining the occurrence of specific behaviors of concern. Generally speaking, a FBA is used when preventative strategies (i.e., well-designed classroom management procedures) are not working for a student and/or when the environmental variables that set the stage for or maintain challenging behaviors are unclear. An effective FBA allows the practitioner to predict when and where the behavior will occur. Thus the goals of conducting a FBA are to be able to describe the behavior, to predict when it will or will not occur, to understand the variables that set the occasion for and maintain behavior, to develop hypotheses about these variables, and to collect data that either support or reject these hypotheses (O'Neill et al., 1997). Ultimately, the information gathered through a FBA allows practitioners to understand problem behavior and develop effective positive behavior support plans.

The FBA information-gathering process makes use of several assessment tools familiar to school psychologists and other school-based practitioners (e.g., interviews, direct observations). The data gathered via such tools is used to determine the function that problem behavior serves for the student in question. Thus the process is used to determine the consequences or outcomes of the behavior, keeping in mind that a behavior may serve multiple functions for the same student depending on the circumstances and that behaviors often serve different functions. Although the specific function a behavior serves may vary both within and across students, what does remain consistent are the typical functions of behavior. These functions are displayed in Figure 4.1 and generally fall into one of three broad categories: (1) to avoid or escape, (2) to get or obtain, or (3) to communicate.

Rationale for FBA in Schools

Particularly relevant to school settings are the three values-based assumptions that underlie the use of FBA discussed by O'Neill et al. (1997). First, the dignity of the person for whom the FBA is being conducted is the primary concern. As such, FBA is founded on the notion that all behavior serves a purpose for an individual, that there is logic to his or her behavior. Second, the overarching rationale for conducting FBA is to teach and develop functional alternative behaviors, not to simply reduce or eliminate problem behavior. Challenging behaviors are learned. Thus teaching functional alternatives is important for both reducing the occurrence of challenging behavior and enhancing student skill development. The function a challenging

> The overarching rationale for conducting FBA is to teach and develop functional alternative behaviors, not to simply reduce or eliminate problem behavior.

behavior serves is critical information to have for intervention development. Third, FBA is a process for examining relations between behavior *and* the environment. FBA considers the broader context in which behavior occurs, and the assessment process is as much an analysis of the environment as it is of the behavior(s) of concern. As such, when conducting a FBA, the student's challenging behavior is examined, along with behaviors of support staff, patterns of support, and relevant structural features of the environment. This information is then used to restructure the physical or social environment or to redesign curricula to make challenging behavior less likely and appropriate behavior more likely (O'Neill et al., 1997). The notion of context is particularly relevant for students with HFA/AS. Oftentimes it is not the behavior itself that is considered the primary problem but, rather, the context in which the behavior occurs. Thus examining contextual variables is critical.

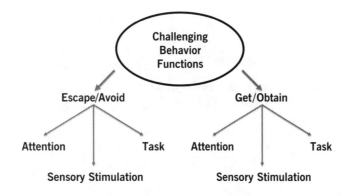

FIGURE 4.1. Challenging behavior functions.

How to Conduct an Effective FBA

When conducting a FBA, information-gathering efforts are focused on describing antecedents, behaviors, and consequences. Antecedents are those things that occur before the behavior and set the occasion for behavior to occur. Antecedents can occur immediately before a behavior occurs (e.g., the student is asked to join others in a game of basketball) or may be more distal setting events (e.g., the student did not sleep well). When conducting a FBA, it is important to consider both types of antecedents, as well as the impact of combinations of them. Several antecedents and examples relevant to students with HFA/AS are shown in Table 4.5. In addition to these antecedents, other ecological events to consider that may be more distant from the occurrence of problem behavior include medical or physical concerns (e.g., asthma, use of medication), sleep routines, diet and eating habits (e.g., food preferences), and daily schedule (e.g., the availability of choices, predictability).

TABLE 4.5. Types of Antecedents and Examples

Antecedent type	Examples
Informational cues	• Verbal or written instructions • Picture cues
Presence or absence of particular people	• Teaching assistant • Particular student(s) • Changes in staffing
The number of people present	• Large group or small group instruction
Particular activities or tasks	• Social play situations • Activities requiring expressive language • Preferred topic or activity related to specific area of interest • Difficult or nonpreferred tasks
Temporal factors	• The amount of time since last meal • The amount of time since the last opportunity practice a target skill • Transitions between activities
Behavior of others	• Peer modeling • Teasing
Changes in internal states	• Drop in blood sugar • Onset of a headache
Cognitive events	• Expectance of success • Anxiety • Thoughts about experiences
Exposure to conditioned stimuli	• Preferred person, topic, or event

Finally, it is also useful to consider and obtain information about those circumstances or settings in which behavior does *not* occur.

Behaviors must be defined precisely so that they may be measured reliably. Precisely defining behaviors means to describe them in clear, measurable, and objective terms. For example, consider this sample definition of aggression:

> *Aggression means that the student strikes another person or object with a body part (e.g., hand, foot) or object (e.g., pencil, ruler) such that a physical mark is left on the person or object. Examples of aggression include punching a person, kicking a hole in a wall, poking a person with a pencil, etc. Non-examples of aggression include giving a high-five, shaking hands, knocking or tapping on a desk or door, etc.*

When describing behaviors, consider including the following elements: (1) what the behavior looks like, or its topography; (2) the intensity (or severity) of the behavior; (3) how often the behavior occurs; and (4) how long the behavior lasts. It is useful to consider whether or not certain behaviors cluster together. Examine whether there are groups or classes of behaviors or a consistent relation between certain behaviors. Keep in mind that although it is useful to describe problem behaviors thoroughly in this manner, it is equally important to put this same level of effort into describing appropriate replacement behaviors to teach. Importantly, FBA is designed to provide enough understanding of the problem behavior to be able to select an appropriate functional replacement behavior to teach, while also restructuring the environment to make inappropriate behavior less likely. Let's say, for example, that the aggression just defined above served the purpose of inappropriate attempts to join in activities or conversation with other students in the class. Then one could define an appropriate replacement as "joining in a game or activity with other students" defined as follows:

> **Importantly, FBA is designed to provide enough understanding of the problem behavior to be able to select an appropriate functional replacement behavior to teach, while also restructuring the environment to make inappropriate behavior less likely.**

> *Joining in means the student initiates or participates in some activity (e.g., game of basketball, completing a puzzle) or conversation with one or more fellow students. Examples include the student calling another student's name to get his or her attention and expressing enjoyment of participation in an activity (e.g., saying, "This is really fun!"). Joining in does not include aggressive behaviors such as pushing or hitting.*

Consequences are those things that happen after the behavior occurs that make the behavior more or less likely to happen in the future. Consequences may be things that we perceive are positive (e.g., obtaining a reward), or they may be things we perceive as aversive (e.g., punishments). However, whether a consequence is positive or negative depends on the impact it has on behavior. If the behavior that precedes the consequence increases in the future, then the consequence is positive. If the behavior decreases in the future, then the consequence was negative. When conducting a FBA it is important to observe what happens after behavior occurs, without preconceived notions about what is reinforcing or punishing to the student but instead allowing the data collected to reveal these relations.

In addition to determining what the consequences are, it also is important to consider how efficient the behavior is in achieving the consequences. If a particular problem behavior is very efficient, a challenge to intervention development is to find an equally efficient appropriate replacement behavior. Likewise, if the behavior has a long history, it may be a greater challenge to change. Finally, in some cases, problem behavior may be a form of communication (Carr & Durand, 1985; i.e., consider the example for aggression and joining in given previously). Efforts to index consequences will need to consider this important facet of behavior.

Specific FBA Data Collection Procedures

As stated previously, several tools are often used when collecting information during the FBA process. Most typically, the process includes interviews and direct observations. Occasionally, systematic environmental manipulations or experimental procedures are necessary to determine the function of behavior and the environmental antecedents and maintaining consequences.

Interviews are used initially to describe ecological events and relevant stimuli that set the occasion for behaviors of concern and to begin to understand the function of the behavior. The interview will help in identifying those elements to target for direct observation (O'Neill et al., 1997). One of the first decisions to make regarding interviews is whom to interview. Those who know the student the best, such as parents or other family members, teachers, and school staff members (one or two) who have daily contact with the student, are all relevant persons to interview.

It is also important that careful consideration be given to interviewing the student whose behavior is of concern. Students may be the most relevant persons to provide information about their preferences, to describe complaints about schoolwork or activities that might otherwise not come to light, to request alternate activities, to indicate what distracts them, and to describe problems with peers (O'Neill et al., 1997). This kind of information may not be available from any other source. Thus, it is crucial that practitioners consider interviewing the student.

When conducting interviews, initial questions are asked to determine a specific list of behaviors of concern. Next, interviewees are asked to describe those behaviors thoroughly, along with what they believe the sequence of behaviors are that may cluster together. In addition, information about what interviewees believe are likely antecedents to the behaviors of concern are obtained. Important information about the efficiency of the behavior, as well as background information on the communication skills and potential reinforcement for the student, are obtained via interviews as well. Specific strategies that parents or teachers have found useful also can be investigated during these interviews. Importantly, the interview is a time during which information about functional alternative behaviors already in the student's repertoire can be obtained. Such information may help better target instruction and determine whether the focus needs to be on teaching a new skill or prompting and reinforcing skills students already have in their repertoires. Finally, the interview is also a good time to determine the behavior's history and any previous attempts to modify or manage the behavior.

Once the interview information is obtained and summarized, it may be that no further information is needed. If a clear pattern is present, then it is possible to proceed with intervention development. However, in most cases, additional data will be needed prior to moving on to intervention development. According to O'Neill et al. (1997), after the interview step, several possible decisions might be made, including (1) to gather more data (e.g., another 2–5 days or 10–15 occurrences of the behavior); (2) to check on data collection integrity; (3) to conduct systematic environmental manipulations; and/or (4) to develop a behavior support plan.

> **Importantly, the interview is a time during which information about functional alternative behaviors already in the student's repertoire can be obtained. Such information may help better target instruction and determine whether the focus needs to be on teaching a new skill or prompting and reinforcing skills students already have in their repertoires.**

Direct observations are a primary means of obtaining information in a FBA and should be linked to the information obtained during the interview. Basic considerations when conducting behavioral observations for the purposes of FBA are to decide when and where the observations should occur, as well as who should do the observing. In general, these observations should be conducted during as many times of day as possible and across various times and settings when the behavior *does* and *does not* occur. It is important to observe at times when the conditions that you believe are functionally related to the behaviors of concern both are and are not present. Personnel who know the student well and work directly with the student should conduct these observations whenever possible.

Data collection should occur over 2–5 days or 15–20 occurrences of the behavior, but the decision about how many days or occurrences ultimately will depend on the consistency and clarity of the relation between behavior and environmental conditions (O'Neill et al., 1997). Most typically, frequency or event recording is used for low-frequency behaviors (e.g., less than 20 occurrences per day). These observations may utilize simple antecedent–behavior–consequence (A–B–C) observation recording forms (see Chapter 9, Figures 9.11 and 9.12, and Appendix Forms 9.7 and 9.8) or a more complex form that includes setting events and perceived functions (see O'Neill et al., 1997). In other cases, a time sampling procedure is a better choice. Chapter 9 of this book contains details on selecting a recording procedure depending on the behavioral dimensions of concern and includes several sample behavioral recording forms.

Keeping in mind the goals of conducting a FBA (i.e., to describe, predict, and determine the function of behavior so that effective support plans can be developed), observations should answer the following questions:

1. How often does the behavior occur?
2. What behaviors occur together?
3. When does the behavior occur the most and the least often?

4. What setting events appear to be related to the behavior?
5. What patterns are there in the consequences that follow the behavior?

Finally, in examining all the data collected, school personnel need to determine whether the function of the behavior can be determined from the observation data obtained. If conclusions are unclear, they should cycle back through some of these processes to revisit hypotheses generated about the conditions under which behaviors of concern occur.

Systematic Experimental Analyses/Environmental Manipulations

For the most part, gathering information for FBA purposes involves collecting interview and observation data. Occasionally, however, formal tests of the relation between environmental variables and the occurrence or nonoccurrence of the behavior are needed. These formal tests are referred to as *functional analysis* (O'Neill et al., 1997; Steege & Watson, 2008). This process for conducting experimental analysis of the contingencies that maintain problem behavior provides a formal test of the relation between environmental variables and the occurrence or nonoccurrence of behavior. Approaches to these experimental procedures include manipulation of antecedents, consequences, or both during typical routines in which problem behavior has occurred. Examples of variables to manipulate might include such things as attention or access to objects, activities, or persons. Essentially, these analyses involve attempts to arrange the environment to increase and/or to decrease behavior in a systematic fashion such that controlling functions of antecedents and consequences can be determined (Steege & Watson, 2008). They are considered the most precise, rigorous, and controlled method of functional assessment.

Although they are largely considered helpful and sometimes necessary, systematic environmental manipulations are expensive in terms of time and personnel resources. They also require safeguards such as those discussed by O'Neill et al. (1997). These safeguards include having adequately trained staff, adequate numbers of staff members, and established protective and emergency procedures. Prior to conducting these manipulations, personnel must have clear hypotheses to test and have adequate justification for any risk involved. Due consideration also should be given to whether or not internal states, which are difficult to control, are relevant to the behavior of concern. Extreme caution should be exercised for potentially dangerous behaviors. In such cases, safety is very important.

Should personnel decide to consider environmental manipulations, before engaging in these procedures, several issues should be examined. The following precautions should be observed (see O'Neill et al., 1997) for a detailed discussion of considerations):

1. Conduct environmental manipulations only when relevant and when important situations can be controlled readily.
2. Consider the risk involved for the student and school personnel.
3. Consider whether the benefits outweigh the costs.
4. Conduct these manipulations only if other data are unclear.
5. Employ review and informed consent procedures.

6. Keep in mind that conducting manipulations may introduce change into the environment that can alter the function of the behavior.

7. Consider that environmental manipulations are not practical or efficient with low-frequency behaviors, which are often the very types of behaviors for which a FBA was pursued initially.

Because of these concerns, systematic environmental manipulations are not typically conducted in school settings and are not covered in great detail here. They are most often done in research settings by highly trained personnel under conditions in which a group of people oversee the protection of human participants in research (e.g., an institutional review board or research ethics committee) and in which informed consent from parents and caregivers is obtained (O'Neill et al., 1997).

In conclusion, a complete FBA process may take several days to several weeks and can be expensive; therefore, practitioners may find that portions of the process are frequently used. Overall, practitioners will want to keep in mind that the intensity of the assessment process should match the complexity of the behavior of concern. In situations in which behavior is serving multiple functions that differ based on the context, or in situations in which behaviors are extreme and cause great distress to the student or caregivers or severely limit the student's future opportunities, then the intensity applied to the assessment process will likely be at its greatest. Ultimately, the information obtained must be useful in building behavior support plans that are designed to increase opportunities for learning, for social inclusion, for access to meaningful activities, and for participation in the community. As such, the interventions will necessarily be comprehensive in nature and attend to antecedents of problem behavior, while also teaching new skills as part of a general problem-solving approach.

ASSESSING SOCIAL SKILLS

Difficulty with social behavior is perhaps the most significant disabling condition that children and youth with HFA/AS encounter. Specifically, these individuals exhibit significant lifelong impairment in their ability to engage in and maintain social interactions and relationships, despite having an interest in wanting friendships (Klin, McPartland, & Volkmar, 2005). Sustained difficulties with social skills not only make developing long-standing interpersonal relationships very challenging for individuals with HFA/AS but also make maintaining employment or functioning independently on a day-to-day basis practically unsustainable. Thus the assessment of social skills in students with HFA/AS should be a foundation of practice. School-based social skills assessment can be conducted using both informal and standardized methods. In the next sections, information pertaining to the assessment of social behavior in children and youth with HFA/AS through the use of interviews, observations, and rating scales is highlighted.

> **The assessment of social skills in students with HFA/AS should be a foundation of practice.**

Interviews

Perhaps the simplest way to begin identifying and targeting social skills is to interview those who know the child best (i.e., parents and teachers). Interviewees should seek information to questions such as:

1. What is the extent and nature of social skills (and related) difficulties?
2. In what settings do the social skills difficulties occur?
3. What specific events influence or predict social skills difficulties?
4. What factors frequent or maintain the social skills difficulties?
5. What is the frequency, duration, and/or intensity of the social skills difficulties?

In addition to interviewing parents and teachers, interviewers are encouraged to talk to the child. The child will provide information related to his or her social interests and motivation, as well as provide an opportunity for the interviewee to observe his or her social interactions. Although educators are encouraged to develop their own questions, several guided interview forms exist that are comprehensive and useful for pinpointing specific social skills difficulties in individuals with HFA/AS. See Forms 4.1, 4.2, and 4.3 in the Appendix for reproducible parent, teacher, and child interviews.

Observations

Directly observing the student provides the most useful and relevant information for developing effective instruction. Direct observations of the individual's behavior provide a measure of social skills difficulties as they occur in naturalistic settings such as the classroom, playground, cafeteria, and/or hallway. Moreover, direct observations provide information related to a child's social performance across multiple settings and multiple persons that cannot be obtained in any other way. First, they allow the observer to notice things occurring within the environment that may be affecting an individual's behavior in that setting. For example, a parent of a student with HFA indicated that her son never mentioned talking with his friends at lunch. Observations of the student quickly revealed that he sat alone, away from his friends. Second, directly observing a child with HFA/AS permits the observer to view the behaviors and reactions of peers. Such observations are useful to determine the ways a child with HFA/AS differs from other students, as well as to establish the degree to which his or her behavior deviates from that of peers (a normative comparison). For example, observations on the playground demonstrated that a student with AS engaged in overly excessive amounts of "sportsmanship" behaviors (saying "way to go" or "nice job" when playing) that was not the norm for his peers. This behavior resulted in the child with AS being ridiculed and ostracized from group activities.

Finally, when conducted concurrently with instruction, direct observations allow one to evaluate whether the social skills training has been effective. Two common direct observation methods are useful for recording social behaviors in school-based settings: anecdotal recording and systematic recording. Brief overviews of these methods as they pertain to social skills assessment follow; detailed information and examples of these methods are provided in Chapter 9.

Anecdotal Record

The intent of an anecdotal record is to provide an account of the elements that occur during a behavior episode as completely as possible (Alberto & Troutman, 2008). Often, detailed notes are taken regarding the behavior and other features of the situation as they occur in "real world" settings. With regard to social skills, an anecdotal record may describe a student's interaction patterns on the playground, as well as information pertaining to the environmental stimuli (e.g., noise levels, social interactions of others, teacher responses). For example, a running record conducted on the playground may indicate that "Clyde walks around the perimeter of the playground and does not interact with other students" or "Amelia walks up to peers, sticks out her tongue, and runs away." Although these examples provide some indication of the social interaction styles of students, they offer limited information regarding how frequently, how long, or why a student engages in such behaviors. Nevertheless, anecdotal records can be useful as a first step aimed at providing information regarding the child's level of social functioning, the environmental characteristics that signal or maintain specific behaviors, and the reactions of others, and they also assist practitioners with the development of target behavior definitions.

Systematic Recording

Educators often want more than a simple description of what behavior occurred and the environmental characteristics that occasioned or maintained that behavior. For example, educators are more interested in knowing how frequently a student interacts with other students on the playground, or how long these interactions last. To provide answers to these questions, more systematic observation is needed. Systematic observation allows educators to observe social behavior across a variety of settings and provides detailed information regarding the frequency (how often) or duration (how long) of target behavior(s). Further, systematic observation allows comparison with peers. Knowing that a student with HFA/AS "joins in" activities three times during a 35-minute period provides very little information without understanding how this rate compares with those of other children.

> Systematic observation allows educators to observe social behavior across a variety of settings and provides detailed information regarding the frequency (how often) and duration (how long) of target behavior(s). Further, systematic observation allows comparison with peers.

The use of systematic recording methods to assess social skills begins with a clear understanding of what behavior is to be observed and recorded (e.g., maintaining a conversation, taking turns). Behaviors are chosen based on information obtained through interviews, FBAs, or anecdotal records. Then a specific system of data collection (e.g., frequency, duration, latency) is selected that best matches the concern. For example, Arlene, a first-grade student with AS, demonstrated limited turn-taking behavior when engaging in free time in the classroom. Because Arlene's teachers were interested in increasing how often Arlene engaged in turn-taking behavior, frequency data were gathered. Initial data collection provided a detailed measure of Arlene's present level of social functioning (baseline) and served as a measure of progress throughout the intervention phase. Although there are many social behaviors that can be targeted for assessment, Table 4.6 provides a list of the more common concerns about behavior of students with HFA/AS in schools.

Rating Scales

Rating scales are helpful in pinpointing additional information about social skills deficits by asking raters to evaluate specific behaviors, such as their abilities to play cooperatively

TABLE 4.6. Common Social Skills Concerns Targeted for Assessment and Intervention

Broad domain	Potential targets	
Social responsiveness/ perspective taking	• Recognizing facial cues of others • Recognizing nonverbal behavior of others • Responding to greetings of others • Responding to invitations to join in • Responding to questions from others	• Understanding the intentions of others • Understanding the thoughts of others • Understanding the interests of others • Expressing sympathy for others • Understanding jokes told by others
Social interactions	• Making/maintaining eye contact • Understanding "body basics" • Interacting with a peer or group of peers	• Inviting others to join in • Introducing oneself • Regulating emotions
Social play	• Engaging in solitary play • Engaging in parallel play • Engaging in cooperative play	• Sharing materials • Participating in group activities • Taking turns
Social communication	• Initiating conversations • Maintaining conversations • Providing compliments to others	• Comprising during disagreements • Ending conversations appropriately • Expressing feelings appropriately
Inappropriate social behavior/blunders	• Maintaining hygiene • Telling inappropriate jokes	• Being a "tattletale" • Making noises, picking nose, farting

Note. Behaviors listed here are only a small sample of social skills behaviors that may be targeted for further assessment and subsequent intervention. This list is intended to provide a list of common areas of functioning.

with peers, to respond to greetings, or to recognize emotions in others. Moreover, rating scales provide an estimate of the severity of problems such as how often inappropriate social interactions occur (e.g., ending conversations abruptly, changing the topic of conversation to fit self-interests). In the context of intervention-based assistance, rating scales serve as a method not only for describing and categorizing behavior but also for evaluating the effects of interventions designed to improve functioning. Although many of the scales highlighted in Table 4.7 can be used to examine broad social skill difficulty in students with HFA/AS (e.g.,

> **In the context of intervention-based assistance, rating scales serve as a method not only for describing and categorizing behavior but also for evaluating the effects of interventions designed to improve functioning.**

Asperger Syndrome Diagnostic Scale [ASDS], Gilliam Asperger Disorder Scale [GADS]), such instruments may not be sensitive enough to identify or evaluate the specific skills sets that likely will be the targets of interventions. However, several social skills rating scale measures are available to school-based practitioners that provide detailed descriptive information on the social interactions, reciprocal social behaviors, and communicative patterns of students with HFA/AS. A few of these measures are described in more detail next, and Table 4.7 provides an overview of the most frequently used social skills rating scales.

The Social Responsiveness Scale (SRS; Constantino, 2002) is a 65-item questionnaire that provides detailed information pertaining to interpersonal and reciprocal social behavior. The SRS can be used for children ages 4–18 and is considered a useful tool for screening and aiding in diagnosis, as well as measuring response to intervention over time. All items on the scale describe an aspect of observable social behavior (e.g., social anxiety, social awareness) that parents and/or teachers rate on a scale of "0" (*never true*) to "3" (*almost always true*). These item scores are then converted into a singular index score that reflects the severity of social skills deficits. A higher score on the SRS indicates greater severity of social impairment. In addition to a total score, five treatment subscale scores are provided that can be useful for designing and evaluating intervention outcomes. Psychometric properties of the scale are strong, demonstrating robust reliability and validity (e.g., Constantino et al., 2003, 2004). In addition, the SRS has been shown to differentiate ASD from other disorders successfully (Constantino, Przybeck, Friesen, & Todd, 2000).

A more general measure of social skill behavior that can be particularly useful for students with HFA/AS is the Social Skills Improvement System (SSIS; Gresham & Elliott, 2008), which has been designed to replace the Social Skills Rating Scales (SSRS; Gresham & Elliott, 1990). The SSIS is a comprehensive approach that can be used as part of a multi-tiered assessment and intervention system for students between the ages of 3 and 18 years. Specifically, the SSIS facilitates universal screening of students at risk for social behavior difficulties, planning interventions for improving these behaviors, and evaluating progress on targeted skills. The SSIS contains the Performance Screening Guide, Rating Scales, Classwide Intervention Program, and in-depth social skills Intervention Guide. Although it was not designed specifically for working with students with ASD, practitioners will find the system extremely useful, as it focuses on key skills that many individuals with HFA/AS lack (e.g., self-control, social engagement, cooperation). In addition, the SSIS offers a

TABLE 4.7. Rating Scales for Assessing Social Skills Difficulties in Individuals with HFA/AS

Measure	Age range (years)	Number of items	Purpose	Benefits	Drawbacks
ASSP	6–17	50	Measures a broad range of social characteristics typically exhibited by individuals with ASD (e.g., initiation skills, reciprocity, perspective taking).	Can be used as an assessment tool to identify social skills interventions and as a formative assessment tool; parents, teachers, or others who have knowledge of the child's social skills can use the scale; focus on autism-specific behaviors.	Has not been standardized; studies investigating the psychometric properties (i.e., reliability and validity) of the measure are yet to be published; unclear how scores will be used.
MASC	8–19	39	Assesses various dimensions of anxiety in children, such as fear of separation, fear of rejection and public performance, physiological arousal, and anxious coping mechanisms.	May be particularly useful for individuals with comorbid anxiety disorders; empirically derived scale.	Children with ASD were not included in the standardization sample; may be of limited utility in school-based settings that do not provide counseling interventions.
SCQ	Above 4	40	Evaluates communication skills and social functioning in children who may have autism or an ASD.	Can be used as a screener and a formative assessment tool; contains a lifetime form (assesses child's entire developmental history) and a current form (assesses child's behavior during most current 3-month period).	Children with ASD were not included in the standardization sample; questions are answered in yes/no format; parents are the only raters; only raw scores are calculated.
SRS	4–18	65	Distinguishes ASD from other childhood disorders by identifying the presence and extent of social skill impairment characteristic of autism.	Provides an overall standard score (T-score); yields five treatment scores (T-scores) that can be used to evaluate intervention outcomes; has separate parent and teacher forms.	Children with ASD were not included in the standardization sample; may not provide any information related to social anxiety.
SSIS	3–18	Varies by form and tool.	Offers screening, targeted assessment, and intervention scripts for a variety of social skill problem behaviors and academic competence.	Contains parent, teacher, and student response forms; is a family of assessment and intervention tools; melds with current multi-tiered assessment and intervention systems; yields standard scores.	Can become cost prohibitive depending on the tools purchased; may not be used to its fullest potential within schools due to complexity of approach.

Note. ASSP, Autism Social Skills Profile (Bellini, in press); MASC, Multidimensional Anxiety Scale for Children (March, 1999); SASC-R, Social Anxiety Scale for Children—Revised (La Greca & Stone, 1993); SAS-A, Social Anxiety Scale—Adolescent (La Greca, 1999); SCQ, Social Communication Questionnaire (Rutter, Bailey, & Lord, 2003); SRS, Social Responsiveness Scale (Constantino, 2002); SSIS, Social Skills Improvement System (Gresham & Elliott, 2008).

balanced assessment of both prosocial and problem behaviors with direct links to interventions. As was true of its predecessor, the psychometric properties of the rating scales used within the SSIS are strong (Gresham & Elliott, 2008).

One measure that is forthcoming, and one worth investigating when it becomes commercially available, is the Autism Social Skills Profile (ASSP; Bellini, in press). The ASSP is a 50-item questionnaire that measures the level of social functioning of children and youth with ASD between the ages of 6 and 17 years. Items on the ASSP coincide with a variety of social characteristics that individuals with HFA/AS typically demonstrate, including perspective taking, initiation skills, social reciprocity behaviors, and nonverbal communication (Bellini, 2008). All items on the scale describe an aspect of observable social behavior (e.g., turn taking, understanding jokes, offering assistance to others) that parents and/or teachers rate on a Likert scale ranging from 1 (*never*) to 4 (*very often*). The ASSP was developed not only as a tool for identifying specific social skills that can then become the targets for intervention but also as a progress monitoring device. Preliminary analysis of the psychometric properties of the ASSP suggests a robust scale with respect to factor structure, reliability, and validity (Bellini & Hopf, 2007). The developer of the ASSP currently is conducting further reliability and validity studies, noting that revisions may be made prior to final dissemination of the scale (S. Bellini, personal communication, October 3, 2007).

ASSESSING EMOTIONAL DIFFICULTIES

Emotional difficulties are common among adolescents but even more prevalent among those with HFA/AS. During adolescence, many students with HFA/AS may begin to demonstrate symptoms of depression and anxiety as they develop insight into their differences from others (Kim et al., 2000; Macintosh & Dissanayake, 2006b; Tonge et al., 1999). Thus these individuals likely are caught in a downward spiral of social withdrawal compounded by inadequate social skills and negative experiences when interacting with peers and/or within community settings. That is, their level of social engagement and desire for relationships decrease as symptoms of depression and anxiety increase. Because of this process, it becomes important for educators to assess the emotional functioning of students with HFA/AS. However, assessment of emotional functioning typically has occurred within schools only when the student is being considered for special education services under the Emotional Disturbance category. Given the complications of emotional problems for later outcomes, it is crucial that school-based practitioners assess the emotional functioning of students with HFA/AS for purposes of educational and lifelong planning.

> **Given the complications of emotional problems for later outcomes, it is crucial that school-based practitioners assess the emotional functioning of students with HFA/AS for purposes of educational and lifelong planning.**

In contemporary practice, the most common method of assessing emotional functioning utilizes self-report measures. A variety of self-report instruments exist, and several measures that are easy to use and that have been proven psychometrically sound should be considered part of the school-based practitioner's tool box. For example, the Children's Depression Inventory (CDI; Kovacs, 1991), an instrument for measuring depressive symptoms in students between 6 and 17 years of age, is perhaps one of the most widely used self-report measures for depression. Unfortunately, the CDI does not have a nationally standardized normative group, and cutoff scores may be too low. Therefore, practitioners should use the CDI conservatively in combination with other methods. Practitioners also may consider using the Reynolds Adolescent Depression Scale—Second Edition (RADS-2; Reynolds, 2004). The RADS-2 is a self-report depression screening measure for individuals between the ages of 11 and 20 years. Items are logically related to most adolescent concerns, and the development and standardization of the instrument are impressive. In addition to these instruments, practitioners may consider the Revised Children's Manifest Anxiety Scale—Second Edition (RCMAS-2; Reynolds & Richmond, 2008) for examining multiple traits of anxiety (including social anxiety) in children and youth 6–19 years. The RCMAS-2 is extremely easy to use, and its technical adequacy is acceptable.

Aside from self-report measures, practitioners also should integrate the use of rating scales and direct observation when assessing emotional functioning of students with HFA/AS. Rating scales are useful when parent and/or teacher ratings of the student's behaviors are desired. For example, the Behavior Assessment System for Children—Second Edition (BASC-2; Reynolds & Kamphaus, 2004), already used by many practitioners in schools, likely will provide perspectives on the student's behaviors and emotions. However, the many complicated aspects of depression and anxiety may not be captured completely with the BASC-2, as ratings of internalizing behavior problems by parents (and by inference, teachers) are not always accurate (Kolko & Kazdin, 1993). However, the Self-Report of Personality (SRP) or the SRP Interview (SRP-I) that accompany the BASC-2 may provide far better information for practitioners. Specifically, the SRP and SRP-I provide insight into the student's thoughts and feelings by asking questions related to traits such as self-esteem, depression, and social stress, among others. The BASC-2 and the accompanying self-report options have an impressive amount of research to support their use and are practical. With regard to direct observation, practitioners should provide some measurable unit (e.g., duration, latency) of the depressive and/or anxious characteristics pinpointed by self-report or through rating scales. Specifically, practitioners would want to measure such characteristics as diminished social activity, avoidance of feared or anxiety-provoking situations, and affect-related expression, to name a few.

CONCLUSION

Assessing students with HFA/AS in schools often can be an overwhelming task. Many students with HFA/AS may present with a combination of behavioral, social, and academic skills problems, all of which require in-depth assessment and subsequent intervention. Traditionally, school-based practitioners have approached the assessment of students with HFA/AS from a psychoeducational standpoint utilizing a very narrow range of traditional standardized assessment devices. However, students with HFA/AS represent a heterogeneous group that exhibit a wide array of strengths and weaknesses. It is imperative that school-based practitioners conduct more comprehensive assessments that evaluate a child's total functioning. To do so requires that school-based practitioners understand the unique patterns of strengths and weaknesses exhibited by children and youth with HFA/AS and then build on their subsequent assessment practices using a combination of traditional and functional practices. Overall, assessment of intellectual, academic, behavior, and social and emotional skills of students with HFA/AS should be viewed through an intervention-focused lens. Comprehensive and meaningful assessments must be conducted that provide detailed information that can guide teams toward the development of meaningful solutions, resulting in improved outcomes for students with HFA/AS.

CHAPTER 5

Improving Academic Skills

STUDENT SNAPSHOT: Corrado

Corrado, a fifth-grade student with AS, receives his education in several inclusion classrooms. Corrado has difficulty with all academic skills, but especially with reading comprehension. In addition, he becomes easily frustrated and begins to yell and scream in class when given academic tasks that require abstract thinking or that require him to make inferences, such as math word problems. He needs ample time to make decisions and to answer questions, and he quickly loses his ability to focus academically if the material is not of interest to him. Due to his poor fine-motor skills, Corrado has illegible handwriting and is unable to staple papers and to cut on a straight line with scissors; therefore, academic tasks need to be assigned accordingly. In addition, Corrado frequently misplaces academic supplies, which, unintentionally, forces his teachers and aides to delay their instruction as they locate his materials. Because Corrado continues to demonstrate difficulty across academic subjects, his parents have requested a team meeting to plan for his future academic success.

OVERVIEW

With increasing numbers of students identified with HFA/AS in general education settings, educators must be increasingly aware of evidence-based strategies for improving educational outcomes for these students. Despite this need, a somewhat limited amount of research exists specifically evaluating interventions designed to improve the academic performance of students with HFA/AS (Delano, 2007b). Nonetheless, based on the existing literature in this domain, several interventions and structured teaching approaches are suggested in this chapter to address the needs of students with HFA/AS. These general strategies and interventions should not be viewed as a one-size-fits-all set of approaches. Rather, educators are encouraged to take a scientific, data-based approach each time an intervention is implemented. Such an approach means that effectiveness is not assumed when implementing interventions. Instead, interventions are examined to determine their effectiveness with individual students each time they are implemented. Although the approaches described in this chapter are evidence-based, meaning there is general research support for their use, there is no guarantee that they will work for any individual

> **Educators are encouraged to take a scientific, data-based approach each time an intervention is implemented. Such an approach means that effectiveness is not assumed when implementing interventions. Instead, interventions are examined to determine their effectiveness with individual students each time they are implemented.**

student with HFA/AS. Thus it is recommended that educators collect data to determine an individual's response to intervention (see Chapter 4 for details on assessment options and Chapter 9 regarding collecting data and evaluating outcomes). This data-based approach to determining intervention efficacy is the best way to ensure positive student outcomes.

One general academic challenge that students with HFA/AS often experience is that their attention may drift and they can become disconnected from activities occurring in the classroom (Silverman & Weinfeld, 2007). Thus they may miss task requirements described by the teacher. In addition, students with HFA/AS have more difficulty maintaining the same amount of information in their working memory than typical peers (Musarra, 2006; Silverman & Weinfeld, 2007). For these reasons, a number of the strategies offered in this chapter rely on visual supports or stimuli. The rationale behind the use of such strategies is that visual stimuli are nontransient. Information is presented and made external for students to review, process, and understand on a time line suited to their learning needs. By contrast, spoken language is a transient form of communication, meaning that spoken information is present for only a short time. Under those circumstances, the relevant information can be more easily missed, misunderstood, or misinterpreted.

This chapter is organized into two major sets of strategies: general strategies and specific strategies. The general strategies are those that cut across academic domains, whereas specific strategies are designed to address a specific academic domain (e.g., mathematics). The general strategies described in this chapter address the following areas: task presentation, teacher communication, priming, assignments, and homework and study skills. Specific strategies described in this chapter address skills of greatest concern to students with HFA/AS in the domains of reading, written expression, and mathematics.

GENERAL STRATEGIES

Task Presentation

Students with HFA/AS may experience difficulties with less structured tasks and with following directions (Church, Alisanski, & Amanullah, 2000). Thus presenting tasks in a structured fashion is the best approach for these students. In part, structuring tasks means, whenever possible, assigning short tasks with a clear end in sight and reinforcing each step of the process (Silverman & Weinfeld, 2007). In addition, tasks should be broken into component parts or small steps. Breaking down tasks is particularly important for complex tasks or those that involve multiple-step directions. Explicit directions for each step of the task also should be provided. Consider the vocabulary task presented in Figure 5.1, in which the student is required to generate and write sentences with new vocabulary words. In this example, each step of the task is broken down and described. A visual prompt to check one's work is provided as well. Finally, both verbal and visual cues are provided with respect to turning in the completed task.

> Tasks should be broken down into component parts or small steps. Breaking down tasks is particularly important for complex tasks or those that involve multiple-step directions.

When using lecture as a teacher presentation format, consider using visual aids such as pictures or graphics or providing lecture outlines or notes ahead of time with critical information highlighted. Providing guiding notes ahead of time serves as an advance organizer for the information to be presented and will assist the student in comprehending the material. Preteaching key vocabulary or important concepts beforehand also can enhance comprehension. Before the lecture, students can be provided with a rationale for the information to be presented that will help them to contextualize it. For example, before presenting a lecture describing a project the students will complete on the salmon life cycle, a teacher might say, "I am going to describe each part of the salmon life cycle before you do a project showing the life cycle. The reason I am going to describe each part of the life cycle first is so that you will be able to easily recognize each phase of the life cycle as you read about it in your research for this project." This rationale can be combined with an explanation of the goals of the lesson and can include visual tools such as concept maps (e.g., a life cycle concept map). To avoid overwhelming students with lecture presentation, a good rule of thumb is to match length of lecture time (in minutes) to the student's age. For a class of 7-year-olds, speak for 7 minutes, then give a break for a hands-on or interactive activity that helps process what they just heard. When using a lecture format, it also can be helpful to intersperse hands-on tasks or activities within the lecture period to help sustain attention and reinforce learning. For instance, with the salmon life cycle example, the teacher could stop briefly after explaining each phase and have students write a key word and/or draw their own representation for that phase directly on a life cycle concept map.

Teacher Communication

The way in which teachers communicate also can be an avenue of support for students with HFA/AS. For example, teachers can use proximity and prompting as a means of providing additional support to students who experience difficulties with executive function skills such as attention to task and organization (Silverman & Weinfeld, 2007). For example, it may be helpful to seat the child with HFA/AS in close proximity to the teacher or, at a minimum, in a location in the classroom where the student and the teacher are in each other's direct line

Materials: Paper, pencil, and word list.

Directions: Complete each step below. Put completed paper in the blue vocabulary box.

STEP	ACTION	CHECK MY WORK
1.	Take out a piece of paper.	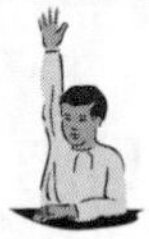
2.	Write your name in the upper right-hand corner.	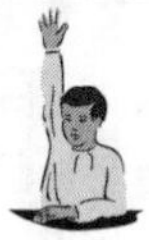
3.	Number the lines on your paper from 1 to 5, leaving two lines between each number.	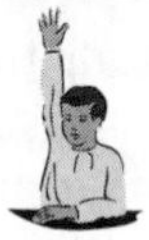
4.	Write each vocabulary word next to each number.	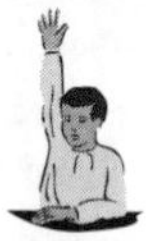
5.	Write one sentence using the first word.	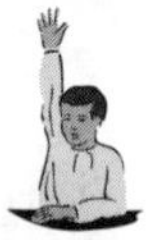
6.	Reread sentence silently to yourself. Does it make sense?	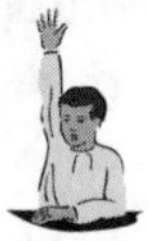
7.	Repeat steps 5 and 6 with remaining words.	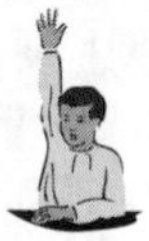
8.	Put completed work in **BLUE** vocabulary box.	Turn in work. 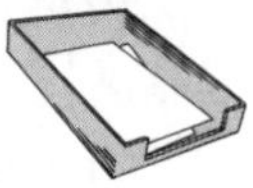

FIGURE 5.1. Vocabulary sentences task.

of sight. This arrangement can facilitate prompting the student to remain focused, as well as increase the opportunities for positive reinforcement. Importantly, proximity allows the use of nonverbal visual cues to the student, which teachers may find more effective for students with HFA/AS. In addition, simplify instructions by reducing the number of steps or words. Beyond oral explanation, write the instructions or steps down for the student. This suggestion is designed to eliminate distracting stimuli and focus student attention, again providing a visual cue that the student can refer back to if needed. Complex directions may need to be

> **Importantly, proximity allows the use of nonverbal visuals cues to the student, which teachers may find more effective for students with HFA/AS.**

repeated. It is recommended that teachers check for understanding when directions are given orally. For example, have the student repeat or perform the first item, task, or problem with the teacher, paraprofessional, or another student.

Priming

Another general strategy that can be used to support the academic success of students with HFA/AS is priming (Koegel, Koegel, Frea, & Green-Hopkins, 2003; Myles & Adreon, 2001). Priming is a means of providing the student with task materials used for teaching prior to the lesson or showing materials that will be used in the lesson before the lesson occurs. Prim-

> **The purposes of priming are: (1) to increase student competence, (2) to familiarize students with material, (3) to decrease frustration and anxiety, and (4) to allow exploration of concepts prior to instruction on them.**

ing also might involve previewing information or activities with which the individual is likely to have difficulty. The purposes of priming are: (1) to increase student competence, (2) to familiarize students with material, (3) to decrease frustration and anxiety, and (4) to allow exploration of concepts prior to instruction on them. In addition, priming is a strategy that links well to what is known about children with HFA/AS, namely that increasing predictability and familiarity significantly decrease confusion and problem behaviors.

Priming is an easy strategy to implement and is portable. Priming can occur immediately before the lesson or activity, the day before, or the evening or morning before. Priming can occur in the classroom or at home. Also, the priming activity can be conducted by anyone familiar with the lesson (e.g., teacher, teacher's aide, parent, etc.). A list or description of the activities that will occur can be one successful way to engage in priming. For example, if the activity is reading, the list should include the reading assignment, the number and type of questions the student will have to answer followed by an example, and whether the reading is to be done individually or in a small group. Other examples of priming activities include: prereading a story, reviewing a visual schedule, practicing with art supplies before doing an art project, talking about and showing a finished product, playing a game related to the activity, videotaping new activities and sites and showing the video before encountering the activity or site (e.g., showing a short video about the natural history museum before taking a field trip there), and using Social Stories™ (see Chapter 7 for a description of Social Stories). Finally, it is important to note that priming is most effective when it is brief, built into the student's routine, and conducted in a relaxed atmosphere in which the student will receive encouragement.

Assignments

Some students with HFA/AS will need additional time to complete tasks, whereas other students with HFA/AS will need tasks to be shortened (i.e., reducing the number of items to be completed). One option for adjusting assignments that is helpful for students with HFA/AS is to divide worksheets into sections and have the students complete them one section at a time. Mark the sections that need to be completed. Give one worksheet or assignment at a time to be completed before moving on to another. This approach will allow more frequent feedback to the student while also reducing the task load. Also, use worksheets keyed to text page numbers or highlight select items to be completed as a way to provide a visual cue. In some cases, it also may be helpful to consider an alternate grading scheme such as using the number correct/number attempted $\times 100 = \%$.

Given that students with HFA/AS tend to spend large amounts of time concentrating on facts that will not be tested and may be considered less important, teachers should consider identifying exactly what material or information for which the student will be responsible. It will be helpful to teach students explicitly to use informational resources such as an index, table of contents, glossary, maps, and so forth. In addition, teach students how to find key words and concepts in directions and instructions (Silverman & Weinfeld, 2007). To provide greater structure in assignments, create task lists or job cards. These task lists or job cards may include such elements as step-by-step instructions, a list of materials needed to complete the task, the amount of time allocated for the task (if applicable), and prompts or information on how to stay engaged in the tasks. A sample of a task list that includes many of these elements can be seen in Figure 5.1. Such task lists or job cards may also color-code content and indicate where work is to be turned in (e.g., a folder or box of the same color; see Figure 5.1). Finally, a model of what is expected on assignments or a specific list of criteria for grading assignments may be helpful. In short, making expectations explicit for the student is key.

> **To provide greater structure in assignments, create task lists or job cards. These task lists or job cards may include such elements as step-by-step instructions, a list of materials needed to complete the task, the amount of time allocated for the task (if applicable), and prompts or information on how to stay engaged in the tasks.**

Homework and Study Skills

Taking Notes

Students with HFA/AS may experience great difficulty with listening and writing at the same time. In addition, poor motor skills can affect both skill and motivation with respect to taking notes. Because note-taking skills increase in importance as students advance in grade (i.e., they are particularly important for middle- and high-school students), attention to teaching these skills directly and/or providing additional support is needed. Ideas that might help alleviate these concerns involve presenting alternatives or options for students to obtain notes through other means. For example, a peer can take notes and then share them with the student with HFA/AS. Students also may be allowed to use the computer or other assistive device to take notes. Another option might be for the teacher to provide the student with notes that have key words or phrases omitted for the student to fill in, thus requiring active engagement during a lecture. A student also could tape-record lectures so that he or she may study from those "auditory" notes rather than from written notes. In a similar manner, taping text and allowing the student to listen to and read it for purposes of repetition can help with retention of material while studying. Finally, skimming and scanning are helpful study skills to teach as a way to help the student distinguish relevant from irrelevant information.

Homework and Assignment Notebooks

When giving homework, provide the student with the written homework assignment or check to ensure that the student has accurately written down the assignment. Once it is taught explicitly, an assignment notebook can be a useful organizational strategy, as well as a place to keep a record of assignments and expectations. Like other assignments, long homework assignments may seem daunting to the student and could create problems with the student's spending an undesirably long period of time attempting to complete it. To alleviate this problem, apply similar strategies to the homework as those applied for other assignments. Break homework assignments down (e.g., fewer math problems per page and in larger font) and/or reduced the total amount of homework required if the student already has mastered the material.

> Once it is taught explicitly, an assignment notebook can be a useful organizational strategy, as well as a place to keep a record of assignments and expectations.

Studying and Taking Tests

Students with HFA/AS often experience difficulties with studying and test taking due to executive function difficulties (i.e., organizational skills, sustaining attention). These issues, combined with the potential to experience increased anxiety, can render test taking a formidable challenge. Empowering students by teaching specific study and test-taking skills can help alleviate these concerns. Instruction in these strategies is particularly important for students in middle and high school.

An example of a studying and test-taking strategy with some research support for its use with students with HFA/AS comes from the *Test-Taking Strategy Instructor's Manual* (Hughes, Schumaker, Deshler, & Mercer, 2002). Materials from this manual were used with four high-school-age students with ASD in a study conducted by Songlee et al. (2008). The manual provides scripted lessons and explicit instruction in the strategies. In their study, the effectiveness of the strategies was examined using a multiple-probe design. Salient features of the strategies taught to the participants included the use of mnemonic devices, positive self-talk, strategies for approaching tests (e.g., "carefully read all instructions"), ways to reduce or chunk information, and strategies for choosing responses on tests (e.g., avoiding absolutes). Results of the study were very positive; students were successful in their application of the strategies as a result of instruction, the results generalized to tests that did not align directly with the strategy, and students' strategy use maintained 2 weeks postintervention.

SPECIFIC STRATEGIES

Reading Support

Typically, though not always, students with HFA/AS have good reading-decoding and word-reading skills. They may even have excellent vocabulary knowledge. However, reading comprehension remains an area of difficulty for many of these students (Nation, Clarke, Wright, & Williams, 2006). One reason it is believed that reading comprehension problems occur is that students with HFA/AS have difficulties with pragmatic language comprehension despite otherwise normal language abilities (Loukusa et al., 2007a; Norbury & Bishop, 2002). These deficits affect the ability to properly apply contextual information when answering comprehension questions. In particular, students with HFA/AS have difficulty focusing on *relevant* contextual information (Norbury & Bishop, 2002). Further, even when students can appropriately use context to answer comprehension questions accurately, they experience difficulty when asked to explain their correct answers. Although evidence suggests that the difficulties students have in answering questions decrease as students develop, students with HFA/AS still lag behind typical peers (Loukusa et al., 2007a). In a study further examining why students gave incorrect explanations, Loukusa et al. (2007b) suggested that these students tend to overgeneralize their own world knowledge. Also, when explaining their answers, students with HFA/AS tend to engage in frequent topic drifts. These topic drifts are more common in younger children with HFA/AS as compared with older children with HFA/AS. Loukusa et al. (2007b) concluded that because of difficulties inhibiting their train of thought, students with HFA/AS continued processing and thinking out loud even after they already had given a relevant answer. The tendency toward topic drift can contribute to difficulties in integrating or synthesizing information as well, further affecting comprehension.

Given this information, instruction should focus on specific skill development and teaching reading comprehension strategies, as well as on increasing student awareness of which skills and strategies are effective in producing correct responses and why. Further, techniques that sustain student attention to cues within the text and that assist with comprehension are important. In the sections that follow, several specific reading support strategies are offered as potential ways to enhance the reading comprehension of students with HFA/AS. Once again, many of the strategies rely on visual supports, and they are organized by those that are generally applied before, during, and after reading.

> **Instruction should focus on specific skill development and teaching reading comprehension strategies, as well as on increasing student awareness of which skills and strategies are effective in producing correct responses and why.**

Before-Reading Strategies

One strategy that may be used before reading is priming background knowledge. The technique of priming was described earlier in this chapter. The purpose of applying this strategy to reading is to help students use what they already know about a topic to understand the information they are expected to obtain from text and to support them in integrating that information into their existing schema about the topic. Priming is a useful strategy for many students, and it is particularly useful for students with HFA/AS who may experience difficulty when they are expected to link information in text to previously learned concepts. To maximize the utility of this strategy while preventing topic drift or overgeneralization of prior knowledge, consider two possible ideas described by O'Connor and Klein (2004). First, instead of prereading questions, use an abstract of the passage to activate prior knowledge that is relevant and accurate with respect to the passage. Second, use graphic organizers as a means of activating or priming background knowledge. For example, a topic wheel can be used to engage the class or group of students in a discussion of what they already know about a topic. Information from students is entered into each section of the wheel. For example, Figure 5.2 shows a topic wheel about salmon that could be used to activate prior knowledge before students read about the salmon life cycle. Additional examples of graphic organizers are presented later in this chapter.

Another useful prereading technique is called a picture walk (Zimmerman & Hutchins, 2003). In a manner similar to priming, students use the picture walk strategy to review illustrations within a story and make predictions about what might happen. The illustrations are used to confirm predictions. The information discussed as part of the picture walk

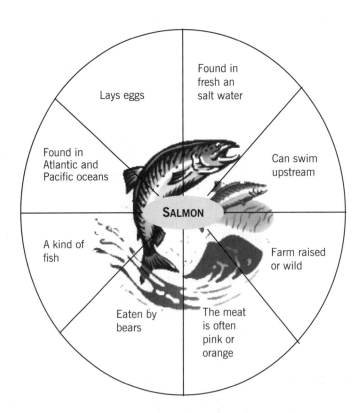

FIGURE 5.2. Sample topic wheel (graphic organizer) used as a prereading strategy.

provides a framework for the additional information the student will obtain while reading the text. Use of the picture walk strategy also can facilitate recall of details when comprehension questions are asked.

Finally, Silverman and Weinfeld (2007) provide additional prereading strategies that can be taught to prevent common problems with comprehension. They suggest that reading comprehension can be enhanced by carefully explaining ambiguous language such as metaphors, similes, idioms, and figures of speech that students might encounter as they are reading. They also suggest explaining the use of sarcasm and jokes with double meanings. Finally, they suggest that the use of nicknames be avoided or, if used, that they be explained to students so that they understand that, even though another name is used to refer to a person, its use does not indicate disrespect.

During-Reading Strategies

Using a think-aloud strategy is particularly helpful when focusing on strategies for predicting, questioning, clarifying, and summarizing (Gately, 2008). Essentially, the think-aloud process involves the teacher making the thought processes involved in each of these strategies explicit for the student. Thus, as text is read, the teacher periodically stops and discusses what he or she is thinking at that moment as it relates to the story. The idea is to make the teacher's thinking and the connection of this thinking to what is being read concrete and obvious to the student. After this type of teacher modeling occurs, students are asked to discuss their thoughts about what they are reading as well as to pose and answer questions.

Another during-reading strategy that may be helpful is goal structure mapping (Sundbye, 1998). This visual mapping strategy is used to help students understand chains of events, how the actions of characters in a story influence one another, and how events are organized in a story. It is particularly useful for students with HFA/AS with respect to their understanding of why a particular character might feel a certain way or engage in a particular action. Using the goal structure map, the student places information on each character and their actions into boxes and maps them out next to each of the other main characters in a sequential order. Then arrows are drawn to show how characters' actions influence other characters' actions.

Another strategy that can support students' reading comprehension as they read is anaphoric cuing, or cuing students to attend to pragmatic signals that inform them to search for a referent in the text (e.g., to search for and determine the referent for a particular pronoun). O'Connor and Klein (2004) determined the effectiveness of a cuing intervention designed to facilitate text understanding with a group of students with HFA/AS. The rationale behind the cueing process is that it allows students to monitor their comprehension as they read and also prompts them to use a rereading strategy, something

> **Another strategy that can support students' reading comprehension as they read is anaphoric cuing, or cuing students to attend to pragmatic signals that inform them to search for a referent in the text (e.g., to search for and determine the referent for a particular pronoun).**

While Bill and Fred were getting ready to leave for lunch, something caught their

attention. As Bill stood looking out his window, **he** noticed people walking around on the
(Bill, Fred, Larry)

roof of the building next door. Bill could not figure out what was going on up on the roof.

What might **they** be doing up there on the roof? As he thought about this . . .
(birds, Fred and Bill, people)

FIGURE 5.3. Anaphoric cuing example.

good readers often do to maintain comprehension. In this intervention, the notion of anaphora as a short way of saying something in the story that has been said before is described to the student. Then, the student reads the passage. Whenever the student comes to one of these "shortcuts" that was encountered in text, three choices are presented underneath the shortcut word (i.e., a pronoun). Students are asked to select the correct referent for the shortcut word. In the O'Connor and Klein (2004) study, data demonstrated that anaphoric cuing increased students' passage comprehension significantly and produced moderate effect sizes. Figure 5.3 provides a framework for designing an anaphoric cuing intervention.

Although it could be time-intensive for teachers to place anaphoric cues into passages students will read, two possible solutions to this problem are suggested. First, the intervention procedure could be automated using computer software. Second, and more practical in the immediate sense, students can be taught to attend to and check pronoun antecedents as they are reading. If this second approach is used, teachers should model the strategy first and then watch students as they apply it and provide them with immediate feedback. For example, students could be taught to identify and highlight anaphora as a prereading strategy and then use those highlighted words as cues while reading.

After-Reading Strategies

The reading comprehension challenges of students with HFA/AS may be further complicated by their difficulties with understanding the emotions and feelings of characters. To help students in this area, emotional thermometers might be used (Westby, 2004). Gately (2008) suggests that using color (e.g., a shaded bar) and descriptive words to represent varying levels of emotional intensity (e.g., a little bit happy, very happy; see examples in Figure 5.4) provides a framework for understanding and describing the emotions of characters within a story. Doing so also can help students understand how a character's feelings affect the choices he or she makes or how they can change as events unfold in a story. This strategy also might be used to assist students in drawing conclusions and making inferences related to feelings and emotions of characters (e.g., why a particular character engaged in a specific action).

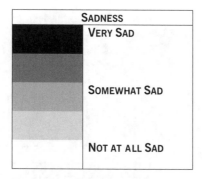
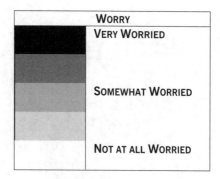

FIGURE 5.4. Sample emotional thermometer.

Strategies during or after Reading

Visual supports for reading comprehension, such as semantic maps and graphic organizers, are useful not only for students who have difficulties answering questions about text, but also for students with HFA/AS. These tools present abstract or implicit information in a concrete manner to relate meaning to text. Semantic maps provide information in a brief, predictable, and systematic manner. They can include information using pictures and/or in written text. Tools such as semantic maps and graphic organizers are useful for students with HFA/AS because they present information in a concrete and consistent manner. The visual representation of information allows students more time to process information presented. Both semantic maps and graphic organizers also help students with HFA/AS analyze and synthesize information. Because these tools show how key concepts are related within an organized framework, they help students to organize and separate relevant from

> Tools such as semantic maps and graphic organizers are useful for students with HFA/AS because they present information in a concrete and consistent manner.... Because these tools show how key concepts are related within an organized framework, they help students organize and separate relevant from irrelevant information.

irrelevant information. These organizers can help students to identify unifying themes and/or common elements across pieces of information, which can be useful when teaching students to generalize. Both semantic maps and graphic organizers also can be used as a scaffold to help with story retell or recall of information from expository text.

Four examples of these visual tools are shown in Figures 5.5–5.8. Figure 5.5 demonstrates an example of a semantic map that provides a visual representation of the history of the automobile. Figure 5.6 shows a graphic organizer that could be used to help students understand the information in a lesson about methods of transportation. These types of visual tools can be used when a teacher is presenting in a lesson or when students are reading from a textbook or discussing in a small group. They can also be helpful for students when recalling information in preparation for a writing activity. Graphic organizers for cause-and-effect text structure and basic narrative story grammar are shown in Figures 5.7

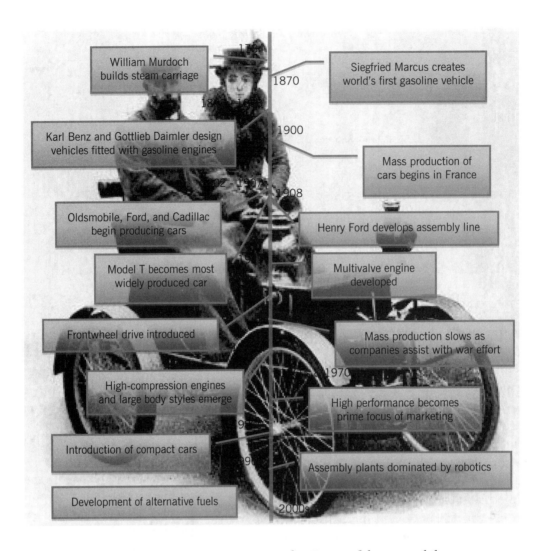

FIGURE 5.5. Semantic map example: History of the automobile.

	TRUCK	**TRAIN**
FEATURE #1	Heavy-duty tires to carry heavy loads	Moves along steel tracks
FEATURE #2	Large bed or trailer to carry loads of goods or materials	Connected series of cars that can carry loads or people
FEATURE #3	Powered by a diesel engine	Powered by a diesel engine or by steam

	BOAT	**PLANE**
FEATURE #1	Watercraft designed to float on water	Fixed wings that keep it in the sky
FEATURE #2	Open or closed compartment to carry loads or people	Closed compartment that carries loads or people
FEATURE #3	Powered by hand, wind, or engine	Powered by a jet engine

FIGURE 5.6. Graphic organizer example: Features of modes of transportation.

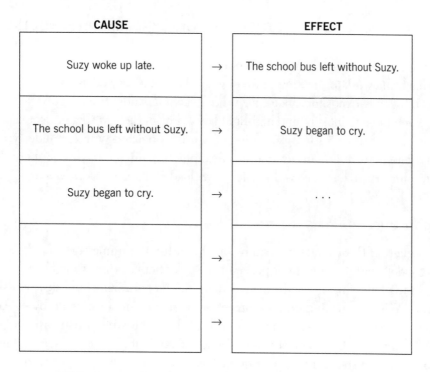

CAUSE		EFFECT
Suzy woke up late.	→	The school bus left without Suzy.
The school bus left without Suzy.	→	Suzy began to cry.
Suzy began to cry.	→	. . .
	→	
	→	

FIGURE 5.7. Graphic organizer example: Cause and effect.

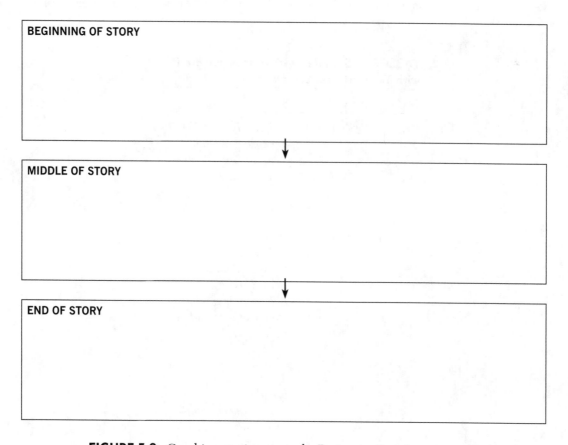

BEGINNING OF STORY

MIDDLE OF STORY

END OF STORY

FIGURE 5.8. Graphic organizer example: Basic narrative story structure.

and 5.8, respectively. Teaching students about story grammar and text structure can provide them with a framework for making sense of what they read, as well as a permanent product from which to study expository material. When teaching students about text structure, it is useful to teach them to look for and highlight key words in the text that indicate a particular text structure (see Table 5.1 for a sampling of words associated with common types of text structure). There are too many examples of graphic organizers to display here; however, myriad graphic organizers are available for download at *www.educationoasis.com*.

Reading Instruction Process

The use of many of these strategies can be taught within the framework of a direct instruction or a model–lead–test teaching procedure. In particular, direct instruction should be provided in the following areas: drawing conclusions, generalizing, and distinguishing fact from fiction. When providing direct instruction, first provide a rationale by explaining to the student (1) why the information is useful, (2) how the student can use the information, and (3) where it fits in with the knowledge the student already possesses. During the teacher presentation stage, the teacher describes and demonstrates the goals of the content and explicitly indicates exactly what the student needs to learn. Information should be broken down into component parts and presented through both visual and auditory stimuli.

TABLE 5.1. Sample Key Words Associated with Types of Text Structure

Text structure	Sample key word(s)
Cause and effect	*As a result . . .*
	Because . . .
	Consequently . . .
	Due to . . .
	Nevertheless . . .
	Therefore . . .
Compare and contrast	*However . . .*
	Although . . .
	Compared with . . .
	In contrast . . .
	Like/similar to . . .
	On the other hand . . .
	Unlike . . .
Descriptive	*Also . . .*
	Another . . .
	Finally . . .
	For instance/example . . .
	Including . . .
	Such as . . .

Instruction should be active with the teacher presenting information, asking questions, and providing corrective feedback.

The process follows a model–lead–test format. When modeling the skills, the teacher must first be sure to obtain the student's attention and then move to showing the student what he or she is supposed to do. At the "lead" or "we do" step, the teacher and the student do the task together, with the teacher providing prompts and support as needed. This step may need to be repeated multiple times before going on to the next step. The final step is the test or evaluation step. At this point, the student is given the opportunity to do the task or skill without teacher support. Throughout the lesson, but in particular at this step, student understanding and use of the skill is assessed. Students also may be encouraged to use self-evaluation strategies at this step.

Remember that students with HFA/AS may know what to do but may not understand what the requirements are for how to do it (i.e., lack of awareness of how to arrive at the correct answer). Thus being provided with explicit instruction and teacher modeling during the initial teaching phase, as well as plentiful opportunities with the "we do" or "lead" stage, is crucial. The goal is for the student to attempt the skill on his or her own with few or no errors. When errors do occur, corrective feedback is provided immediately, along with another opportunity to demonstrate correct application of the strategy with support first if needed. Importantly, explicit instruction should lower the probability of students' practicing mistakes.

Writing Support

Students with HFA/AS may need support with writing tasks. At times, students with HFA/AS may produce writing samples that are brief and less complex than those of typical peers (Myles et al., 2003). Part of what may be contributing to these outcomes is that students with HFA/AS may have poor fine-motor skills. Likewise, students with HFA/AS often experience problems with visual–motor speed, in particular when using a pen or pencil (Silverman & Weinfeld, 2007). Both of these issues make the physical task of writing more difficult. They also may render written products illegible to the teacher. Process issues (e.g., topic drift, poor organization) and difficulties with pragmatic language also can affect content and quality of the written product. For example, students with HFA/AS often have difficulty internalizing a future context on which to plan and organize their actions (Silverman & Weinfeld, 2007). Thus students with HFA/AS may need support for both the mechanics of writing tasks and for the content-related aspects of writing tasks.

Dealing with Handwriting Mechanics

Students with HFA/AS may need explicit instruction in how to hold a pencil or pen with an appropriate grip in addition to instruction in the formation of letters (Silverman & Weinfeld, 2007). *Handwriting Without Tears*, created by Jan Olsen, takes a developmental approach to handwriting and includes basic exercises in top-to-bottom and left-to-right sequencing, as well as figure–ground discrimination (see *www.hwtears.com* for description and usage).

Other tools and supports that might help with the mechanics of handwriting include paper with raised lines, pencil grips, mechanical pencils, and markers that require minimal pressure (Silverman & Weinfeld, 2007). Consulting with an occupational therapist to find out about access to and use of materials to support the student in this domain of functioning can pay large dividends in the long run.

In addition to these instructional elements and support tools, it is useful to consider whether or not handwriting is really necessary or required to accomplish the goals of the lesson. If handwriting is not crucial to the goals of the lesson, then teachers might consider alternative means to achieve the same functional outcome. For example, can the student provide verbal responses instead of written ones? Alternatively, simple accommodations can be used to help minimize the physical demands of writing, such as (1) allowing students to write using the writing style that is easier for them (i.e., print vs. cursive); (2) allowing students to use a computer, typewriter, or other assistive technology; and (3) having an aide or volunteer write for the student (i.e., through the process of dictation). Using tests with multiple-choice response formats rather than short answers is another option. Finally, consider alternatives that might be used for student projects other than written work (e.g., posters, charts, models, and minipresentations).

> **Simple accommodations can be used to help minimize the physical demands of writing, such as (1) allowing students to write using the writing style that is easier for them (i.e., print vs. cursive); (2) allowing students to use a computer, typewriter, or other assistive technology; and (3) having an aide or volunteer write for the student (i.e., through the process of dictation).**

Writing Process and Content

With respect to formulating content for writing activities, individuals with HFA/AS often have difficulty formulating their thoughts spontaneously or have difficulties accessing memory. As a result, simple story starters may not be enough for a student with HFA/AS to produce an adequate written product. The student likely will need extra preparation in order to write a sufficient written product from a prompt. This extra preparation might include providing a story outline that the student can follow or using priming activities prior to engaging in the writing assignment (see earlier discussion of priming). Using visual organizers such as semantic maps also may help. Finally, the use of self-management strategies for editing will help to produce better writing. Examples include mnemonic strategies and checklists to ensure correct spelling, grammar, and punctuation. A sample checklist for writing tasks is shown in Figure 5.9.

> **The use of self-management strategies for editing will help to produce better writing. Examples include mnemonic strategies and checklists to ensure correct spelling, grammar, and punctuation.**

One specific intervention that incorporates the use of self-management and has recent research to support its use with students with HFA/AS is self-regulated strategy development (SRSD) instruction (Graham, Harris, MacArthur, & Schwartz, 1991; Graham & Harris, 2005). This intervention focuses on teaching specific writing strategies (e.g., plan-

ELEMENTS OF GOOD WRITING	MAKE A CHECK (✓) IF PRESENT/ COMPLETE
Topic sentence provided.	
Supporting information provided.	
All sentences relate to topic.	
All sentences make sense.	
Sentences sequenced appropriately.	
Conclusion provided.	
Punctuation checked and is correct.	
Spelling checked and is correct.	

FIGURE 5.9. Sample checklist for writing activities.

ning, monitoring, making revisions) using an explicit instructional procedure, along with scaffolding, to support students' use of the strategies. Part of this explicitness means that the instruction ensures that the student has the background knowledge to use the strategy. Thus, during the beginning stages of instruction on any particular strategy, the student is taught the necessary background knowledge to apply the strategy. For example, if the strategy is to use descriptive words, then initial instruction would focus on what descriptive words are and how they are used when writing. During this beginning stage, the rationale for the strategy is explained to the student. Modeling the use of the strategy, including the use of self-talk, is incorporated as well. Students are taught self-reinforcement and positive self-talk as a means of replacing negative statements about their writing skills. Practice with immediate feedback is provided prior to independent use of the strategy.

Two recent studies have evaluated the use of SRSD for students with HFA/AS. One study (Delano, 2007a) showed positive effects of this intervention as part of a broader video-delivered intervention package. Another study by Delano (2007b) using SRSD alone further demonstrated the efficacy of this strategy for a 12-year-old student with AS. In this implementation of SRSD, picture prompts designed around the student's special interest were used. Using a single-subject multiple-baseline design, Delano (2007b) demonstrated improvement in the student's use of three specific strategies; using action words, using descriptive words, and making revisions. Improvements were maintained in a 2-week follow-up as well. Finally, the overall quality of the student's writing improved. Therefore, it appears that SRSD is an effective writing intervention that incorporates many strategies discussed thus far (e.g., direct instruction, visual cues).

Math Support

Most students with HFA/AS have average math skills compared with typical peers (Chiang & Lin, 2007). In a practical sense this means that, in most cases, instruction in math can proceed as it does for typical students. Nevertheless, suggestions for supporting students with HFA/AS are offered here based on what is known about the overall learning support needs of these students, as well as the difficulties they are likely to encounter with word problems.

Math Task Presentation

Because students with HFA/AS often learn best with visual supports, access to manipulatives provides a visual and tactile means of learning math facts. Having students complete computation problems on graph paper can help keep numbers in the correct place value column when completing math problems; turning lined paper on its side can provide a similar form of support. Both of these options allow the student greater independence in completing math problems. Sometimes, difficulties in math occur because the number of problems presented on a worksheet is overwhelming to the student. To avoid this problem, worksheets can be divided into sections, and the student can be given one section to complete at a time. Figure 5.10 shows an example of a math worksheet divided into three sections. At the end of each section there is a visual prompt for the student to seek feedback from the teacher. Alternatively, the print on the worksheet may be enlarged and copied onto several pages. These multiple enlarged sheets are not presented all at once. Rather, the student completes one and then turns it in to the teacher in exchange for the next one. Not only does this format chunk the task into more manageable pieces, but it also allows the student to encounter more frequent feedback and positive reinforcement for work completion from the teacher.

> Sometimes, difficulties in math occur because the number of problems presented on a worksheet is overwhelming to the student. To avoid this problem, worksheets can be divided into sections, and the student can be given one section to complete at a time.

Navigating Word Problems

> Word problems can be challenging for students with HFA/AS because of their abstract nature. Efforts should be made to teach students with HFA/AS the types of word problems they will encounter, as well as explicitly teaching the algorithm or steps needed to solve them.

Word problems can be challenging for students with HFA/AS because of their abstract nature. Efforts should be made to teach students with HFA/AS the types of word problems they will encounter, as well as explicitly teaching the algorithm or steps needed to solve them. Teach the student to learn strategies, such as how to follow a problem-solving routine or algorithm, but also teach him or her some variations in those routines in order to allow flexible responding when needed.

Students may need to be taught to look for key words or cues in the word problem that indicate the appropriate action steps. A list of sample key words related to various mathematical operations is found in Table 5.2. Sample problems, their associated key words, and the required operations are shown in Table 5.3. During a lesson focused on teaching a

258 − 245	218 − 177	57 + 51	452 − 282	29 − 28
80 − 24	339 − 13	235 + 197	403 + 65	164 − 133

Stop and check
with the Teacher

357 − 110	457 − 377	224 + 145	43 + 41	473 + 266
241 + 28	334 + 12	143 + 127	460 − 97	91 − 79

Stop and check
with the Teacher

242 − 204	419 − 364	243 − 202	255 − 240	148 + 125
132 + 75	239 − 19	103 + 58	315 + 107	97 − 25

Stop and check
with the Teacher

FIGURE 5.10. Divided math worksheet with prompts to check in with the teacher.

problem-solving strategy using key words, the teacher could provide modeling using a chart like the one shown in Table 5.3 but with several word problems listed in the first column. On the first story problem, the second and third columns would be completed for the student as an example. The teacher can use this example to show the students how to highlight and then list key words and the required operation(s). Remaining problems listed on the chart can be used for teacher modeling and independent student practice. The number of problems used for modeling will depend on student success in identifying key words and the required operation(s). This strategy is similar to the reading comprehension strategy in which students are taught signal or key words to help them determine the text structure. Some other strategies to use with word problems are to draw a picture, make a chart, or use a table. These strategies capitalize on visual cues. Finally, word problems can be made more relevant or interesting to a student with HFA/AS by incorporating content that is related to the student's special area of interest.

TABLE 5.2. Sample Key Words Associated with Various Mathematical Operations

Mathematical operation	Key word(s)
Addition	*Increased by . . .* *More than . . .* *Combined together . . .* *Added to/together . . .* *Altogether . . .* *Sum . . .* *Find the total . . .* *How many . . .*
Subtraction	*Fewer/less than . . .* *Reduced by . . .* *Decreased by . . .* *What's the difference . . .* *Make a comparison . . .* *How many/much more . . .*
Multiplication	*Of . . .* *Times . . .* *Every . . .* *Multiplied by . . .* *Find the total . . .*
Division	*Per . . .* *Each . . .* *Out of . . .* *Ratio of . . .* *Percent . . .*

TABLE 5.3. Sample Story Problems, Key Words, and Required Operation(s)

Story problem	Key words	Operation(s)
Jeff rode his bicycle 5 miles to the skateboard park. He found a shortcut on the way home that was only 3 miles long. **How many** *miles did Jeff ride* **altogether**?	*How many . . .* *Altogether . . .*	Addition
Max wants to buy an iPod that costs $149. He has $25 saved. **How much more** *does he need to save? If he wants to save the remaining money needed in equal amounts over 4 weeks so he can buy the iPod in time to take it to summer camp, how much money must he save* **per** *week to buy the iPod?*	*How much more . . .* *Per . . .*	Subtraction Division

Use of Timed Tasks and Tests

Timed tests or activities often are a key component of math instruction. Unfortunately, students with HFA/AS may not understand timed tasks and the need to be efficient when completing them (Silverman & Weinfeld, 2007). In fact, these students "may not have the same sense of internal time monitoring or subjective time as other kids" (Silverman & Weinfeld, 2007, p. 61). To better prepare students for these kinds of tasks, teachers will want to ensure that students with HFA/AS fully understand the task requirements prior to using these timed tasks in the classroom. Thus, this may be yet another domain in which the use of priming might be helpful. In addition, the teacher may decide to mark where the student was at the end of the time limit to assess his or her fluency compared with that of classmates.

> **Timed tests or activities often are a key component of math instruction. ... To better prepare students for these kinds of tasks, teachers will want to ensure that students with HFA/AS fully understand the task requirements prior to using these timed tasks in the classroom.**

CONCLUSION

A number of general and specific strategies for enhancing the academic success of students with HFA/AS were described in this chapter. The strategies described highlight the specific learning needs often encountered when teaching students with HFA/AS. Many of the strategies make use of visual cues, a high degree of structure, and explicit instruction. Although the specific strategies focus on the academic domains of reading, math, and written expression, they can be adapted for use in content areas such as science, social studies, and history. Teachers and other educators are encouraged to use and adapt these strategies based on data collected with their own students, with the goal of increasing positive school outcomes for students with HFA/AS.

CHAPTER 6

Providing Behavioral Supports

STUDENT SNAPSHOT: Liam

Liam, an 8-year-old with HFA, displays behaviors that are intensely rigid and repetitive in nature. In general, he is always the first one to notice changes made to the classroom, such as the admittance of a new student, the hanging of a poster on the wall, or the addition of a novel box of math manipulatives. Rather than just taking note of changes, Liam insists on touching everything and asking the teacher why such changes had to be made. Moreover, Liam obsesses over small details that his typically developing classmates often overlook, and he insists that things be done in a certain manner. He places his crayons and pencils in a specific basket and his worksheets on a certain shelf. In gym, Liam has to use the same ball every day, otherwise, he refuses to participate. When walking down the hallway, he obsessively reads all of the numbers of the doorways, rechecking them twice before continuing on his way. If allowed, many of Liam's behaviors and routines can take hours to accomplish, significantly interfering with the school day.

OVERVIEW

Problematic behaviors in children with HFA/AS span a wide range and tend to vary according to the child's development and intellectual ability. Although stereotyped, repetitive behaviors (e.g., body rocking or hand flapping) do occur in individuals with HFA/AS, they occur infrequently and most likely arise during highly stressful, unpredictable situations or when the child does not understand the expectations for behavior. Most often, children with HFA/AS engage in rigid patterns of behaviors and/or display restricted patterns of behaviors in the context of an all-absorbing preoccupation with a circumscribed topic of interest (Howlin, 1998; Myles & Simpson, 2003). Eventually, the frequent occurrences of such behaviors likely interfere with teaching and can irritate even the most tolerant of educators. As such, educators must proactively plan for effective behavioral support by utilizing a series of prevention and direct intervention approaches. Within this chapter, effective and easy-to-implement strategies are provided to inform practitioners of behavioral support strategies that lead to positive student outcomes.

> **Although stereotyped, repetitive behaviors ... do occur in individuals with HFA/AS, they occur infrequently and most likely arise during highly stressful, unpredictable situations or when the child does not understand the expectations for behavior.**

EFFECTIVE BEHAVIORAL SUPPORT

To be most effective, behavior support strategies for students with HFA/AS (1) are assessment based and hypothesis driven, (2) emphasize environmental change and skill building, and (3) involve multiple intervention components. Overall, effective strategies for improving the behavior of students with HFA/AS build on or shape behavior. The rationale for such a focus is that positive, educative interventions build skills in students with HFA/AS who likely have restricted behavioral repertoires. As such, simply applying behavior reduction strategies (e.g., time-out) is less desirable because it likely does not result in lifelong behavior change that improves the student's quality of life. Thus, prior to implementing any behavioral intervention strategies, thought must be given to what the student will be taught, what outcome behaviors are desired, where the behaviors need to occur, and how those behaviors function such that they replace (functionally speaking) any inappropriate behaviors in which the student engages. In this way, the behavioral intervention process becomes, in large part, a teaching endeavor.

> **Students with HFA/AS typically have high levels of stress, and the application of punishers or the use of aversive stimuli may increase the likelihood of problematic behaviors (not to mention foster negativity between the adult and child).**

Supporting the behavioral needs of students with HFA/AS rarely should include the use of punishment (e.g., time-out). Moreover, aversive stimuli (e.g., placing a child in a room that he or she cannot exit) should never be used, especially in school settings. Students with HFA/AS typically have high levels of stress, and the application of punishers or the use of aversive stimuli may increase the likelihood of problematic behaviors (not to mention foster negativity between the adult and child). When used with students with HFA/AS, punishment and aversive stimuli only encourage avoidance, escape, and strong emotional backlash, as well as modeling inappropriate behaviors as solutions to problems. Instead, practitioners should follow three guidelines for effective behavior support: (1) *prevent* inappropriate behaviors from occurring, (2) *teach* effective replacement behaviors, and (3) *reinforce* appropriate behaviors that encourage positive student outcomes and simultaneously promote independence.

PREVENTATIVE APPROACHES

Despite the common and frequently referenced areas of behavioral difficulty in students with HFA/AS, appropriate support and education can dramatically increase their independent functioning. Because many of the difficulties that students with HFA/AS display stem from a lack of understanding or a misinterpretation of the world, preventative actions can decrease the occurrence of inappropriate behaviors considerably and without need for additional individualized approaches. Carefully planned environmental and visual strategies help children with HFA/AS understand the world, help them accept change, and increase their independent functioning (Myles & Simpson, 2003). Such preventative strategies include environmental modifications, choice and preference, and visual supports. A brief description and examples of each follow.

Environmental Modifications

Classroom Layout

> **Students with HFA/AS function best in classrooms that are not only well organized and predictable (Attwood, 1998, 2007), but also minimally decorated and simply arranged.**

Students with HFA/AS function best in classrooms that are not only well organized and predictable (Attwood, 1998, 2007), but also minimally decorated and simply arranged. Thus everything from the arrangement of desks to the layout of bulletin boards should be simple and uncluttered (Moore, 2002). Such efforts give the student with HFA/AS the kind of structure and predictability necessary to function effectively in the classroom, as well as increasing the probability of maintaining the student's attention to academic tasks. If desks are grouped, groups should be kept to a maximum of four or five students (Moore, 2002). Also, under such circumstances, it may be best to seat the student with HFA/AS toward the outside of the group. Similarly, if desks are arranged in rows, the student with HFA/AS should be seated near the end of the row. While facilitating social interactions, such desk arrangements allow the student with HFA/AS to have some distance from others when overstimulated, as well as allowing the teacher to reach the student easily if any problems arise.

In addition to a simple classroom design, a variety of visuals may be provided to help students with HFA/AS stay focused and on task. For example, part of keeping the classroom structured and predictable is the establishment of a small number (e.g., three to five) of briefly stated classroom rules. Once established, rules should be posted where they are visible to all students (Paine, Radicchi, Rosellini, Deutchman, & Darch, 1983). In addition to clearly posting rules, providing the student with HFA/AS with a visual schedule of activities for each day may be helpful (Moore, 2002; Kunce & Mesibov, 1998). Such visual schedules can be written or picture based, depending on the needs of the child. Regardless of the method, research on visual schedules suggests that they increase on-task behavior for students with HFA/AS (Bryan & Gast, 2000). Schedules may be used for activities in a single classroom (i.e., at the elementary school level) or for activities across various classrooms (i.e., for middle school and high school). In a classroom setting, it is best to post the schedule in a clearly visible location (e.g., on the student's desk or on the chalkboard or whiteboard). Students may carry a printed copy of the schedule for use across classes. Schedules also may provide information on daily, weekly, or monthly activities for the student with HFA/AS (Kunce & Mesibov, 1998). The use of posted rules and schedules allows students with HFA/AS to anticipate what is expected of them academically and behaviorally.

Home Base

Another example of effective environmental modifications for students with HFA/AS is called Home Base (Dunn, Saiter, & Rinner, 2002). Home Base provides the student with a quiet place to go when the classroom becomes too stressful, or it can be an area in which to plan or review information (Myles & Adreon, 2001; Myles & Southwick, 2005). Although there are no specific criteria for selecting a location for Home Base, care should be taken to select an environment that will allow the student to work quietly or provide a place to calm down when he or she is highly stressed (Myles, 2005). Examples of locations for Home Base can include a resource classroom, a favorite teacher's classroom, the principal's or behavior specialist's office, or anywhere within the school that is comforting to the student and allows close supervision of the student's behavior. Home Base is not a time-out! Rather, it is a location to which the student can go so that loss of instructional time is minimized. Table 6.1 provides a list of common uses for Home Base during different times of the school day. The key to using Home Base as a preventative approach is to teach the student the times at which he or she should go there, not that it is a place for escape. This likely will involve some sort of cuing strategy supported by an external source (e.g., teacher or aide) that can be faded over time as the student becomes more proficient at self-monitoring and using Home Base independently.

TABLE 6.1. Uses of Home Base during Different Times of Day

Beginning of the school day	End of the school day	As needed
• Preview the day's schedule • Provide an overview of schedule changes • Prime for upcoming activities • Provide transition time and activity from bus to school • Provide time and place to organize materials • Support social skills instruction	• Work on homework • Organize unfinished assignments, books, and supplies • Complete assignment sheets • Modify curriculum (e.g., break assignments down into smaller, more manageable chunks)	• Preventative: at the first sign of student stress • Immediately after challenging activities: (1) as a cool-down activity and/ or (2) to provide time to interpret

Choice and Preference

Historically, individuals with developmental disabilities have had very little choice regarding the events that affect their lives. More recently, there has been a push to allow children to exert greater control through choice making. Choice making refers to the process of allowing a child to select an activity among several available alternatives. For example, a child with HFA/AS may be given the choice of whether to complete math or reading work first during independent seatwork time. The expectation is that the student will complete tasks for both academic areas, but the choice regarding which one to do first is student directed. Related to choice making is the concept of preference. Preference refers to those objects, particular tasks, and activities that an individual finds most appealing and naturally rewarding. When choice making and preferences are incorporated, children with HFA/AS may exert more control over their lives and thus reduce some of the odd behaviors that result from anxiety.

Over the past two decades, an increasing body of research has demonstrated the beneficial effects of allowing choice-making opportunities for children with various developmental disabilities, including children with HFA/AS. For example, incorporating choice making into daily tasks has resulted in increased task engagement, decreased disruptive behavior challenges (Moes, 1998; Peterson, Caniglia, & Royster, 2001), and increased homework completion (Moes, 1998). Likewise, incorporating individuals' preferences into activities has been shown to decrease problematic behaviors and increase time engaged in academic and social contexts (e.g., Vaughn & Horner, 1997).

Visual Supports

Visual supports are one of the best strategies for preventing problematic behaviors from occurring and are much more effective than using constant verbal reminders. Specifically,

> **Visual supports are one of the best strategies for preventing problematic behaviors from occurring and are much more effective than using constant verbal reminders.**

visual supports consist of clip art or media pictures, photographs, and/or lists that prompt or remind children with HFA/AS to engage in a particular behavior or that prepare them for an upcoming activity or task. Because children with HFA/AS often have difficulty understanding the world in which they live, and because they need frequent reminders, visual supports provide the structure and predictability necessary for effective functioning in a variety of settings (e.g., classrooms, community). That is, visual supports allow children with HFA/AS to anticipate upcoming events and any expectations regarding setting or task requirements, thereby creating a sense of security and reducing anxiety. Visual supports can be used in a variety of forms, such as schedules, rules, or other graphically represented cues, to support the inclusion and education of children with HFA/AS. In addition, visual supports should be used to introduce all new activities and tasks, as well as for regular daily activities (Moore, 2002). Brief descriptions of the most common visual supports and examples of each are provided next (for a comprehensive list and examples of visual supports, see Moore, 2002).

Daily Schedules

A daily schedule simply is an illustrative representation of the planned activities for the day. Such schedules can be created to represent the schedule of an entire school day, activities that will occur during a specific class period, or time frames for community involvement during a field trip. The manner by which this information is provided should be individualized to the student's developmental level. For example, for very young children who may not yet be proficient readers, pictures only may be appropriate. For older students who have a solid grasp of reading, a combination of words and pictures or entirely words may be more fitting. Moreover, schedules should be adapted that consider the student's characteristics and preferences to the greatest degree possible (Myles, 2005). Although schedules frequently include specific times for certain activities (e.g., reading from 10:00 to 10:30), some students may find this particularly difficult to handle. For instance, Luke, a teenager with AS, often became agitated if an activity accidently ran slightly longer (or shorter!) than the time frame projected on his schedule. At times, such accidental behavior prompted a temper tantrum that resulted in a loss of teaching time for Luke and the class. In such a case, a schedule that simply provided a list of the order of activities was more suitable and led to far fewer occurrences of problematic behavior. Daily schedules can be as simple or as complex as needed, as long as the student benefits from their use (see Figures 6.1 and 6.2 for examples).

Change-in-Routine Cards

Many times within school-based settings, a change to a routine schedule must occur. This is particularly common in middle and high school environments when periods are eliminated or shortened due to assemblies or abbreviated school days (e.g., inclement weather days).

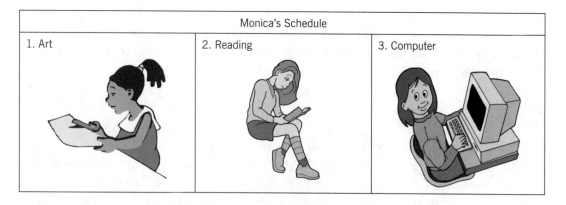

FIGURE 6.1. Sample daily schedule (elementary grades).

Time	Class	Location
7:20–7:40	Homeroom	Room 101
7:40–7:44	Hall time	Hallway, walk to class
7:44–8:40	Algebra	Room 108
8:40–8:44	Hall time	Hallway, walk to class
8:44–9:40	English	Room 118
9:40–9:44	Hall time	Hallway, walk to class
9:44–10:44	Reading	Room 103
10:44–11:40	Lunch	Cafeteria
11:40–11:44	Hall time	Hallway, walk to class
11:44–12:40	Physical Education	Gym
12:40–12:44	Hall time	Hallway, walk to class
12:44–2:05	Resource Room	Room 211
2:05–2:09	Hall time	Hallway, walk to class
2:09–2:20	Homeroom	Room 101
2:20	Dismissal	Go to bus #45

FIGURE 6.2. Sample daily schedule (middle/high school).

In addition, changes in routine may occur when a substitute teacher is asked to cover for a teacher who is ill or when a change from outdoor to indoor recess occurs due to rain. Regardless of the nature of the change, students with HFA/AS likely will interpret such events as confusing and exceptionally frustrating. This increase in anxiety can become maddening for some, leading to explosive behavioral meltdowns. To prevent the likelihood of a behavioral meltdown, educators can create a change-in-routine card that prompts the student about the change and allows him or her time to calm down. In fact, a change-in-routine card can be used at the beginning of the school day in conjunction with Home Base. Although there will be times when it is impossible to forewarn students (e.g., a fire alarm), when a schedule change is known, creating a card to reflect the alteration is far more effective than allowing a student to be surprised on his or her own.

Checklists

Checklists can be used for a variety of purposes for students with HFA/AS. Not only do they provide structure and predictability for the student, but also they help him or her to remain focused. Most often, checklists are used for students with HFA/AS to prompt academic steps required for an assignment or steps for completing a certain task. For example, Figure 6.3 provides an example of a checklist that could be used to prompt a student about the steps

> ☐ Place one number above the other number so that the tens-place digits and ones-place digits line up.
>
> ☐ Add the ones-place digits.
>
> ☐ Carry the tens-place digit to the top of the tens column.
>
> ☐ Add the numbers in the tens-place column (don't forget the carry over).
>
> ☐ Place your answer below the line and to the left of the ones-place column.

FIGURE 6.3. Sample independent seatwork checklist.

for completing an independent work assignment. A checklist also can be used to prompt a kindergarten student with the tasks necessary when arriving in the classroom on school days (see Figure 6.4). Figure 6.5 provides an example of a checklist of the steps necessary for a student during independent reading time in the classroom. Aside from the several examples provided, checklists prompt students with HFA/AS to follow a sequence of steps that assist them in functioning appropriately within school (Moore, 2002). When creating checklists, it is important to include all of the steps that are required, but care should be taken to limit the number of words.

Expectations/Rules Cards

Visuals that provide students with prompts for the expected behaviors and rules within a classroom or other location within a school can be particularly effective for preventing problematic behaviors. As is the case with daily schedules and checklists, rules cards may be used for a variety of purposes. For example, Figure 6.6 demonstrates a sample rule card that was attached to Justin's desk; he was a student with HFA who had particular difficulty remembering to raise his hand and be called on by the teacher when answering questions. Figure 6.7 demonstrates an example of using photographs to create a checklist of rules for using a standard ATM machine.

Stress Cards

A particularly useful form of visual support that may be effective for students prone to behavioral meltdowns and temper tantrums is a stress card. Stress cards serve as a preventative measure as well as a coping strategy that students with HFA/AS can learn to use in order to calm their senses, reduce anxiety, and eliminate their feelings of frustration as they learn to control their emotions (see Figure 6.8). I (F. J. S.) used a stress card as a preventative approach for a middle school student with AS who frequently displayed uncontrollable outbursts in class (e.g., screaming, kicking, throwing objects). The purpose of the approach

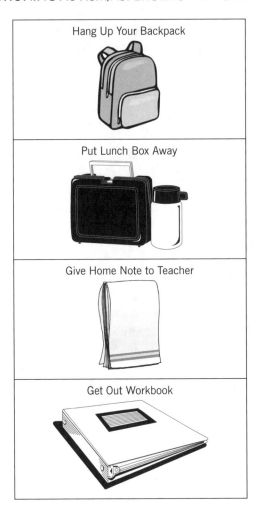

FIGURE 6.4. Sample morning routine checklist.

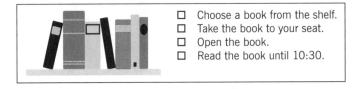

FIGURE 6.5. Sample independent reading activity checklist.

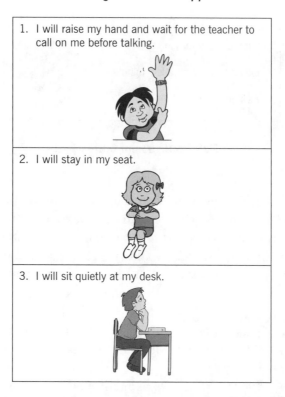

1. I will raise my hand and wait for the teacher to call on me before talking.

2. I will stay in my seat.

3. I will sit quietly at my desk.

FIGURE 6.6. Personal rule card.

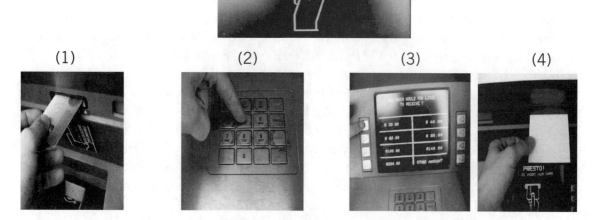

FIGURE 6.7. ATM rules card.

Stress Card

1. I am feeling stressed!

2. I need to leave for a few minutes.

3. I will return when I am calm.

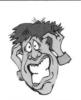

FIGURE 6.8. Sample stress card.

was to allow the student a brief moment to turn his stress card in to his teacher, signaling that he was upset and about to lose control of his emotions. The student would then leave the classroom with permission and report to his Home Base area (the behavior specialist's office). While at Home Base, the student would engage in a series of calming routines that he was taught and then return to class. To ensure the effectiveness of such an approach, the student was awarded points for returning to class. Specifically, he received only 1 point for using his stress card but 25 points for returning to class that period, 15 points for the next period, and so on. In essence, the intervention was predicated on keeping the student in class (and prevented the use of Home Base as a place to escape). However, the stress card was used as a visual approach to remind the student of his choice to leave the class without reprisal or subsequent disciplinary actions due to inappropriate (and dangerous!) behavior.

> Stress cards serve as a preventative measure as well as a coping strategy that students with HFA/AS can learn to use in order to calm their senses, reduce anxiety, and eliminate their feelings of frustration as they learn to control their emotions.

First . . . , Then . . . Boards

In order to perform a desired behavior, some students with HFA/AS may need a reference to an immediate motivator. To accomplish this task, educators can use *First . . .* (or *When*), *Then . . .* boards. *First . . . , Then . . .* boards provide students with HFA/AS clear expectations and help motivate and assist them with task completion. These boards are particularly useful for engaging students with HFA/AS in nonpreferred activities. To create a *First . . . , Then . . .* board, take a laminated sheet of paper or card stock (a small, dry erasable marker board works perfectly) and divide it into two sections, with the word *First . . .* on one side and *Then . . .* on the other (see Figure 6.9). When using a *First . . . , Then . . .* board, place a picture of the activity (or activities) the child needs to complete under "first." Similarly, place a picture of the rewarding or preferred activity under "then." The *First . . . , Then . . .* format allows the child to focus on the current activity by providing incentive for completion. This strategy can be used during standardized assessments (e.g., *First . . .* Blocks, *Then . . .* Play-Doh), academic activities (e.g., *First . . .* Reading, *Then . . .* Recess), or other home/community environments (e.g., *First . . .* Eat Your Peas, *Then . . .* Video Game).

First	Then

FIGURE 6.9. Sample First . . . , Then . . . board.

DIRECT INTERVENTION STRATEGIES

Preventative actions in and of themselves are necessary but sometimes not sufficient to produce changes in the behavioral functioning and development of children with HFA/AS. Therefore, more specific interventions that are designed to increase the skill, frequency, or quality of behaviors emitted by children with HFA/AS may be necessary. Within the remaining sections, strategies for teaching replacement behaviors and providing effective reinforcement are discussed. It is suggested that educators utilize a combination of preventative strategies and the following behavioral interventions to maximize positive outcomes for students with HFA/AS.

Teaching Replacement Behaviors

Most often, students with HFA/AS do not engage in inappropriate behaviors with malicious intent. In fact, the majority of problematic behavior that students with HFA/AS display is the result of a loss of control of the environment and/or feelings of unpredictability. Persistent problem behavior displayed by students with HFA/AS is best understood as a skill deficit (i.e., the student lacks the skills necessary to regulate emotions and control behavior). Given this perspective, building basic skills and competencies is critical for producing long-lasting and durable behavioral change. To best meet the persistent behavioral needs of students with HFA/AS, a comprehensive functional behavioral assessment (FBA) should be conducted (see Chapter 4 for detailed information pertaining to FBA). As described previously, a FBA provides detailed information for developing effective intervention plans. In reference to behavioral skills, an effectively executed FBA will target specific skills that will allow the student to meet his or her goals in a more efficient, effective, and appropriate

> Persistent problem behavior displayed by students with HFA/AS is best understood as a skill deficit (i.e., the student lacks the skills necessary to regulate emotions and control behavior). Given this perspective, building basic skills and competencies is critical for producing long-lasting and durable behavioral change.

manner (Horner, Sprague, & Flannery, 1993). Quite often skills that need to be taught are replacement behaviors.

Replacement behaviors can best be conceptualized as skills that provide access to a desirable outcome through the use of a socially appropriate and functional alternative rather than by engaging in some form of inappropriate behavior. For example, a student with HFA/AS may desire access to a ball during recess. His current method for obtaining the ball is to run up to any student who is playing with a ball, yell "mine," and run away with the ball. A more socially appropriate replacement behavior that is functionally equivalent (i.e., the student gets the same outcome—the ball) is to ask for the ball or to create a sharing plan with another student. The emphasis here is a skill deficit. It is the skill deficit that needs to be directly targeted and the skill specifically taught to the student. To teach the targeted replacement behavior, instruction must occur systematically. Systematic instruction involves (1) using effective instructional cues, (2) breaking skills down into their component parts and teaching discretely, (3) employing appropriate teaching methods (e.g., prompting, shaping), and (4) rewarding appropriate behaviors consistently. For students with HFA/AS, systematic instruction should incorporate the use of pictures, videos, and multiple models to teach the replacement behavior. Once a target replacement behavior and strategies for systematically teaching the skills associated with that particular behavior are identified, strategies to increase replacement behavior are necessary. For students with HFA/AS, these strategies ideally will involve contingent positive reinforcement.

Providing Contingent Positive Reinforcement

The Power of Reinforcement

Within the context of applied behavior analysis (ABA), reinforcement is used to increase the likelihood of behavior recurrence. At the core of any behavioral support plan is the inclusion of reinforcement to teach and enhance positive, adaptive behaviors. When it is used *immediately* following the desired target behavior and when it is *contingent* on the emission of that behavior, reinforcement can be a powerful tool for behavior change. Two forms of reinforcement exist: positive reinforcement and negative reinforcement. Whereas positive reinforcement involves adding something positive following a desired behavior (e.g., attention, access to items or activities, edibles), negative reinforcement involves the removal of something deemed aversive following a desired behavior (e.g., allowing for a break contingent on completing a certain amount of work). Rhode, Jenson, and Reavis (1993) suggest using the following "IFEED rules" when implementing reinforcement: reinforce the individual _I_mmediately following the desired behavior; reinforce the individual as _F_requently as possible; be _E_nthusiastic when delivering praise and other reinforcers; make _E_ye contact when delivering reinforcement; specifically label or _D_escribe

> When it is used *immediately* following the desired target behavior and when it is *contingent* on the emission of that behavior, reinforcement can be a powerful tool for behavior change.

the behavior being rewarded. To be most effective, educators are encouraged to remind students of the rewards they can earn just prior to the activity (e.g. *"First . . . , Then . . . "*).

Identifying and Selecting Rewards and Motivators

To maximize the efficacy of the reinforcement system for teaching and strengthening emerging behaviors, it is critical to select rewards and motivators that are deemed desirable by the student with HFA/AS. Given the importance of this element, parents, educators, and other community partners are encouraged to take time to assess possible rewards and motivators. Rewards and motivators for students can be identified through four primary means: (1) observing the student in applied settings to determine what he or she finds rewarding; (2) asking the student to verbally identify potential rewards; (3) using reinforcer surveys or checklists; and (4) using sampling procedures to select potential rewards (Alberto & Troutman, 2008; Rhode et al., 1993; Yell, Meadows, Drasgow, & Shriner, 2009).

Observing a student with HFA/AS in both structured and unstructured settings (e.g., during free time, during center-based activities) can be a powerful and simple mechanism for identifying potential rewards. An assumption of ABA is that if individuals continue to engage in a particular behavior, it means that they are receiving some form of reinforcement to drive recurrence. It easily follows that if students repeatedly engage in a particular activity or continually use an item during a play activity, they likely find it highly rewarding. It is common for parents and teachers to assume that some activities or objects in or with which students with HFA/AS engage cannot possibly be rewarding to the student (e.g., watching the same movie over and over again, reading the same book or passage repeatedly). However, it is essential to remember that when selecting rewards, the task is to identify *what the student deems rewarding—not to place value or judgment on that particular item or activity.*

Although observing a student can provide valuable information, it may fall short of truly capturing what motivates an individual with HFA/AS. Therefore, asking the student what he or she likes may be another effective approach to identifying potential rewards. However, there are a few cautions when using this approach in isolation. Whereas many students with HFA/AS are honest about their wants, needs, and desires, some students with HFA/AS may lack the self-awareness necessary to identify such items or activities appropriately. It also is possible that a student may become conditioned to answer in a scripted manner to end the potentially uncomfortable dialog with a stranger (e.g., school psychologist, speech–language pathologist), thus delivering a response that is invalid. For these reasons, it is not recommended that this particular technique be used in isolation when identifying potential motivators for students with HFA/AS.

An invaluable and particularly effective tool for identifying potential rewards is to use a preexisting survey or checklist with the target student. A variety of these forms are available in textbooks and can be found easily using an online search engine. However, a major disadvantage of using such "canned" surveys or checklists, particularly with students with HFA/AS who may possess unique areas of interest, is that the preexisting product may not include the types of reinforcers relevant (or of interest) to the target student. Instead, educators are encouraged to create their own checklist or survey that matches the curiosities of the student with HFA/AS. Such an approach often can be based on those items and activities identified during observations of or interviews with the child. In addition, educators can use the Jackpot Online Reinforcement Survey tool (see *www.jimwrightonline.com/php/jackpot/jackpot.php*) to create an individualized reinforcement survey for any student.

A less common approach to identifying and prioritizing rewards and motivators for students with HFA/AS is to use one of three sampling procedures: (1) single-item presentation, (2) choice–forced-choice presentation, and (3) multiple-stimulus presentation (Alberto & Troutman, 2008). With the single-item-presentation approach, items are presented one at a time until they are selected by the student a predetermined number of times, thus indicating preference. A limitation of this approach is that it does not allow for relative preference to be systematically determined. With the choice–forced-choice approach, each item is presented at least once paired with each of the remaining items. Such an approach allows the student to select one of the two options with each presented pair. This process may be repeated until the teacher can determine a rate of selection or level of preference (e.g., if a particular item is selected 75% of the time when randomly paired with competing items, it may be deemed highly preferred; Alberto & Troutman, 2008). Finally, the multiple-stimulus presentation approach involves the simultaneous presentation of items; once the student selects an item, it is removed. This process continues until either all items have been selected or the student no longer responds, and it may be repeated to confirm a student's relative preferences.

When selecting potential reinforcers for use with students with HFA/AS, it is important to consider two key factors. First, it is important to remove subjective value or judgment when attempting to identify potential rewards and motivators for students with HFA/AS. Many students with HFA/AS may identify items that would not be rewarding to typically developing individuals. However, use of such rewards likely will result in greater behavioral change because the student is motivated to have access to them. Second, it is important to reconsider the common assumption that verbal praise is rewarding to *all* students. Whereas verbal praise may be an effective means of reinforcement for *many* students (Rhode et al., 1993), *some* individuals (e.g., older students and young adults) may find public praise embarrassing and unpleasant, thus resulting in a decrease in desired behavior (i.e., praise becomes a form of punishment; Bowen, Jenson, & Clarke, 2004).

When educators and related professionals conduct a FBA in an applied setting, they often conclude that the hypothesized function of many disruptive behavior(s) is escape or avoidance (Cowan & Sheridan, 2009). That is, for many students, the most powerful form of reinforcement is the ability to escape or avoid nonpreferred activities. This observation particularly is true for students with HFA/AS. Because individuals with HFA/AS may find many seemingly harmless tasks (e.g., social interactions during "down time," assignments that do not align with their perseverative topic) to be aversive (Myles et al., 2004), school-based practitioners may want to select reinforcement strategies that utilize escape contingent on a predetermined amount of engagement in the nonpreferred task or activity (i.e., "*First . . . , Then . . .*").

Differential Reinforcement Strategies

With differential reinforcement strategies, the student is provided with reinforcement when engaging in appropriate behaviors (thereby not reinforcing the student's inappropriate behaviors). In doing so, the student learns to respond differentially based on the cues (discriminative stimuli) that are present. There are four general types of differential reinforcement strategies: (1) differential reinforcement of incompatible behavior (DRI), (2) differential reinforcement of alternative behavior (DRA), (3) differential reinforcement of low rates of behavior (DRL), and (4) differential reinforcement of other behavior (DRO). Each of these approaches is discussed in greater detail next.

DRI is useful when educators want to replace an inappropriate behavior with an appropriate functional equivalent that the student cannot engage in at the same time (i.e., one that is topographically incompatible). For example, sitting in one's seat would be reinforced as a replacement behavior for walking around the classroom, because these behaviors are incompatible (i.e., both behaviors cannot occur at the same time). Another example might be requiring a student with HFA/AS to join in an activity with peers rather than turning around and walking away. Similar to DRI, DRA provides reinforcement for an alternative form of a behavior that is more socially desirable. Perhaps the best example to illustrate this approach is teaching a student to ask for a ball or create a sharing plan rather than grabbing the ball from another student. For both DRI and DRA, the desirable behavior results in reinforcement each time it occurs (Miltenberger, 2007). Also, with both DRA and DRI, if the appropriate replacement behavior is not occurring at least some of the time, you will need to spend time teaching the student what is expected before using either of these approaches (Miltenberger, 2001). Finally, likely the greatest challenge with DRI and DRA is choosing a replacement behavior that is functionally equivalent and is nearly as efficient at obtaining reinforcement as the behavior one is trying to replace. Conducting a FBA (see Chapter 4) can be an important step toward addressing this challenge.

DRL is useful when you do not want to eliminate a behavior completely but rather want to shape the frequency or timing of particular behaviors. For example, if a student with HFA/AS talks about dinosaurs frequently because it is a topic of special interest, one would not want to completely eliminate those discussions (after all, the student is being social!). Rather, it would be important for the student to learn to discriminate an appropriate frequency for the topic to be discussed. In cases such as this,

> **DRL is useful when you do not want to eliminate a behavior completely but rather want to shape the frequency or timing of particular behaviors. For example, if a student with HFA/AS talks about dinosaurs frequently because it is a topic of special interest, one would not want to completely eliminate those discussions (after all, the student is being social!).**

DRL might be a very useful intervention strategy. To implement DRL, educators first must identify a criterion level of performance to be reached. For example, the student would have to engage in no more than three instances of discussing dinosaurs before lunchtime. This example illustrates full-session DRL (Miltenberger, 2001). Another option with DRL is to use what is referred to as spaced responding DRL (Miltenberger, 2001). With spaced responding, a specified amount of time would have to elapse after one incident of talking about dinosaurs before reinforcement would be available for again talking about them (e.g., 30 minutes).

The three aforementioned approaches utilizing differential reinforcement can be described as educative in nature. That is, each of these differential approaches focuses on teaching the student appropriate ways of interacting that increase his or her social desirability. DRO, an approach that involves reinforcing a student if an undesired behavior is *not* displayed during a designated period, is considered to be less educative. For example, consider a student with HFA/AS who frequently disrupts the teacher with inappropriate questions during instruction that are reinforced through teacher attention. To apply this intervention technique, the teacher would need to ignore those questions and ensure that the student receives no other reinforcement. In addition, the teacher would need to reinforce the student for a predetermined amount of time that elapses without interruptions. One of the challenges with this intervention is determining the appropriate amount of time that must elapse for the student to be reinforced for not engaging in the inappropriate behavior. Though used less often in recent published research due to the level of effort involved in implementing this procedure, it can be made more efficient when combined with self-monitoring procedures (Tiger, Fisher, & Bouxsein, 2009). In particular, this combination is useful for students with HFA/AS, as it provides a greater level of individual control over the intervention in addition to the time saved. Tiger et al. (2009) found that the use of DRO and self-monitoring was effective in reducing skin-picking behaviors to near-zero levels for an adolescent student with AS.

For all of the differential reinforcement strategies, it is best to select behaviors to increase that are in the learner's repertoire, that the learner emits regularly, that will increase skills, and that the natural environment will support (e.g., for which peers will provide naturally occurring reinforcement). For example, when using a differential reinforcement strategy to increase a student's joining in games and activities, the likelihood that the student will continue to engage in this behavior increases substantially if the natural reinforcement of peers' accepting the student into the game or activity occurs. In addition, educators should select appropriate reinforcers based on the student's preferences, as well as those that are stronger than the reinforcement available for the inappropriate behavior.

Contingency Agreements and Behavioral Contracts

A contingency agreement is a formal means of setting up the expectation that X amount of Y behavior will result in a specified reward. Essentially, it is a two-way contract—verbal or written—stipulating that if one party (e.g., the student) emits a specified desired behavior (or a lower rate of a disruptive behavior) and if this emission follows the terms of the agreement, a second party (e.g., the teacher) will deliver a predetermined amount and type of reward. The core components of a contingency agreement include reference to the behavior of interest, the conditions, the criterion, and the reward (Alberto & Troutman, 2008). Perhaps one of the greatest strengths of contingency agreements is their flexibility in terms of specified behaviors and rewards. For example, as applied to a student with HFA/AS, a contingency agreement may be developed whereby if the student writes a creative short story about the topic of the teacher's choice, he or she can then develop a story about his area of interest and share it with his or her class. The specifics about the length of each story may be negotiated between the student and the teacher. Alternatively, a father may work with his daughter with HFA/AS to jointly determine that if she plays with the toys selected by her sister for 15 minutes, she may select the activity in which they will engage for the subsequent 15 minutes. A verbal contingency agreement may be most useful when the intervention period is in the immediate or near future.

Although a contingency agreement may come in the form of a verbal plan, it is quite common for educators to develop a written behavioral contract following negotiation. Several advantages to using a written contract for students with disabilities exist: (1) it serves as a permanent product of the teacher–student negotiation, which helps prevent forgetting the plan or renegotiation during critical times; (2) it allows the student to have an active role in the development of the contingency agreement; (3) the contract itself reflects a form of individualized instruction; and (4) when implemented regularly, it can serve as a means of enhancing self-management in students with ASD (Alberto & Troutman, 2008; Mruzek, Cohen, & Smith, 2007). Furthermore, behavioral contracts have proven effective in both increasing desired behavior and decreasing disruptive behavior across a variety of learners and environments (Rhode et al., 1993; Ruth, 1996), including with students with autism (Mruzek et al., 2007). In addition to their proven efficacy as a stand-alone intervention, there is research to suggest that behavioral contracts may be quite powerful when implemented as part of a multicomponent behavior modification program (De Martini-Scully, Bray, & Kehle, 2000; Musser, Bray, Kehle, & Jenson, 2001).

Rhode et al. (1993) suggest several ways to enhance the effectiveness of a behavioral contract. To begin, they suggest that the student be involved actively in negotiating the details of the contract (e.g., determining the consequences for specific behaviors), especially for higher functioning and older students. In addition to actively involving the student and basing the contract on a specific behavior relevant to that student, Rhode and colleagues suggest that a specific reward be designated for a predetermined behavior criterion. This level of detail serves as a guidepost for both the student and the teacher. Finally, they recommend that the teacher comply with the specifics of the contract (i.e., it is ineffective to change the conditions or expectations once the contract is in effect). Once all of the elements are determined and negotiated, they are written into a contract for both parties to sign. Having the plan in writing prior to beginning the intervention may enhance both treatment fidelity and efficacy.

One way to custom-tailor the contract to enhance self-management skills—a common deficit in individuals with autism (Mruzek et al., 2007)—is to include a progress monitoring system somewhere in the contract (Rhode et al., 1993). Including such a system allows all parties, including the student, to monitor the student's progress toward meeting the conditions of the contract, which may enhance motivation for everyone involved. A final element to consider when designing a contract is to determine whether or not to incorporate a penalty clause (i.e., a reductive consequence for misbehavior or failure to meet the established goal or criteria). As with all interventions reviewed in this volume, it is highly recommended that members of the educational team consider the use of a reductive consequence only after the faithful implementation of a positive behavior support system enriched with multiple reinforcement opportunities.

Token Economies

Perhaps one of the most widely used approaches in education is the token economy system. It has been estimated that approximately 90% of teachers of students demonstrating disruptive behaviors have used some form of a token economy system to teach and enhance adaptive behaviors in the educational setting (Rosenberg, Wilson, Maheady, & Sindelar, 2004). Token economy systems have proven effective in teaching multiple types of skills (e.g., academic, social, vocational) across a variety of settings (e.g., general education classrooms, self-contained classrooms, vocational settings) to students with differing ability levels (Kehle, Bray, Theodore, Jenson, & Clark, 2000; Rathvon, 2003). Furthermore, they have proven effective in both individual and group-based applications. Given teachers' familiarity with token economy systems, coupled with the versatility associated with their implementation, token-based reinforcement systems remain at the forefront of evidence-based interventions for children who require individualized supports to be successful in educational settings. However, there are some basic tenets of the token economy system that warrant discussion to assist parents, educators, and related service providers in maximizing their utility as related to enhancing adaptive behaviors in students with HFA/AS.

> **Given teachers' familiarity with token economy systems, coupled with the versatility associated with their implementation, token-based reinforcement systems remain at the forefront of evidence-based interventions for children who require individualized supports to be successful in educational settings.**

The first assumption of the token economy system is that it is a *reinforcement-based* intervention that involves the use of a *token* (e.g., poker chip, laminated coupon, play money) *delivered* by the adult (e.g., parent, teacher) *contingent* on a student's *demonstration of* a predetermined *positive behavior* (e.g., remaining on task, engaging a peer in conversation). The token—which may be thought of as a "placeholder" for some form of delayed reinforcement—is later exchanged for a backup reinforcer that has more value to the student (e.g., time on the computer, access to art supplies, time in the office assisting administrators). The use of a token as a *placeholder* has several advantages over the immediate delivery of a particular reward (Yell et al., 2009). For example, tokens may be delivered quickly and discreetly to avoid the disruption of academic engagement in the classroom (Yell et al.). In addition, the delivery of the token can be used to bridge the gap between the desired behavior and the delivery of reinforcement under conditions when immediate delivery of a reward may be disruptive (e.g., earned computer time during direct instruction). A related advantage is that over time the student learns a form of self-regulation, as he or she is actively taught through systematic delayed gratification that reinforcement is not always readily available. This process serves students well as they engage in more advanced academic tasks in preparation for postsecondary education and employment.

To implement a token economy system with fidelity, it is critical that the token be delivered *contingent* on the student's demonstration of a discrete positive behavior that is identified and operationalized prior to the implementation of the system. Regardless of whether the educational team is targeting one or multiple behaviors, it is essential that the team identify, operationalize, and specify each desired behavior that can earn the student access to the token. The connection between the token (and reinforcement) and a specific positive behavior is the mechanism through which students learn to demonstrate adaptive behaviors in the classroom (Alberto & Troutman, 2009). It also is recommended that the interventionist use the same type of token each time, according to the appropriate schedule of reinforcement (i.e., on a continuous schedule to begin, then moving to an intermittent schedule once the behavior is consistent; Alberto & Troutman, 2008; Rathvon, 2003). These elements help ensure that the student makes the connection between the desirable behavior and the reward he ultimately receives in exchange for the token.

A variety of tokens have proven effective in behavior modification (Rathvon, 2003), and this lends versatility when developing child-specific interventions. Coupons represent a common form of tokens, as indicated in the positive behavioral support literature (Sugai et al., 2000). The use of tokens that have unique meaning for the target student may well enhance the robustness of the intervention, especially for children with HFA/AS demonstrating perseverance with a specific topic or theme. In a related study, Charlop-Christy and Haymes (1998) discovered that on-task performance was greatly enhanced in children with autism through the use of a token economy incorporating the children's objects of obsession as tokens, as compared with the use of typical tokens. The implication here is that incorporating the student's unique area of interest may serve as a strong motivator as applied to the token (i.e., placeholder) for children with thematic obsessions. This research may shed new light on how tokens are selected for children with HFA/AS.

Additional elements related to the successful implementation of a token economy system prescribe that the backup rewards be available on a predictable schedule and deemed desirable by the student earning them (Rhode et al., 1993). In addition, it is important to decide when and where students may exchange tokens for backup reinforcers. This level of predictability enhances the success of the token economy system and may be particularly relevant for students with HFA/AS who tend to thrive on predictability in schedules. Another major aspect of the token economy system is to determine in advance the costs associated with various rewards. It is recommended that a variety of reinforcers be available across a range of cost levels. This may help avoid satiation within the context of the delivery of backup reinforcers (Rhode et al., 1993). Although individuals with HFA/AS may be more likely to work efficiently to gain access to the same powerful reward repeatedly throughout the intervention period, it also may be beneficial to expose the student with HFA/AS to a variety of reinforcers so as to expand his or her limited range of interests. In addition to satiation, it is important to consider deprivation. That is, it is critical to reserve some forms of reinforcement exclusively for use within the token economy system. If the student has regular access to a reward throughout the day, that item or activity may lose power over time as a motivator.

As discussed earlier within the context of the development and implementation of contingency agreements and behavioral contracts, the individual implementing the token economy system must consider the potential costs and benefits associated with incorporating a reductive consequence as part of the treatment. As indicated earlier, it is highly recommended that interventionists consider the use of a reductive consequence only after the faithful implementation of a positive behavior support system enriched with multiple reinforcement opportunities. If the token economy system is implemented with integrity but the student continues to demonstrate disruptive behaviors in the classroom, the educational team may opt to incorporate a response-cost system. By definition, response cost involves reducing a maladaptive behavior through the removal of a specific amount of previously earned reinforcement following the emission of a predetermined negative target behavior (Alberto & Troutman, 2009; Yell et al., 2009). Within the context of a token economy system, the team determines which behavior(s) will constitute the removal of a previously earned token, how much each incident of behavior will cost the student, and how the system will be implemented.

When implementing a response-cost system, the team should consider several recommendations . To begin with, it is important for the team to control the distribution ratio such that the student does not end up "in the hole" with regard to earned tokens, as this may result in a loss of motivation to try to earn access to desired backup reinforcers (Alberto & Troutman, 2009). It also is important to consider whether or not the individual implementing the response-cost procedure can do so without agitating the student to the extent that there are more costs than benefits associated with the procedure (i.e., the response-cost procedure ends up increasing the number of disruptive behaviors observed in the classroom). Research supports the efficacy of token economy systems with and without a response-cost feature. It is ultimately up to the intervention team to determine whether or not to incorporate a reductive consequence.

Although there are several excellent resources to assist practitioners in setting up a token economy system (e.g., Alberto & Troutman, 2008; Rhode et al., 1993), perhaps one of the most thorough sets of guidelines is derived from Yell and colleagues (2009). Specifically, Yell et al. (2009) suggest the following steps: (1) identify target behaviors, (2) select tokens, (3) choose backup reinforcers, (4) decide how tokens will be delivered, (5) determine a system whereby students can exchange tokens for backup reinforcers, (6) decide how to address problem behaviors, (7) determine how to fade the system, (8) develop a data collection and progress monitoring system, and (9) teach the token economy system to the student(s). One of the primary disadvantages of the token economy system is the complexity of the system, which requires much time and energy to develop, implement, monitor, and maintain. However, if used with fidelity, the token economy system has the potential to yield powerful outcomes in terms of promoting and enhancing positive, adaptive behaviors in students experiencing difficulties in the educational setting. Furthermore, they are versatile to the extent that they may be modified for use across the universal, targeted, and individual levels of intervention.

Self-Management

Self-management strategies are those by which the student is taught to manage his or her own behavior. In essence they involve engaging in a controlling behavior to alter the future occurrence of the behavior one desires to change (i.e., target behavior; Miltenberger, 2001). To apply self-management strategies, a systematic process to ensure success that includes both teaching the appropriate behavior and how to record the behavior is used. It also involves successfully teaching the student tools to use that involve the manipulation of either antecedents (i.e., posting a reminder cue; having a checklist to follow) or consequences (i.e., delivery of reinforcing self-evaluative remarks) (Miltenberger, 2001). Self-management interventions also may be combined with contingency contracts or token economy systems, as indicated previously. Because of their flexibility, self-management interventions are useful for both academic and social behaviors that might be targeted for students with HFA/AS. For example, Callahan and Rademacher (1999) successfully used a self-management intervention to increase independent academic behavior, including on-task behavior, for a second-grade student with HFA. In another study, Wilkinson (2005) found that the combination of conjoint behavior consultation (Sheridan, 1997) and self-management increased both on-task behavior and compliance with teacher requests and classroom rules.

Self-management is an attractive intervention strategy because it builds the student's skills and can increase student self-sufficiency. This benefit is particularly attractive for students with HFA/AS because, quite often, students with ASD have poorly developed self-management skills (Wilkinson, 2008). Self-management interventions frequently are recommended to address behavioral concerns of students who have difficulty learning self-regulation skills (Wilkinson, 2005). In addition, students with HFA/AS also experience difficulties internalizing social rules, which can result in their behavior being intrusive and disruptive to the classroom (Wilkinson, 2005). The use of self-management strategies also can increase classroom efficiency, as they may alleviate or minimize the power struggles that can accompany the use of external behavior change procedures and are aligned with the value of structure and locus of control for students with HFA/AS (Simpson & Myles, 1998). Thus self-management interventions are ideally suited for students with HFA/AS. Finally, self-management interventions are easily learned and easy to implement consistently in classrooms, making them ideal for use in inclusive settings (Wilkinson, 2005).

> **Self-management is an attractive intervention strategy because it builds the student's skills and can increase student self-sufficiency.**

Often, self-management involves a combination of goal setting, self-instruction, self-monitoring (i.e., behavioral recording), self-evaluation, and self-reinforcement (Snell & Brown, 2005). Self-monitoring can be particularly helpful in maintaining behavior change in part due to reactivity. Generally speaking, the reactivity due to self-monitoring will result in behavior changing in the desired direction, a desirable clinical outcome (Cooper, Heron, & Heward, 1987). According to Wilkinson (2008), there are 10 steps to designing a self-management program in general education settings. Wilkinson notes that each of these steps is subject to modification considering the specific needs of the student. A general summary of these steps, along with essential elements and important considerations for each one is given in Table 6.2.

Techniques and tools used with self-management strategies include cues such as notes or picture cards, checklists, opportunities to change the stimulus (e.g., walking away from

TABLE 6.2. Steps for Self-Management Programs, Essential Components, and Considerations

Step	Essential components	Considerations
1. Identify target behavior(s).	• Clearing operational definition (e.g., one the student understands and can track accurately), including examples and nonexamples.	• Focus on appropriate replacement behaviors for challenging or disruptive behavior. • Consider FBA data to understand problem behavior context and select an appropriate functional equivalent (Smith & Sugai, 2000).
2. Decide how often self-management will occur.	• Recording procedures (i.e., interval or frequency). See Chapter 9 of this volume for details on these recording procedures. • Determining cues to be used to indicate that student should record behavior.	• For high-frequency behaviors it may be necessary to engage in self-monitoring more frequently to provide increased opportunities to engage and be reinforced for the appropriate replacement behavior.
3. Meet with the student and develop the self-management plan.	• Explaining rationale for self-management. • Setting goals. • Determining rewards and schedule.	• It is best to involve student and caregivers (parents) in the process of developing the plan, including goal setting.
4. Prepare self-monitoring forms and/or checklists.	• Obtaining or developing forms that match target behaviors.	• Consider the student's skill level when developing checklists.
5. Model and practice.	• Modeling the entire self-management process (i.e., accurate self-observation, recording, and evaluation) followed by student practice and performance feedback.	• Enough practice for the student to obtain mastery is needed for successful implementation of the self-management plan.
6. Implement the plan.	• Cuing self-monitoring procedures during designated times.	• Some plans may incorporate an accuracy check (i.e., student record must match the teacher record most of the time) to determine whether review of procedures and target behaviors is needed.
7. Review progress.	• Meeting with the student and deciding whether the goals were achieved.	• These meetings may be daily or more frequent depending on the target behaviors and the needs of the student.
8. Provide rewards.	• Providing incentives agreed on at Step 3.	• Consider discussion of rewards and motivators presented at the beginning of this chapter.
9. Send home self-recording sheet for parent review.	• Sending checklists or self-monitoring forms home for parent review and signature.	• It is highly desirable to have ongoing communication with the parents about student progress and the success of behavioral intervention plans.
10. Fade the intervention.	• Reducing and eventually fading use of external cues. • Reducing the time self-management procedures are used across the school day.	• Fading of interventions increases independence and maintenance and generalization of behavior change.

an upsetting event), and physical aids. Although several types of cues may be used in self-management interventions, care must be taken that they are nondisruptive to the classroom, that they can be faded easily, and that they are suited to the student's needs and preferences. For example, silent cues (e.g., a timer with a vibrating alarm or a watch with a quiet alarm function) may be better suited to students with HFA/AS than a teacher's verbal cues. Simple checklists also are useful tools in self-management interventions.

CONCLUSION

Students with HFA/AS may display a wide array of inappropriate and problematic behaviors at various points within their education. However, this behavior most often is not intentional and is the result of the student having limited control of the environment. To best meet the needs of students with HFA/AS, preventative approaches that employ environmental manipulation and the use of visuals should be incorporated. In fact, many preventative approaches will decrease problematic behaviors without the need for more individualized behavioral supports. However, there are occurrences when preventative approaches no longer are effective and more reactive behavioral strategies are necessary. Through a combination of preventative approaches, teaching of replacement behaviors, and contingent positive reinforcement, many of the behavioral issues of students with HFA/AS can be alleviated. In essence, interventions that build and enhance student skills and address the function of challenging behavior will have the greatest likelihood of enhancing positive outcomes for students with HFA/AS.

CHAPTER 7

Enhancing Social Skills

> **STUDENT SNAPSHOT: Enzo**
>
> Enzo is a 10-year-old student with AS who has always had difficulty with social interactions. He frequently invades others' personal space to the point at which individuals are uneasy around him or avoid contact with him altogether. Although he dislikes it when both adults and peers touch him, Enzo frequently touches others. When in a crowd or in line, he attempts to make contact with as many people as possible. He regularly grabs girls' backsides or chests, which is increasingly becoming a problem. Enzo is so fanatical about touching others that, during class, he will run across the room simply to touch the hand of another student before quickly returning to his seat. Additionally, Enzo has the propensity to blow air in other people's faces, kiss their hands, and press his body up against theirs. Enzo also will walk up to unfamiliar individuals and smell their clothing, hair, or skin without asking. In addition to such inappropriate social behaviors, Enzo has difficulty understanding the social conventions of play, such as taking turns or following rules. For instance, when Enzo's classmates are playing kickball or shooting hoops at recess, he will steal the ball and run away with it. Although Enzo thinks he is being funny, his classmates typically do not find this amusing and refuse to let him get near them. Enzo does not understand why his peers reject him. On several recent occasions, Enzo has been sitting at lunch or recess alone, crying.

OVERVIEW

Children and adolescents with HFA/AS may be anywhere from withdrawn to active on a continuum of social behavior. At times, they may prefer to spend time alone or may appear to have little awareness of or interest in others. In some instances, individuals with HFA/

126

AS may attempt to interact with others in abnormal, socially clumsy, or unacceptable ways (e.g., excessively sharing facts about washers and dryers). Despite individual variability, the social skills of individuals with HFA/AS typically are characterized by a failure to (1) recognize and orient to stimuli and cues (e.g., body language, gestures, facial expressions, tone of voice) within their social world; (2) understand how their own behavior may affect the thoughts and feelings of others; and (3) engage in shared relationships with peers and adults. Very often, individuals with HFA/AS demonstrate a desire to interact with others despite not understanding how to engage and/or respond socially. Therefore, educators must incorporate social skills instruction as part of any educational routine.

PROGRAMMING FOR SOCIAL SKILLS IN SCHOOLS

Within schools, a systemic approach to assisting the social development of individuals with HFA/AS is essential. Even when social skill development is made an educational priority, it remains a broad and somewhat ambiguous area to cover. It is important that educators make careful decisions regarding what areas of social skill development to focus on for each student with HFA/AS as well as what types of instruction or instructional programs will best support the individual's targeted needs. Not every social skills program will be right for every child with HFA/AS or for every educational environment. It is important that educators assess all the variables and make an informed decision about which type(s) of social skill instruction to embark on. Questions to ask before implementing any social skills intervention may include:

1. Are you looking for a student-specific program or are you looking for a schoolwide program?
2. What are the student's areas of strength and need?
3. What resources within the school are available?
4. Is social skill development a priority?
5. What are the parents' goals and desired outcomes for social skill development?

Answers to these and many other questions will be important in choosing the strategies that are the best fit to achieve desired outcomes.

School-based efforts to enhance the social development of individuals with HFA/AS should provide a multi-tiered approach. That is, social skills interventions should focus on a combination of schoolwide, small-group, and individualized supports. Within each of these areas, explicit teaching of basic social behavior(s), emotional understanding, and social problem solving

> School-based efforts to enhance social development of individuals with HFA/AS should provide a multi-tiered approach. That is, social skills interventions should focus on a combination of schoolwide, small-group, and individualized supports.

must occur. Furthermore, students should be provided with opportunities to participate and interact in a wide variety of integrated environments in which appropriate opportunities, peer models, and functional reinforcers are available (Pierangelo & Giuliani, 2008). Examples of common social skills strategies that have been demonstrated to work well with children and youth with HFA/AS within each tier of support are provided, as well as brief descriptions of common elements for putting such interventions in place.

SCHOOLWIDE (PRIMARY) APPROACHES

Schoolwide Positive Behavior Support

Schoolwide positive behavior support (SWPBS) is a proactive, systems-level approach to creating a positive culture within a school. Specifically, SWPBS involves the application of evidence-based strategies that increase safety and decrease inappropriate behaviors within a school building by teaching and supporting positive (and appropriate) social behavior (Kincaid, Childs, Blase, & Wallace, 2007; Simonsen, Sugai, & Negron, 2008). When using an SWPBS model, schools develop a systemic approach to handling behavioral concerns that are common or meaningful to their particular building. This whole-school approach includes developing a data-based decision-making process for referring students who behave inappropriately, identifying and directly teaching behavioral expectations and rules to students at all grade and ability levels, and implementing a schoolwide reward and reinforcement system that promotes the continuation of proactive social behaviors (Kincaid et al., 2007; see *www.pbis.org* for a review of SWPBS and related contemporary scholarship).

Unlike traditional behavioral systems that wait for a student to misbehave or act inappropriately and then react by applying a form of punishment, SWPBS incorporates a three-tier approach that encourages prosocial behavior with *all* students and that prevents social and/or academic failure (Sugai et al., 2000; Sugai & Horner, 2002). Such support often consists of three levels of intensity: (1) primary (schoolwide) support, (2) secondary (group/classroom) support, and (3) tertiary (individual) support (see Figure 7.1). Primary support includes the development and direct teaching of prosocial behavioral expectations to *all* students. As one common example of such support, a school may establish three to five school rules to promote safety within the building, use class time to teach all students the expected behavior associated with these rules, and ask teachers to provide reinforcement when they observe a student or students demonstrating one or all of the expected behaviors. Secondary supports include supplemental instruction for those students who are not responding positively to primary prevention efforts (those students who are at risk for more serious problem behavior). Intervention or instruction provided within the secondary level is more intensive and presented within a small-group setting (8–10 students). Most often, regular school-based personnel (e.g., teachers, guidance counselors) implement the majority of secondary-level interventions with a high degree of success. Specific strategies and/or practices that qualify as secondary supports include a variety of "social skills groups," "friendship clubs," and/or "anger management groups." Tertiary supports focus on the needs of individual students who continue to demonstrate patterns of behaviors that are dangerous and disruptive and/or that result in social isolation or exclusion. In such cases, student support services personnel (e.g., school psychologists, behavior specialists) conduct a FBA

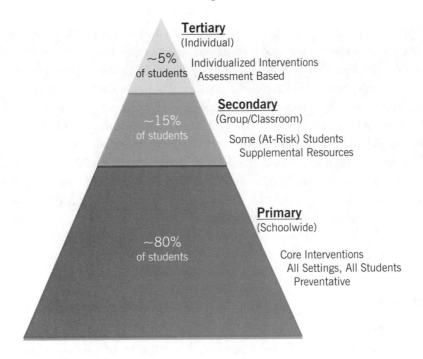

FIGURE 7.1. Three-tiered model of schoolwide positive behavior support.

and create a behavior intervention plan (BIP) tailored to the individual's specific needs. Following assessment, these individuals work collaboratively with educators to implement and monitor individualized interventions.

Schools that have implemented SWPBS not only report a significant reduction in the number of discipline referrals, suspensions, and expulsions but also increases in academic behaviors and outcomes of students (Horner, Sugai, Todd, & Lewis-Palmer, 2005). Aside from these general effects, early research indicates that students with significant needs, including students with HFA/AS, also benefit from participating in SWPBS (e.g., Freeman et al., 2006; Turnbull et al., 2002). Students with HFA/AS not only benefit from various levels of support but also become part of the school community because of their participation (Gould & Pratt, 2008). Using universal and secondary preventative actions within an SWPBS system likely will reduce many of the behavioral concerns of students with HFA/AS. For example, learning behavioral expectations and rules of the school likely will reduce occurrences of tardiness, name calling, or other inappropriate nuisance behaviors that may be irritating to teachers and result in negative consequences for the student. In addition, students with HFA/AS may learn global strategies during small-group instruction for dealing with anger, ways to ask for help, or methods for sharing toys

> **Aside from its effects on students with HFA/AS, SWPBS likely will encourage nondisabled peers to develop respect and receive reinforcement for engaging in prosocial behaviors toward students with HFA/AS during unstructured activities (e.g., lunch, recess).**

appropriately on the playground. Aside from its effects on students with HFA/AS, SWPBS likely will encourage nondisabled peers to develop respect and receive reinforcement for engaging in prosocial behaviors toward students with HFA/AS during unstructured activities (e.g., lunch, recess). Such a positive climate not only benefits students with HFA/AS individually but also encourages positive peer interactions that likely will maintain throughout all levels of school and provide students with HFA/AS opportunities to practice in naturally occurring contexts. Granted, primary and secondary strategies may not be enough to overcome all of the behavioral and social difficulties students with HFA/AS exhibit, and subsequent tertiary interventions may be necessary (e.g., visual supports, communication/social skills training). However, if preventative actions are implemented that decrease many of the common behavioral problems demonstrated by students with HFA/AS, fewer students and problems would then need to be addressed at a higher, more intensive level of support (Gould & Pratt, 2008).

Character Education

"Character education" (CE) is an umbrella term used to describe curricula designed to increase the prosocial behavior of students, as well as to promote a sense of community in schools (Lickona, 1991). Typically, CE includes concepts such as social-emotional learning, violence prevention, and conflict resolution and mediation. Over the course of the school year, large-group instruction is provided to *all* students to address common "character traits" such as caring, trustworthiness, respect, citizenship, and responsibility. At times, instruction may involve class meetings, buddy programs that pair older and younger students together, and family and community involvement activities. By conducting a variety of instructional approaches and activities, educators can help students develop ethical values that are good for society (Lickona, 1991).

The Character Education Partnership (CEP) currently targets three specific areas necessary for effective character education: (1) social skills training, (2) training in self-awareness and self-management, and (3) social problem solving and decision making (Berkowitz & Bier, 2005). In addition to these three characteristics, effective CE takes on a systemic, schoolwide approach that engages school staff as a community with a collective responsibility to guide the education of *all* students (Lickona, Schaps, & Lewis, 2007). Similar to SWPBS and other school-based prevention programs that create a communal approach to change, implementation of effective CE programs is purported to increase prosocial behaviors of students and to result in decreased rates of inappropriate behaviors (e.g., bullying), suspensions, and expulsions.

Despite the potential value of CE programs, the existing literature regarding their efficacy is limited. To date, only a handful of empirical studies demonstrate the utility of CE programs. For example, DeRosier and Mercer (2007) demonstrated that the LifeStories for Kids series, a school-based storytelling intervention, was effective at reducing rates of direct aggression and immature–impulsive behavior of students. In addition, the All-Stars Character Education program also has been scientifically evaluated (Harrington, Giles, Hoyle, Feeney, & Yungblugh, 2001) showing that participating students evidenced a significant reduction in aggressive, antisocial behavior compared with control students. Although support for CE programs is emerging, limitations of the extant research exist (e.g., lack of random assignment of students to treatment groups, limited sources of direct data collection, no data regarding whether reported effects persist over time). Thus it may be premature to suggest that CE is an evidence-based approach.

Overall, implementation of SWPBS, CE, and/or other schoolwide initiatives likely will be useful for providing buildingwide expectations for behavior, as well as having some effect on students with HFA/AS. Moreover, SWPBS and CE programs are often already in place in many schools, to some degree, and they can serve as an excellent form of primary intervention (schoolwide instruction) for teaching positive student behavior. Including students with HFA/AS at the schoolwide level may decrease many problem behaviors without the need for intensive, individualized supports (Gould & Pratt, 2008). However, such approaches may not teach specific social skills directly to children with HFA/AS.

Large-Group Social Skills Instruction

Social skills training (SST) programs have a well-documented literature base supporting their use as part of a schoolwide initiative (e.g., Skiba & Peterson, 2003; Sugai & Lewis, 1996; Walker, Colvin, & Ramsey, 1995). Many large-scale SST programs address some of the same concerns as SWPBS and CE approaches, and, in fact, many of the same character traits that are part of a comprehensive SWPBS or CE program are included in large-scale SST programs (Consortium on the School-Based Promotion of Social Competence, 1996; Merrell & Gimpel, 1998). Although not meant intentionally to remediate the specific social skills deficits of students with HFA/AS specifically, many large-scale school-based SST programs can assist with reducing the number of social skills deficits experienced by these students, as well as increasing their behavioral functioning. The reason is that students with HFA/AS (as well as students with other disabilities, such as attention-deficit/hyperactivity disorder [ADHD], social anxiety disorder) need to be taught the skills needed to succeed in school, no matter how routine the skill may appear.

Large-group or schoolwide SST combines daily academic instruction with skill-based lessons on specific social skills. That is, teachers find small increments of time (e.g., 15–30 minutes) to infuse social skills instruction into daily academic content without removing students from the classroom (Korinek & Popp, 1997). Incorporating SST into whole-class instruction has several advantages. First, combining SST and other academic content is time and cost efficient. There is little need for extra personnel (e.g., resource teachers, student services personnel), and instruction occurs during down times within classrooms. Second, classrooms are increasingly diverse, and the disparate life experiences and ranges of social skills that *all* children possess vary greatly (Gresham, 2002; Meier, DiPerna, & Oster, 2006). Because social skills are critical for attaining academic and behavioral success (Lane, Wehby, & Cooley, 2006), efforts to provide *all* students with an equal opportunity to learn academic and nonacademic skills are critical. Third, the lessons learned and practiced within the classroom setting are more likely to generalize to other environments in which students with HFA/AS will need them most (Gresham, Sugai, & Horner, 2001). Finally,

> Because many students with HFA/AS receive their instruction within general education settings and may not qualify for special education services, educators cannot assume that these students will receive social skills instruction elsewhere. Instead, teachers must look for effective ways to teach students with HFA/AS social skills within inclusive contexts.

because many students with HFA/AS receive their instruction within general education settings and may not qualify for special education services, educators cannot assume that these students will receive social skills instruction elsewhere. Instead, teachers must look for effective ways to teach students with HFA/AS social skills within inclusive contexts.

Currently, two evidence-based curricula are available that may assist educators in providing schoolwide SST as part of a treatment approach for students with HFA/AS. For example, the Strong Kids program (Merrell, 2007a, 2007b) provides easy-to-implement, scripted lessons aimed at promoting social-emotional competence and resilience in children and adolescents. Each class activity within the Strong Kids program takes 30–45 minutes to complete and can fit into a variety of lessons. Specifically, students learn how to (1) understand emotions, (2) manage anger, (3) relieve stress, and (4) solve interpersonal problems. Current research on the Strong Kids program suggests that students who participate demonstrate significant gains in social-emotional understanding and coping skills (Gueldner, 2006) and decreases in symptoms of behavior problems (Isava, 2004). Moreover, the social-emotional skills taught as part of the Strong Kids curriculum appear to maintain following instruction (Harlacher, 2008), demonstrating the preventative utility of this program (see *strongkids.uoregon.edu* for a review of the Strong Kids programs and related contemporary scholarship). A second research-based schoolwide SST approach that would be effective in teaching students with HFA/AS foundational social skills is Second Step (Committee for Children, 1986). Similar to the Strong Kids curriculum, Second Step teaches social-emotional understanding and allows students time to practice vital social skills such as empathy, emotional regulation, and social problem solving (see *www.cfchildren.org/programs/ssp/overview/* for a review of Second Step and related contemporary scholarship). Contemporary research examining the efficacy of Second Step suggests that students exhibit lowered levels of aggression (McMahon & Washburn, 2003) and increased levels of prosocial skills and behaviors (Edwards, Hunt, Meyers, Grogg, & Jarrett, 2005; Frey, Nolen, Edstrom, & Hirschstein, 2005; McMahon, Washburn, Felix, Yakin, & Childrey, 2000) after receiving instruction.

A host of other large-group strategies that combine social skills training with affective education also are available that would be particularly useful within inclusion settings as preventative approaches. The benefit of such programming is that it provides education and practice to allow students not only to learn prosocial skills but also to manage their emotions, resolve conflict nonviolently, and make responsible decisions. Similar to the previously mentioned strategies, social-emotional programs require little time to implement but can be of benefit to all students, not just those with HFA/AS. Such programs include Do2Learn and Wings for Kids, among others. A comprehensive review of the available programs is beyond the scope of this book. However, interested readers will find valuable information pertaining to social-emotional learning and related curricula at the Collaborative for Academic, Social, and Emotional Learning (CASEL; *www.casel.org*).

There are many important considerations when developing and implementing large-group SST. First, it is necessary to examine the degree to which personnel within the school are committed to supporting the program. To be successful, administrators, teachers, para-professionals, and other educational staff members must share responsibility for implementing the program and monitoring the program's effectiveness. Second, preparation of key individuals responsible for implementing the large-group SST needs to occur. Specifically, educational staff should receive training on (1) the need for a large-group SST, (2) components of the SST, and (3) the logistical issues of implementing SST, such as when the training will begin, how long it will last, and who is responsible for coordinating the program. In addition, time and energy should be spent preparing those staff members responsible for directly teaching social skills on the specific training components of the program.

Oftentimes, large-group SST is too subtle for individuals with HFA/AS to understand completely. For example, a behavior specialist was frustrated that a student with AS with whom she was working, Joey, was "failing to making adequate social progress," even after repeated lessons from a well-known program were presented to him in the classroom. The reason was that the five lessons on "being a good friend" consisted of using "storytelling" and board games to teach. Although such an approach may be appropriate for many kids, Joey failed to learn because he did not receive direct instruction on the specific skills he needed to make and keep friends and reasons why he should use the skills. When large-group SST or other schoolwide approaches do not appear to be working, more focused, small-group approaches may be necessary.

SMALL-GROUP (SECONDARY) APPROACHES

Social Skills Groups

Historically, the most common approach for conducting SST with individuals with HFA/AS has been through small groups. In fact, many schools and agencies across the country purchase a variety of social skills curricula and establish small groups for children and youth with HFA/AS in hopes of increasing their social skills. However, the simple act of purchasing programs, creating groups, and conducting lessons, in and of itself, is no guarantee that an individual (or group of students) with HFA/AS will learn and demonstrate social skills. In truth, research has demonstrated that traditional small-group SST programs have only minimal effectiveness in teaching social skills that extend to more naturalistic environments

> **The simple act of purchasing programs, creating groups, and conducting lessons, in and of itself, is no guarantee that an individual (or group of students) with HFA/AS will learn and demonstrate social skills.**

(Gresham et al., 2001; Quinn, Kavale, Mathur, Rutherford, & Forness, 1999). Now, this statement should not suggest that incorporating small-group SST into the educational plan of a student or students with HFA/AS is not essential—it is! Rather, it suggests that the effective approach to teaching social skills needs to be more systematic than simply purchasing a curriculum and running a group.

Systematic social skills instruction involves carefully planning lessons by identifying target skills and goals, carefully outlining and implementing instructional procedures for teaching necessary target skills, evaluating the effectiveness of instruction, and adjusting instruction based on data (Gresham et al., 2001; Hurth, Shaw, Whaley, & Rogers, 1999; Westling & Fox, 2000). That is, systematic instruction provides a structured teaching plan that educators follow. Too often, educators adopt the most recent social skills curriculum and force children with HFA/AS to learn global skills (e.g., "friendship" skills) rather than matching instructional strategies to the type of skill deficit(s) exhibited (Bellini, 2006; Quinn et al., 1999). Without a high degree of specificity in instructional planning, most small-group SST will have minimal effects, if any at all. Considerations for effective small-group SST include four simple and very basic steps (see Table 7.1): (1) identify and target specific social skills, (2) distinguish between a skill deficit and a performance deficit, (3) provide direct, systematized instruction, and (4) monitor student progress. A brief description of each of these steps follows (readers interested in a systematic procedure for planning and implementing small-group SST should refer to Bellini, 2008).

Identify and Target Specific Social Skills

Prior to conducting a social skills group, considerable time and effort should be made to identify and target specific skills for instruction. The identification of social skills deficits can occur as part of an evaluation conducted by student services support personnel in schools, such as school psychologists, counselors, autism consultants, and/or speech and language pathologists. These professionals collect information from teachers, as well as through observations of student behavior. However, some evaluations may not be comprehensive enough to capture the true nature of the social skills difficulties that individuals with HFA/AS may possess. Therefore, a more thorough assessment should be conducted. Such an evaluation provides detail regarding strengths and weaknesses in students' social skills, and, more important, it provides data that link directly to goals and objectives for

TABLE 7.1. Steps for Small-Group Social Skills Programming

Steps	Purpose
1. Identify/target specific social skills.	• Tells you what you need to teach.
2. Distinguish between skill and performance deficits.	• Determines the focus of your intervention.
3. Provide direct, systematized instruction.	• Teach skills in a meaningful and purposeful manner.
4. Monitor student progress.	• Determines whether or not the instruction is effective for the student.

social skills instruction. Strategies to identify and target social skills deficits include the use of interviews, rating scales, and direct observations. (Readers should refer to Chapter 4 for a thorough description of social skills assessment.)

Distinguish between a Skill Deficit and a Performance Deficit

Once skills have been identified to include within a social skills group and a thorough assessment of the child's functioning has occurred, it is essential to determine whether the social skills difficulties the child experiences are the result of a skill deficit or a performance deficit (Elliot & Gresham, 1991). Although information related to skill and performance deficits was discussed in previous chapters, a brief review is warranted here. Assessments may reveal that the individual with HFA/AS has a *skill deficit*, or simply does not have a particular skill or the necessary foundations of behavior to function in or adapt to his or her environment. For example, a child with HFA/AS may not know how to join a conversation with two or more people without interrupting. Therefore, it is necessary to teach specific skills. A *performance deficit* refers to the fact that an individual knows the skills necessary to perform the behavior but does not use them consistently. Using the same example, a child may have the skills to join in a conversation without interrupting but fails to use them. In this case, it will be important first to isolate the variables that impede performance (e.g., anxiety) and then to provide support, encouragement, and reinforcement for appropriate behaviors. From the information provided, failure to differentiate between a skill deficit and a performance deficit may very well determine the success of instruction because the interventions differ greatly for each.

> **Failure to differentiate between a skill deficit and a performance deficit may very well determine the success of instruction because the interventions differ greatly for each.**

Provide Direct, Systematized Instruction

Prior to teaching individuals within a social skills group, several critical variables must be explored that ensure that instruction is direct and systematic. First, group leaders need to identify and select appropriate materials for instruction. Several curricula designed for teaching social skills to individuals with HFA/AS are available and briefly described in Table 7.2. Each of these curricula provides lesson plans and activities for sequencing instruction. Second, group leaders must train members of their instructional team. Specifically, coleaders or volunteers who assist with implementing small-group SST need to be trained on the components of the lessons, implementation strategies, and use of prompts and reinforcement (Bellini, 2006). Third, leaders need to determine whether typically developing peers or individuals with other social skills difficulties (e.g., children with ADHD and social anxiety) will be included in the group. It is our opinion that including typically developing peers and/or peers with similar deficits (but who are capable of demonstrating basic social advances) provides more opportunities to practice skills and offer feedback. Fourth, leaders of small-group SST need to identify when, where, and for how long groups will meet. There is no one place that is better than another, and SST can occur in classrooms or

TABLE 7.2. Available Social Skills Curricula for Individuals with HFA/AS.

Title	Author	Publisher
Social Skills Training for Children and Adolescents with Asperger Syndrome and Social Communication Problems	Baker (2003)	Autism Asperger Publishing Company
Building Social Relationships: A Systematic Approach to Teaching Social Interaction Skills to Children and Adolescents with Autism Spectrum Disorders and Other Social Difficulties	Bellini (2006)	Autism Asperger Publishing Company
Super Skills: A Social Skills Group Program for Children with Asperger Syndrome, High-Functioning Autism, and Related Challenges	Coucouvanis (2005)	Autism Asperger Publishing Company
S.O.S. Social Skills in our Schools: A Social Skills Program for Verbal Children with Pervasive Developmental Disorders and Their Typical Peers	Dunn (2005)	Autism Asperger Publishing Company
Navigating the Social World: A Curriculum for Individuals with Asperger Syndrome, High-Functioning Autism, and Related Disorders	McAfee (2002)	Future Horizons
Promoting Social Success: A Curriculum for Children with Special Needs	Siperstein & Rickards (2004)	Brookes Publishing

resource rooms and even on the playground. It is more important to consider the resources needed to conduct the group. For example, if part of the curriculum incorporates video clips, access to a television or computer (for digital clips) is necessary, as well as an appropriate location in which to view them. Finally, efforts to manage behavior must be considered in order to maintain control in groups. Most successful groups incorporate a token economy that awards points or tokens for appropriate behaviors such as attending, participating, or completing homework. Participants can then exchange their points or tokens for desirable objects as a reward. A response cost also can be incorporated into the group (e.g., students lose points for noncompliance), but efforts should be made to minimize the points a student loses within the group.

Direct, systematic instruction refers to teaching skills in a purposeful and meaningful manner. In order for SST to be effective, students with HFA/AS first need to know how or why learning social skills is necessary (Myles, 2005). Remember, individuals with HFA/AS often have little awareness or social understanding. Therefore, part of teaching social skills to them requires providing a distinct rationale (Myles, 2005). Rationales for teaching social skills should include why the information is important or useful and how the student can use the information taught within the lesson(s). Moreover, teaching efforts need to provide students with information regarding what skills are going to be taught, what activities will be used to teach the skills, and the length of time of instruction within each group session.

After a strong rationale has been provided and students within the group appear to understand the dynamics of the group, systematic instruction can occur. Each lesson or skill that is taught must follow this sequence: (1) discussion of skills and/or review of previous skills, (2) modeling of the skill (showing the student what to do) by group facilitators and students, (3) role-playing the skill with real-life examples provided by students, and (4) constructive evaluation of role-play performance by peers and group facilitators. For a complete description of the methods used in systematic instruction, see any of the available curricula mentioned in Table 7.2.

Monitor Student Progress

Evaluation of the effectiveness of small-group SST is essential, as it allows not only the demonstration of success of instruction but also accountability. Methods to monitor student progress are similar to those used to assess social functioning (use of rating scales and direct observations). However, educators should overrely on observational data that ties specifically to the skills taught as part of the SST. As was mentioned previously, observations provide a direct measure of how a child is functioning in naturalistic contexts. That is, observational data are collected during unstructured activities such as recess without teacher prompting or reinforcement. Although a discussion regarding systematic data recording methods is important, it is beyond the scope of this chapter. Specific strategies for designing efficient observation data systems useful for measuring social behaviors are provided in Chapter 9, as are methods for interpreting such data.

> **Evaluation of the effectiveness of small-group SST is essential, as it allows not only the demonstration of success of instruction but also accountability.**

Peer-Mediated Approaches

Very often, the interests of individuals with HFA/AS are viewed by their peers as strange or atypical. As a result, the child with HFA/AS may be disliked and intentionally left out of activities or opportunities to interact with his or her peers. However, efforts can be made to decrease social isolation by recruiting peers who have developed skills needed to assist others when they struggle in a social situation (Aspy & Grossman, 2007). Peer-mediated approaches are efforts that attempt to increase the networks of friends that children and adolescents with HFA/AS have, as well as to assist in providing them with opportunities to learn and practice a variety of social skills within naturally occurring contexts (e.g., playground, cafeteria). For example, peers may facilitate or teach basic social interaction skills and new social activities (how to play a new game) or provide opportunities to become socially connected with others. Overall, most peer-mediated approaches provide

> **Peer-mediated approaches are efforts that attempt to increase the networks of friends that children and adolescents with HFA/AS have, as well as to assist in providing them with opportunities to learn and practice a variety of social skills within naturally occurring contexts (e.g., playground, cafeteria).**

structure for students with HFA/AS, which adds a sense of predictability. Moreover, many peer-mediated approaches likely will help to increase acceptance of students with HFA/AS. A description of some common strategies, empirical research on them, and their application to school-based settings follows.

Circle of Friends

A Circle of Friends network is a group of students who meet on a regular basis to help an individual who is socially disconnected. Essentially, this group looks after one other and helps individuals with HFA/AS to build relationships with peers and increase their overall sense of belonging within the social world. In addition to promoting the social connectedness of individuals with HFA/AS, Circle of Friends networks often result in improvements in peers' acceptance of individuals with disabilities (Frederickson & Turner, 2003).

To date, the research support related to Circle of Friends is mixed. Whereas some research has demonstrated that the implementation of a Circle of Friends network has been effective at increasing appropriate social interactions during unstructured activities in schools (Miller, Cooke, Test, & White, 2003) and improving spontaneous social initiations (Gold, 1994; Kalyva & Avramidis, 2005), other studies have found no benefits of weekly Circle of Friends meetings (Frederickson, Warren, & Turner, 2005). Because the effectiveness of this strategy has not been empirically demonstrated, educators should view the use of Circle of Friends networks with some caution. However, the application of a Circle of Friends network may be beneficial when used as part of a systemic (tiered) approach to remediating the social skills difficulties experienced by individuals with HFA/AS.

> **The application of a Circle of Friends network may be beneficial when used as part of a systemic (tiered) approach to remediating the social skills difficulties experienced by individuals with HFA/AS.**

If a Circle of Friends network is used, it is recommended that educators follow a few simple steps to ensure safeguards for students with HFA/AS. First, individuals who make up the Circle of Friends should be selected carefully. Although it may be easy to ask for volunteers willing to be part of this intervention, selection of appropriate candidates likely will increase positive outcomes. For example, peers who are selected generally should be compliant with school rules and interested in helping the student with HFA/AS and should have similar interests to those of the target student. Second, peers who participate in the circle should receive training to help them understand the characteristics of the target student, as well as how to deal with specific behaviors that may arise. With a little planning and minimal commitment, a Circle of Friends network can make a big difference in the life of an individual with HFA/AS, as it opens up the opportunities for social inclusion.

Integrated Play Groups

To teach appropriate social and play skills, Wolfberg (2003) and Wolfberg and Schuler (1993) emphasized the use of a support system that teaches typically developing peers to improve the social play skills of children with ASD. This support system, called integrated play groups (IPG), is a method whereby environments are physically arranged to foster social interaction, communication, and play experiences between children with HFA/AS and typical peers. Moreover, typically developing peers are trained to use a variety of skills, including getting a friend's attention, asking to play, sharing, and giving compliments (Bass & Mulick, 2007). In IPG, small groups composed of three to five students regularly play together under the guidance of an adult facilitator (called the *play guide*). During these times, the play guide encourages the target child to interact with typical peers. The peers then use their skills to engage the target child in activities. The IPG model is believed to increase the motivation of individuals with HFA/AS to socialize and play with peers, as well as to increase the likelihood that peers will be more accepting of students with disabilities.

Although the current research support for IPG is limited, the few studies that exist can be regarded as promising (Bass & Mulick, 2007). In their first study, Wolfberg and Schuler (1993) demonstrated that IPG resulted in reduction of stereotyped and isolated play and increased the amount of social play (e.g., sharing toys, sharing common focus on one activity) in several students with ASD. IPG has also been used to increase pretend play (Yang, Wolfberg, Wu, & Hwu, 2003), to prolong interactions with peers, and to improve the use of social language (Wolfberg & Schuler, 1999). More recently, Lantz, Nelson, and Loftin (2004) demonstrated the effectiveness of IPG in improving turn-taking behaviors and sharing of emotional expression for a 6-year-old boy with autism in a preschool setting. Although this preliminary research is suggestive of an effective strategy, more empirical investigations are needed prior to considering IPG an evidence-based approach. However, preliminary results suggest that this approach may be beneficial as part of a treatment package for improving the social skills of individuals with HFA/AS.

Creating and conducting IPG takes some effort, and a certain amount of training is necessary for facilitators to be effective (see Wolfberg, 2003, for advanced information on creating IPG). All IPG are composed of *guides*, *expert players*, and *novice players* (see Table 7.3 for definitions of roles). Each group should contain three to five members, with a higher ratio of expert players (Wolfberg, 2003). Groups that are smaller than this do not provide the variety of peers with whom novice players will interact, and large groups may be difficult for guides to manage. Once composed, IPG meet at least two times per week

TABLE 7.3. Role Definitions for Participants in Integrated Play Groups

Role	Definition

Guide	• IPG facilitator who:
	  • has experience working with children with autism spectrum disorders.
	  • has been trained in implementing IPG.

Expert players	• Typically developing peers who have good social, communication, and imaginative play skills.
Novice players	• Children with ASD (or those who demonstrate similar social skills needs).

with the same players over a period of 30 minutes to 1 hour. IPG can meet in schools, child development centers, after-school centers, homes, or any other naturally integrated environment. The children participate together in these groups in a developmentally appropriate play activity that is facilitated by a guide (i.e., parent or professional) trained in IPG (Wolfberg & Schuler, 1999).

The main purpose of IPG is for facilitators to first structure opportunities for novice and expert players and then to guide (and challenge) novice players' participation in new or complex forms of play. The IPG program includes four specific methods for guiding play (Wolfberg & Schuler, 1999). First, the guide must be adept at *monitoring play initiations*. That is, the play guide must be able to recognize, interpret, and respond to spontaneous and imaginative play sequences that fall within the novice player's ability level. Second, and perhaps the most important method within the IPG sequence, the guide assists the group by *scaffolding play* consistent with the child's zone of proximal development. For example, Wolfberg and Schuler (1999) note that the guide may first act as an interpreter, helping players understand one another. Later, the guide may model specific behaviors, direct play sequences for the group, and provide scripts. The objective is to push novice players a little beyond their current abilities so they can learn new skills. As the children become more competent in their play, the guide diminishes his or her level of support. Third, the guide provides *social communication guidance* to both expert and novice players in order to facilitate appropriate social exchanges. Typically, guides will direct both experts and novices on how to cue, initiate, maintain, and expand social interactions (e.g., "Do you want to play?" "My turn–Your turn"). Fourth, the guide engages in *play guidance* during activities. Specifically, the guide needs to make sure that novice players are engaging in play routines and activities by using strategies such as parallel play, mirroring, and role playing (to name a few). Taken together, these methods for guiding play facilitate both social and imaginative play in children with HFA/AS so that they can participate in their peer culture more fully.

Peer Buddies

The peer buddy systems that are typically used within schools are passive in nature. That is, there is no actual training that peers receive, nor are specific skills directly taught by the peer to the target student. Rather, the intervention is dependent on the natural transmission of social skills from a more socially competent peer to the student with HFA/AS (Roeyers, 1996). Peers simply act as a support and provide students with HFA/AS assistance on an as-needed basis. For example, Joshua, a third-grade student with AS, is frequently prompted by his peer buddy, Susan, to engage in appropriate teacher-pleasing behaviors such as beginning an academic worksheet, lining up for recess, and remaining quiet during independent seatwork. The peer buddy's (Susan's) responsibility in this example is more as a role model than as a teacher. In this sense, peer buddy systems operate through proximity control (Odom & Strain, 1984), whereby the student with HFA/AS is expected to learn by watching and interacting with his or her nondisabled peer.

Despite the intuitive nature of the passive peer buddy approach, research has yet to demonstrate consistent positive findings for improving specific social interaction skills of individuals with HFA/AS. This is not to say that peer buddy systems cannot be, or are not, helpful in prompting students with HFA/AS to engage in appropriate behaviors. A host of clinical examples and talking with educators quickly affirm the positive outcomes of using a peer buddy system within a classroom. However, the use of peers in

> **Despite the intuitive nature of the passive peer buddy approach, research has yet to demonstrate consistent positive findings for improving specific social interaction skills of individuals with HFA/AS.**

close proximity to a child with HFA/AS is unlikely to lead to significant improvement in specific social behaviors that maintain and generalize across a variety of settings (Odom & Strain, 1984; Roeyers, 1996). That is, although a peer buddy may promote positive behaviors during class time, it is unlikely that such behaviors will be used spontaneously to engage in social interactions with other children in a different location within the school or in a variety of home and community settings. The reason is probably that the proximity approach does not specify specific goals or social skills for the buddy to facilitate in the child with HFA/AS. In order to increase the likelihood of an individual's with HFA/AS learning specific social skills that maintain and generalize to a variety of school and community settings, a more direct teaching model, such as peer tutoring or SST, should be implemented.

If the decision to develop a peer buddy program is made, a few helpful tips will ensure a greater likelihood of success (see Table 7.4). Prior to starting the program, it is necessary to take time and effort to recruit general education participants. Two common strategies can assist in the process of selecting peers: sociometrics and teacher nomination. Sociometrics simply refers to asking peers to rate one another in regard to desirable social qualities. Peers rate each other on qualities such as sharing, saying kind words, following rules, and playing nice. Those peers who rank highest in such qualities likely are the best individuals to support, model, and accept the needs of an individual with HFA/AS. For very young children whose literacy skills are not yet developed, pictures can be used for this process. Specifically, a head shot of each child in the classroom is taken. Then each child is asked to put their classmate's pictures into one of three piles: "I like to play with," "I don't like to play with," and "I don't know them." Once each child has completed this exercise and the results are tallied, the students who were most frequently put in the "play with" pile will be good candidates to consider initially for the program. Another way to conduct a sociometric survey with older children is to use a survey form (see Form 7.1 in the Appendix for a reproducible version) on which peers are asked to identify student(s) in their class who display preferred characteristics (e.g., are fun to play with, share toys, are nice to talk to). Whatever method is selected, the sociometric process should be conducted in a positive manner so that peers will not feel distress for indicating preference for one child over another.

Another method for selecting peers is teacher nomination. Common qualities that teachers should look for in peers include good attendance, average to above-average grades, and an ability to get along with others. It is important that educators nominate students who are capable of interacting positively with other students, not just adults. A student who is overly dependent on adult approval or who likes to act similarly to an adult is likely to become overly directive and adult-like during peer buddy situations. This places the stu-

TABLE 7.4. Steps for Starting a Peer Buddy Program

Steps	Description/strategies
Establish importance and get buy-in.	• Discuss the importance and rationale for creating a peer buddy system for students with HFA/AS. • Meet with school administrators. • Talk with teachers individually regarding the need for a peer buddy program. • Present information on peer buddy programs at a faculty meeting.
Notify parents.	• Send an introduction letter home to parents. • Provide information in the letter regarding the reciprocal benefits of peer buddy programs. • Include a permission slip.
Recruit peer buddies.	• Recruit typically developing peers to be peer buddies. • Employ sociometrics and teacher nomination to recruit socially competent peers. • Identify volunteers to assist with peer buddy program.
Conduct orientation.	• Train peer buddies on expectations for participation. • Discuss HFA/AS with typically developing peers. • Include the concept of "people first" language. • Provide detailed information regarding activities in the peer buddy program. • Share positive examples of productive lives of people with HFA/AS. • Model what you want to see.
Set up the program.	• Identify locations and times when peer buddies will be used. • Select environments that both peers regularly access. • Define and establish purposeful opportunities for interaction.
Evaluate the program.	• Examine the effectiveness of the peer buddy program. • Conduct feedback sessions with typical peers and individuals with HFA/AS. • Meet with other teachers to share information/observations. • Plan a parent night for sharing information.

dent in a tutoring role and likely will detract from the development of true friendships that can come from associating with peers in close proximity.

After peers have been carefully selected, it is necessary to choose settings in which the peer buddy program will occur. Some schools may choose to start the peer buddy program in a special education classroom (commonly referred to as reverse mainstreaming). Although it is very easy to get a peer buddy program up and running in such a setting, special education classrooms often fail to provide opportunities for the benefits of a peer buddy program to generalize to other inclusive settings, not to mention that many of the students with HFA/AS likely will be educated within general education environments. If the goal is to promote friendship and improve social functioning, then settings and activities should include occasions in which both peers and individuals with HFA/AS occupy the same inclusive locations within the building. While the peer buddy program is taking place, monitor the effectiveness of the approach. Strategies may include: (1) holding buddy feedback sessions with the individual with HFA/AS and peers, (2) meeting with teachers to share information and observations, and (3) conducting a parent night for information sharing.

INDIVIDUALIZED APPROACHES

Social Stories™

Social Stories are individualized short stories that can be used to assist persons with HFA/AS in interpreting and understanding challenging or confusing social situations (Gray, 2003). The objective of Social Stories is to describe social situations in which an individual might have difficulty identifying relevant social cues or expected behaviors, and provide strategies for negotiating those situations effectively (Gray, 2000, 2003; Scattone, Tingstrom, & Wilczynski, 2006). Specifically, Social Stories (1) describe targeted situations, concepts, or skills by answering relevant wh- questions (where, when, who, how, and why), (2) describe how to effectively think about or problem solve the targeted situation, and (3) create connections between past, present, and future experiences by having the reader make logical guesses about what may happen using prior knowledge (C. Gray, personal communication, October 15, 2009). In this sense, Social Stories are often "how-to" books for understanding and responding to difficult social situations or contexts (Sansosti, Powell-Smith, & Kincaid, 2004). Some may be tempted to think, at least from this description, that Social Stories are simply task analyses used to prompt a specific order of responses or set of skills. However, a well-written Social Story *describes* more than it directs (Gray, 2000), assisting individuals with HFA/AS in *understanding* their social world and applauding their current achievement and efforts.

During the past decade, the clinical support for the use of Social Stories in homes, schools, and other community settings has been quite strong (Chapman & Trowbridge, 2000; Scattone et al., 2006). In fact, simply talking to clinicians, advocates, and various school-based student support personnel (e.g., school psychologists, speech–language pathologists, behavior analysts) would lead one to believe that Social Stories are a "tried and true" intervention for remediating the social deficits of individuals with ASD. However, current empirical support for the use of Social Stories can best be described as incomplete. Although prior research investigating the effects of Social Stories has demonstrated successful outcomes in reducing repetitive and tantrum behaviors

> **Current empirical support for the use of Social Stories can best be described as incomplete.**

(Kuttler, Myles, & Carlson, 1998; Lorimer, Simpson, Myles, & Ganz, 2002; Reynhout & Carter, 2007), decreasing disruptive classroom behaviors (Scattone, Wilczynski, Edwards, & Rabian, 2002), increasing the frequency of social interactions (Norris & Dattilo, 1999; Sansosti & Powell-Smith, 2006; Scattone et al., 2006; Thiemann & Goldstein, 2001), and increasing appropriate play (Barry & Burlew, 2004), a host of methodological concerns and confounding treatment variables raise questions regarding the true efficacy of Social Stories as an evidence-based practice. In their comprehensive review and synthesis of the existing research, Sansosti, Powell-Smith, and Kincaid (2004) found that the majority of studies that were conducted lacked experimental control, showed weak treatment effects, and were confounded by a variety of treatment variables making it difficult to determine whether Social Stories alone were responsible for changes observed in target behaviors. Despite this somewhat discouraging review of the literature, Sansosti et al. (2004) provided preliminary indication that Social Stories may be a practical option for a number of individuals with HFA/AS due to a small number of studies demonstrating a high rate of success across a variety of educational contexts.

Developing a Social Story is similar in scope to other approaches to creating individualized student supports. First, a specific target behavior or a difficult social situation is identified by a teacher or parent. Once a target situation or behavior is identified, the second step involves identifying the salient features of the context or setting. For example, information should be gathered on where the situation occurs, who is involved, how long it lasts, how it begins and ends, and what occurs. These steps are similar in scope to completing a FBA previously discussed in Chapter 4. Finally, this information is used to write the content of a Social Story.

Carol Gray and Team Social Stories recently have updated their detailed guidelines describing how Social Stories should be written and implemented. Stories should be comprised primarily of *descriptive sentences* (objective statements of fact), with additional descriptive information offered as needed in the form of *perspective sentences* (describing thoughts, feelings, and/or beliefs of others), *affirmative sentences* (enhance the meaning of surrounding sentences), and *partial sentences* (fill-in-the-blank sentences to help the reader predict logical outcomes). Social Stories also contain *sentences that coach*, which identify appropriate responses for the reader and other relevant individuals (see Table 7.5 for a description of sentence types and ratios). It is necessary for school-based personnel to

TABLE 7.5. Social Story Sentence Types and Ratios

Sentence Types (Gray, personal communication, October 15, 2009)

Descriptive: Objective statements that identify contextual variables in the target situation.

Perspective: Describe reactions and feelings associated with the target situation.

Affirmative: Enhance the meaning of surrounding sentences.

Partial: Prompt the reader to predict outcomes by filling in a missing word or phrase.

Sentences that coach: Identify suggested responses for the reader or relevant others.

Sentence Ratio

Two descriptive, perspective, affirmative, and/or partial sentences for every sentence that coaches in the story.

Note. New standards for as indicated by the forthcoming Social Stories 10.1.

understand the specific guidelines for the creation of Social Stories. A review of the extant literature has demonstrated that Social Stories are commonly written without regard for the specific guidelines outlined by Gray, which may be responsible for the limited amount of research supporting their efficacy (F. J. Sansosti, 2008). To address these concerns (and perhaps to contribute to the literature base), school-based personnel are encouraged to engage in a variety of professional development activities that will ensure that Social Stories are being created accurately. Perhaps the most successful way for educators to gain the necessary skills is to attend workshops and trainings provided by Carol Gray or Team Social Stories. Educators may wish to engage in their own learning through a variety of training materials that are available through the Gray Center for Social Learning (interested readers are encouraged to visit *www.thegraycenter.org*). These materials, including videos, DVDs, and books, are likely to assist a variety of professionals in structuring and developing accurate Social Stories.

After a complete and thorough FBA has been conducted and a subsequent story has been created, school-based personnel should consider the manner in which Social Stories will be presented to the child. Traditionally, Social Stories have been read to or by the participant(s). This method often entails the teacher's reading the story with the child, followed by the child's reading the story independently. If reading is an area of difficulty for the child, additional implementation approaches may be considered. Gray (2000, 2003) suggests that Social Stories can be recorded on a cassette (or CD) and presented with a tape (CD) player for students who demonstrate reading difficulties or cannot read. Using this method, the child follows along in his or her storybook while the story is being read aloud from the recording (an auditory signal is incorporated to prompt the child to turn the page of the story). In addition to these approaches, the content of Social Stories can be presented by way of computers (e.g., Hagiwara & Myles, 1999; Sansosti & Powell-Smith, 2008) or paired with visual symbols, pictures, and video modeling (e.g., Sansosti & Powell-Smith, 2008).

Video Modeling

Video modeling is a method that can be used to teach a variety of social, academic, and self-help skills to individuals with HFA/AS who have well-developed imitation skills. Specifically, video modeling involves having the child with HFA/AS watch a video-recorded demonstration of a model engaging in a specific series of actions or verbalizations and then imitating the model (Bellini & Akullian, 2007; Charlop-Christy, Le, & Freeman, 2000; MacDonald, Clark, Garrigan, & Vangala, 2005). By modeling the target behavior(s) on video in a systematic and discrete manner, the child learns to memorize and imitate these behaviors for use in appropriate settings.

The rationale for video modeling is based largely on Albert Bandura's social learning theory. In his influential work, Bandura (1977, 1986) demonstrated that a vast array of behavior is learned primarily by observing and then imitating the action of others. Further, Bandura showed that watching others receive consequences for their behaviors serves as a guide for the viewer. For example, if Michelle observes others in her class receiving praise for sitting quietly and working independently, she likely will sit quietly and work in order to receive the reinforcer. As a result of this phenomenon, an individual spontaneously will imitate behaviors they have observed in others within settings other than the one in which the behavior originally was observed. Unlike their peers, children and adolescents with HFA/AS rarely learn skills vicariously. Instead, individuals with HFA/AS benefit from visually cued instruction that incorporates repetitive opportunities to model behavior (National Research Council, 2001; Quill, 1997). In this way, video modeling offers a way for students with HFA/AS to acquire a wide array of behaviors.

To date, video modeling has been used with a wide variety of students with a ASD and is an area full of possibilities for teaching specific skills to students with HFA/AS. Specifically, video modeling has been demonstrated to increase social initiations (Nikopoulos & Keenan, 2004), perspective taking (Charlop-Christy & Daneshvar, 2003), and play skills (D'Ateno, Mangiapanello, & Taylor, 2003). Furthermore, video modeling techniques have been employed within school-based settings to teach correct spelling sequences (Kinney, Vedora, & Stromer, 2003), social interactions (Maione & Mirenda, 2006; Sansosti & Powell-Smith, 2008), compliment giving (Apple, Billingsley, & Schwartz, 2005), and pretend-play skills (MacDonald et al., 2005). Video modeling techniques also have been found to result in quicker acquisition of skills and are more cost- and time-efficient than live (in vivo) modeling (Charlop-Christy et al., 2000). Clearly, the research support for video modeling is strong, and many opportunities exist for incorporating the use of video within educational environments.

Developing a video model may appear to be a complicated task, but it actually is quite easy. Recent advances in technology, combined with the ability to purchase affordable video equipment, make creating a video model an uncomplicated task, even for the most technologically illiterate. To create a video model, an educator first will need access to a video camera (preferably a digital camcorder), a computer (for editing and displaying digital video files), or a TV and VCR (challenging, but effective). Although a video model can be created using a camcorder that records to tapes or DVD disks and can be presented on a television, the process of editing likely will be more difficult, and the final product may not be as appealing esthetically. We recommend (and describe the procedures for) using a digital camcorder and computer combination because it permits editing and creates an attractive final product that many individuals with HFA/AS will find motivating. In particular, educators who have access to or work with Apple computers will find developing video models to be tremendously easy because software for editing and presenting a video is not only available but also exceptionally user friendly.

> **Recent advances in technology, combined with the ability to purchase affordable video equipment, make creating a video model an uncomplicated task, even for the most technologically illiterate.**

Given that the appropriate equipment is available, it is essential for the user to test his or her skills with the gear. First, get to know the digital camcorder. Does it record to a MiniDV tape, or is the video captured and stored in memory? Does the external microphone pick up sounds well enough to hear when recorded? How do clips transfer from the camcorder to a computer? Most digital camcorders manufactured in the past decade are easy to use and offer plug-and-play capability. Second, experiment with basic video editing software such as iMovie (included on all Apple computers) or Windows Movie Maker (included on recent versions of Windows). Specifically, it is important to understand how to transfer clips to the video editing software and to engage in basic editing and saving of clips that are compatible with all computers. Once a comfort level with the equipment is established, it is time to begin developing a video model.

Specific steps for creating and implementing a video model are similar to other strategies discussed in this chapter (see Table 7.6; see Neumann, 2004, for more extensive information on how to make video models). First, identify a target skill based on information obtained through interviews, rating scales, and/or direct observations. Second, break down the identified target skill into smaller, teachable units (a task analysis). Outlining the independent parts of the skill to be taught is important because it allows educators to determine the sequence of skills or steps the model will demonstrate. Third, write a script and plan for recording the model appropriately. Fourth, identify and train the model(s) who will

TABLE 7.6. Steps for Creating a Video Model

Steps	Description/strategies
Identify skill.	• Select a skill to be taught by the video model. • The target skill should be based on information obtained from assessments.
Break skill down.	• Break the target skill down into smaller teachable units. • Identify component steps associated with the target skill and plan for instruction (task analysis).

Write a script.	• Write a script for the video model.
	  • Use information from task analysis to create a storyboard for the model.
	  • Ask others to verify that all steps were included.

Train model(s)/ practice.	• Train models to engage in the skill.
	  • Ensure that models appear believable in their delivery.
	  • Skills should be modeled that can be imitated by an individual with HFA/AS.

ACTION!	• Record the model and edit the video clip.
	  • Allow plenty of time for multiple recordings. It may take several takes before a good video clip is created.
	    • The total intervention should be 2–3 minutes in length (sometimes shorter).
	  • Edit portions of the video as appropriate.

Implement/ monitor.	• Implement the video modeling intervention and monitor effectiveness.
	  • Use the video model as deemed appropriate for the individual.
	  • Monitor the effectiveness of the intervention frequently.

appear on the video. Models can be adults or peers, and the selection likely will be based on the type of skill displayed in the video. We prefer to use peers as models to increase the generalization of the skill(s). Fifth, record the video and transfer files for editing. Edit the video clip as deemed appropriate. For example, unwanted parts or segments with an excessive time lag may be deleted. More technically savvy individuals may decide to incorporate word captions, embed other cues (such as arrows to indicate objects or displays of emotions), or use special features to emphasize the use of the skill(s).

After these steps are completed successfully, the video model is ready to present to the student and to monitor for effectiveness. Implementation of a video model is relatively straightforward, and only a few considerations are necessary. From a very basic level, determination of when, where, and how often the individual with HFA/AS will review the model is needed. More advanced implementation strategies may include feedback sessions with an educator. For example, an educator may want to watch the video model with the student and provide feedback about what is happening in the video while it is playing. Similarly, an educator may have the student review the video model and pause the clip to ask questions to check for understanding. It also may be helpful to have the student practice the skill after reviewing the clip. Regardless of the extra steps considered, educators need to monitor the effectiveness of the video model intervention.

Power Cards

Oftentimes, children and adolescents with HFA/AS are uninterested in new or different experiences or are so engrossed in their own special interests that motivating them to learn is a daunting task (Gagnon, 2001). As is true with most learners, motivation may be increased by incorporating an individual's special interest hero as a motivating tool. A Power Card is a visual-based strategy that incorporates the special interest of an individual with HFA/AS to assist him or her in understanding social situations, teaching appropriate social interaction skills, and/or performing steps in a routine through characters (Gagnon, 2001).

Power Cards are small, typically the same size as a business card or trading card. On the front of the card are pictures or other visual cues that represent the student's special interest and that are motivating. The other side of the card contains a brief script incorporating a character (usually a hero) most closely related to the individual's special interest. This script provides detail about a specific problematic situation or target behavior and includes a portrayal of how the hero solves a problem similar to one experienced by the student. Typically, the solution to the problem situation is broken down into three to five steps on the back of the card for the student to review and follow. Because of their size, Power Cards can be carried, easily attached (using Velcro) to the inside a book, notebook, or locker for easy access, or placed on the corner of a child's desk (Gagnon, 2001; Myles, 2005).

The Power Card strategy is based on the principles of priming and modeling. Priming is a technique used to increase structure and predictability by preparing an individual through exposure to a situation, skill, or lesson in advance. For example, in order to prepare Brandon, a third-grade student with HFA/AS, for a school field trip to an animal park, his teacher described the sequence of events using a series of pictures (e.g., riding the bus from school, seeing animals, eating lunch, riding the bus back to school). Modeling is another type of visual strategy that is frequently used with individuals with HFA/AS to teach understanding and sequencing of behaviors. Specifically, models depict a sequence of events for the student to imitate. For example, Brandon's teacher could have shown a video of other students leaving the school building, observing and petting the animals in the animal park, eating lunch at a picnic table, and riding a school bus back to school. Power Cards employ both priming and modeling, as they are typically presented to an individual prior to an activity (priming) and depict a hero or host of characters solving a social problem (modeling). An example of a Power Card is provided in Figure 7.2.

> **Power Cards employ both priming and modeling, as they are typically presented to an individual prior to an activity (priming) and depict a hero or host of characters solving a social problem (modeling).**

In recent years, empirical support for Power Cards has begun to emerge. For example, Myles, Keeling, and Van Horn (2001) demonstrated in two case studies that Power Cards resulted in marked improvement in student behaviors. More recently, Keeling, Myles, Gagnon, and Simpson (2003) demonstrate that a Power Card intervention depicting the Power Puff Girls was effective in increasing the sportsmanship behaviors of a 10-year-old girl with autism. Specifically, decreases in the participant's frequency of screaming behaviors when she lost a game were observed, and the changes generalized across multiple settings. From the extant literature, it appears that Power Cards may be a creative (and portable) intervention for positively managing problem behaviors of individuals with HFA/AS by teaching appropriate replacement skills.

Creating a Power Card is relatively easy and does not require advanced technical skills. First, educators must identify the special interests and/or heroes of the students. If personnel are unsure of the student's special interests, a brief interview with parents, peers, and the student (if applicable) will quickly provide this information. In addition, observations of the student may provide insight into his or her special interests. Second, educators will need to write the character sketch. Each Power Card begins with a reference to the hero, followed by the steps to carry out the strategy or new behavior. Typically, initial information is presented describing how the hero places value on the expected behavior, followed by a list of key elements for solving a particular social problem (see Figure 7.2). It is important to consider the comprehension level of the student when writing the script, making sure that the student can understand the information that is provided. Third, the script and appropriate pictures are put together on a business-size card and printed for the student. Cards can then be laminated, attached to desk, notebooks, or lockers, or carried by the student.

THE FUTURE OF SOCIAL SKILLS INTERVENTIONS

Although the strategies that have been outlined within this chapter are effective and often assist in increasing the social behavior of individuals with HFA/AS, recent interest has focused on the viability of computers (such as computer-assisted instruction or computer-

(Front of card)

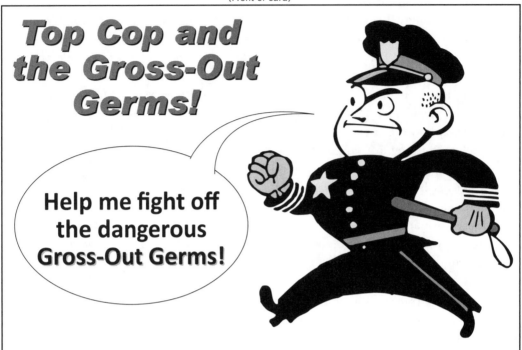

(Back of card)

How Top Cop Fights the Gross-Out Germs

Top Cop is a crime-fighting superhero, and his job is to protect his friends from dangerous enemies. He helps friends make good choices and take care of themselves. Top Cop also takes good care of himself, so he can stay safe and strong. Before any big job, Top Cop always gets himself clean with soap and water. Washing gets rid of Top Cop's other enemies, the Gross-Out Germs!

Top Cop thinks <u>everyone</u> should wash their hands before starting any new activity. Top Cop wants you to remember three things so <u>YOU</u> can help him fight the Gross-Out Germs.

1. Go to the sink and line up as soon as you hear your teacher say, "Wash Your Hands!" *Top Cop doesn't wait to fight Gross-Out Germs, and neither should you!*
2. Wash your hands with soap and water for maximum germ-fighting power!
3. Dry your hands with a paper towel, so you're ready for your next crime-fighting mission.

Washing your hands when you're asked will help you keep Gross-Out Germs away and will help you be ready for your next mission.

FIGURE 7.2. Power Card example.

based learning) to teach skills directly. There is a strong reason to believe that teaching via computers will result in improved outcomes for students with ASD (and HFA/AS in particular) because these individuals often find computers intrinsically motivating (Moore, 1998). For example, Heimann, Nelson, Tjus, and Gillberg (1995) demonstrated that students with autism not only learned more vocabulary words via computer-assisted instruction but also enjoyed learning more when they were taught by the computer than by a teacher. In addition, the use of computers likely creates an environment for learning that appears to individuals with ASD as less threatening. Therefore, infusing computers into the daily curriculum, rather than using them solely as a form of reward or recreation during independent leisure time, should become a priority in research and practice.

> **Infusing computers into the daily curriculum, rather than using them solely as a form of reward or recreation during independent leisure time, should become a priority in research and practice.**

With regard to teaching social skills, a variety of computer-based strategies can be employed. First, computers can be used to teach basic discrimination tasks to children with HFA/AS. For example, computers could provide information related to recognizing basic emotions. Within this format, a student may be presented with a collection of photographs of emotions and prompted to select photographs that correspond with feeling words. Second, computers can be used to create a multimedia intervention that provides the student with an opportunity to read about and observe social interaction events. For example, Sansosti and Powell-Smith (2008) demonstrated positive outcomes of a multimedia intervention for individuals with HFA/AS that used PowerPoint to display video modeled Social Stories. Using this intervention, participants followed along with the story as it was read to them by the computer and watched a video clip demonstrating the appropriate social interaction behavior. Third, computers offer a unique opportunity to teach social problem solving through the use of interactive videos and/or educational games. An interactive game could be created whereby a series of social scenarios are presented and the user selects how to solve the problem from a number of alternatives. Based on his or her choice, an additional video clip appears that displays the consequences of choosing that particular solution. Finally, Internet-based virtual worlds, such as Second Life, may be used to provide individuals with HFA/AS opportunities to facilitate and practice social interactions in an environment that is perceived as less intimidating than that of real world. Research on the use of virtual environments is beginning to emerge, but recent results appear promising (e.g., Mitchell, Parsons, & Leonard, 2007; Moore, Cheng, McGrath, & Powell, 2005).

CONCLUSION

The quintessential characteristic of HFA/AS is having difficulty with basic social interactions. Although many individuals with HFA/AS possess a desire to engage socially, they often lack the skills necessary to be successful. As a result, these children and adolescents often engage in social behaviors that are commonly described as obtuse, awkward, and inappropriate. Moreover, their social skills difficulties frequently span home, community, and school settings. Due to the pervasiveness of their social skills difficulties, it is essential that supports for increasing social skills of children with HFA/AS are included as part of the educational plan within schools. To best meet the needs of individuals with HFA/AS in schools, educators must incorporate a systemic, multi-tiered approach to teaching social skills. Such an approach begins with schoolwide supports that provide structure for students with HFA/AS and, at the same time, provide education to *all* students within a building. Strategies at the systems level include incorporation of schoolwide positive behavior supports, character education, and large-group social skills instruction. In addition to systemic approaches, educators should provide small-group interventions to children and adolescents with HFA/AS to teach specific skills and offer opportunities to practice with typically developing peers. Despite educators' best intentions to develop systemic and small-group approaches, individualized interventions likely will be necessary. A variety of individualized approaches have been suggested that provide students with HFA/AS with the specific lessons for understanding and responding to the social world. Aside from the typical strategies that have been offered, educators need to be aware of recent developments in computer-assisted instruction. Using computers may be the final frontier of research that offers educators and, more important, individuals with HFA/AS successful approaches for learning and practicing social skills. A collective understanding of the tried and true methods combined with new approaches will ensure social success of students with HFA/AS.

CHAPTER 8

Using the Individualized Education Program as a Vehicle for Problem-Solving Service Delivery

with JENINE M. SANSOSTI

OVERVIEW

Children and adolescents with HFA/AS manifest a variety of strengths, weaknesses, talents, and support needs. Although students with HFA/AS typically demonstrate difficulties related to socialization, communication, and repetitive interests/behaviors, the specifics of their needs within each of these domains are highly variable from one student to the next. Thus the importance of developing individualized, assessment-driven plans of instructional support for children with HFA/AS cannot be understated. However, the growing volume of hearings and court cases disputing the validity of educational programs for students with ASD over the past 30 years illustrates that developing individualized programs can be a daunting task for school personnel (Yell, Katsiyannis, Drasgow, & Herbst, 2003).

The development and monitoring of written educational plans for students with disabilities has been required since the inception of federal special education legislation in 1975 (Public Law 94-142, the Education of All Handicapped Children Act [EHA] of 1975) and continues to be a dominant aspect of special education service delivery today. The

Jenine M. Sansosti, PhD, NCSP, is a school psychologist in the Preschool Program of the Berea City School District in Berea, Ohio. She has school-based experience in working with individuals with ASD at all age and grade levels. Prior to her current position, Dr. Sansosti was a consultant and research associate at the Center for Autism and Related Disabilities at the University of South Florida (CARD-USF), providing technical assistance and professional development to school districts and consultative behavior support for parents of children with ASD. Her research interests include educator–parent attitudes, beliefs, and decision-making strategies regarding inclusive placements for students with ASD, as well as utilizing response to intervention (RTI) in public and community preschool settings.

Individuals with Disabilities Education Improvement Act of 2004 (IDEA, 2004) mandates that each child receiving special education services shall have an individualized education program (IEP) that delineates (1) the student's present levels of academic and functional performance, (2) measurable goals for increasing the student's level of functioning within a period of no longer than a year, (3) services and supports needed to obtain those goals, (4) how progress on said goals will be measured and reported to parents, and (5) the least restrictive environment in which these services can be provided. The IDEA (2004) further stipulates that the IEP must be collaboratively designed, implemented, and monitored by a broad IEP team minimally composed of the student's parent(s), a representative from the school district, a general education teacher (if the child is, or will be, participating in general education), a special education teacher, and a person who can interpret instructional implications of evaluation results.

Since the passage of Public Law 94-142 in 1975, the overarching purpose of the IEP has been to ensure that students with disabilities receive a free, appropriate public education, or FAPE (EHA, 1975; IDEA, 2004). Unfortunately, special education law does not offer a substantive definition of FAPE to guide school districts in its implementation. Instead, Congress wrote IDEA and its predecessors with a heavy emphasis on procedural requirements that schools must follow when providing students with special education, believing that these requirements would safeguard a student's right to a FAPE by ensuring that parents were meaningfully involved in developing and implementing their child's educational program (Womack, 2002). Examples of parental safeguards include prior written notice, parental consent, opportunity to examine records, independent educational evaluation, and the right to request an impartial due-process hearing.

As a result of this procedural focus, the President's Commission on Excellence in Special Education (2002) found that, in practice, "IEPs are not actually designed or used for individualized education; instead they are focused on legal protection and compliance with regulatory processes" (p. 16). Because educators have been compelled to focus on stringent procedural requirements, the instructional aspects and expected results of the IEP have become less a priority. Paradoxically, the quest to ensure procedural compliance can render school districts vulnerable to litigation because their IEPs may fail to provide FAPE, program resulting in student progress, and/or meaningful data to document progress (Yell et al., 2003). Yell and colleagues (2003) offer the following guidelines, gleaned from a review of ASD-specific special education litigation from 1990 to 2002, for developing legally correct and educationally appropriate programs for students with ASD:

> **Because educators have been compelled to focus on stringent procedural requirements, the instructional aspects and expected results of the IEP have become less a priority.**

1. School districts must meet the procedural requirements of IDEA, including responding to and involving parents and meeting critical evaluation/IEP timelines.
2. School districts must ensure that individuals evaluating students with ASD have sufficient training and experience specific to ASD and its educational implications.

3. IEPs must address all areas of need that are identified in the evaluation. Furthermore, IEPs must lead to both meaningful programming for students' academic and nonacademic needs and appropriate placement in the least restrictive environment.

4. School districts should adopt empirically validated instructional strategies and programs. Ongoing training and support for developing research-based instructional programming is critical to maintaining high-quality service delivery for students with ASD.

5. School districts can meet the FAPE standards by collecting data and demonstrating that data were used to guide sound instructional decisions. IEPs should be developed and revised through the collection of meaningful data that document both student progress toward IEP goals and the program's overall efficacy.

Clearly, because procedural requirements of IEPs will continue to be a necessary consideration for the foreseeable future, educators simultaneously can serve the best interests of students with HFA/AS and safeguard their districts from litigation by going "back to basics." That is, educational teams should spend the bulk of their time and effort on identifying the outcomes they desire for individual students with HFA/AS and clearly specifying in the IEP how they plan to attain and measure them.

IEP AS PROBLEM-SOLVING VEHICLE

Rather than viewing the IEP as a *product* to be rewritten once a year in compliance with federal and state timelines, it may be more useful to consider the IEP as a vehicle for facilitating the ongoing *problem-solving process* for students with disabilities. The problem-solving process is likely to be a familiar model to both "rookie" and "veteran" educators alike. Over 30 years of applied and clinical research supports the use of the problem-solving model as an evidence-based, systematic approach for examining and responding to a variety of educational problems, ranging from individual student learning difficulties to building- and even district-level challenges (Tilly, 2008). From a student-focused perspective, the problem-solving model (referenced in Chapter 3 and depicted in Figure 8.1) requires that educators review student strengths and weaknesses and clearly identify areas of educational need (*problem identification*), analyze the root cause of student weaknesses (*problem analysis*), identify evidence-based instructional interventions that address student needs and their root causes (*plan implementation*), and frequently collect data to monitor student progress and evaluate the effectiveness of interventions (*plan evaluation*). In recent years, the problem-solving model has received renewed attention as the primary vehicle for analyzing and addressing the needs of students who demonstrate academic and/or behavioral difficulties through an intervention-based, multi-tiered service delivery framework (Batsche et al., 2005; Tilly, 2008). Use of problem solving in conjunction with this framework tends to focus on early identification of students at risk for academic and/or behavioral failure and offers a systematic, data-based approach for addressing student needs. Therefore, a student's

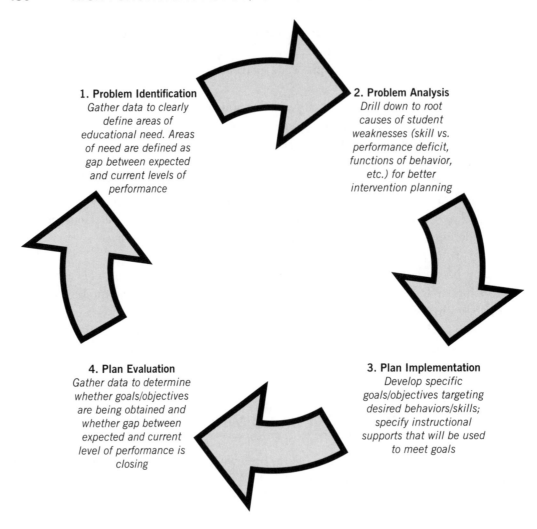

FIGURE 8.1. Problem-solving model applied to IEP process.

failure to demonstrate a positive response to a series of increasingly intensive research-based instruction and intervention may be used, in part, as evidence of a disability (Batsche et al., 2005).

Unfortunately, Yell et al.'s (2003) review of ASD-specific special education litigation suggests that the problem-solving process often comes to an abrupt end once a student is found eligible for special education services. Problem solving is inextricably linked to the required elements of the IEP specified by IDEA (2004) and promotes the outcomes focus and accountability for which the President's Commission on Excellence in Special Education clearly advocated. Yet once a problem in student learning or behavior is identified and certified, IEP teams often fail to provide the services needed to provide FAPE or to promote meaningful student progress (e.g., extended school year services, speech–language services, behavioral programming) and do not collect data to evaluate students' educational progress (Yell et al., 2003). Clearly, when districts cease problem-solving efforts at the point of problem certification, they run the risk of creating IEPs that are big on lofty goals but that fall short in terms of creating true educational progress. Failure to adequately program, monitor, and promote substantive learning for students with HFA/AS not only is a legal vulnerability for school districts, but also represents a failure to provide the truly "special" education that those students with HFA/AS who qualify for services may need to overcome the limitations of their disability.

> **Clearly, when districts cease problem-solving efforts at the point of problem certification, they run the risk of creating IEPs that are big on lofty goals but that fall short in terms of creating true educational progress.**

In the sections that follow, the problem-solving process is reviewed as it applies to the development and ongoing refinement of educationally appropriate IEPs. Several caveats are necessary to guide the reader through the following sections. First, it is important to note that although IDEA (2004) stipulates that all IEPs contain the same basic information, state departments of special education have created their own specific templates for IEPs with different names for its constituent sections (e.g., present level of performance, or PLOP; present level of educational performance, or PLEP; student profile, etc.), which are organized in differing sequences. What follows is a general discussion of IEP sections as specified by IDEA (2004). Second, because IEPs must, by definition, be individualized and specific to students' unique needs, the following guidelines for using IEPs as a problem-solving vehicle are not recommended exclusively for educators working with students with HFA/AS. Rather, *any* high-quality, legally defensible IEP should contain each of the elements of the problem-solving process, whereas specific instructional or data collection strategies described in a particular IEP should be based on that student's individual needs and best-practice recommendations for educating students with HFA/AS. For an extensive list of specific skills that should be considered when developing an IEP for a child with ASD, the interested reader is referred to Wilczynski, Menousek, Hunter, and Mudgal (2007).

STEP 1: PROBLEM IDENTIFICATION— DESCRIBING PRESENT LEVELS OF PERFORMANCE

An oft-repeated axiom of the problem-solving model is, "One cannot begin to solve a problem without first understanding it." When it comes to supporting the educational needs of students with HFA/AS or any other disability, educators must first clearly identify what those specific needs are for each individual student. In other words, educational problems must first be thoroughly described by gathering data from a variety of sources and informants. Only after student needs have been adequately defined and analyzed (see Step 2) can specialized instruction and special education programs be designed to tackle those needs. When student learning needs are ill defined (e.g., "Abe struggles with writing"), educators will be hard pressed to develop an instructional program that effectively targets the precise skills the student needs to develop. Thus the introductory section of an IEP is typically a summary of assessment data gathered during the problem-identification phase of the problem-solving process, with careful attention to the specific skill or performance deficits that impede the student's educational functioning. In many states and districts, this opening section is referred to as present levels of performance (PLOP). Some states' IEP formats require that the student's assessment results and other data be summarized in one overall PLOP statement at the beginning of the IEP; in other locales, data on student's functioning in each major area of need (e.g., communication, social skills, reading comprehension) is summarized in a domain-specific PLOP statement that precedes each IEP goal.

Before a PLOP statement can be created, however, the first step in developing a legally defensible, educationally appropriate, and *truly individualized* IEP involves assessment of student functioning to thoroughly describe (and analyze) student needs. Although the need to use assessments to inform interventions and services should not come as news to school-based practitioners, research from the past 25 years of special education service delivery suggests that educators continue to struggle with adequately linking assessment data to IEP goals and services. Fiedler and Knight (1986) found that 0–25% of diagnostic recommendations are translated into IEP goals. Moreover, Nutter, Algozzine, and Lue (1982) found that when comparing IEPs across disability areas, only small differences in these IEPs could be found and thus could not be assumed to be individualized. Comprehensive recommendations and considerations for the assessment of students with HFA/AS are described in Chapter 4, but a general best-practice guideline for compiling comprehensive summaries of student functioning is to gather information from a variety of data sources (observation, interview, rating scales, direct assessment) and informants (parents, teachers, student, related services personnel, guidance counselors, private service providers, etc.). For the initial IEP, information gathered from classroom-based interventions and the student's initial psychoeducational evaluation should be used to develop the PLOP. For subsequent annual reviews, however, PLOPs should be developed from progress monitoring data on previous IEP goals and ongoing formative assessment. Additional norm-referenced or high-stakes assessment data (i.e., summative evaluation) in triennial reevaluations can be an additional source of information, but the best IEPs are those that are derived from ongoing progress monitoring. Indeed, IDEA (2004) now requires that the PLOP statement itself specify "a description of how the child's progress toward meeting the annual goals. . . will be measured" (Gartin & Murdick, 2005, p. 328).

> Although the need to use assessments to inform interventions and services should not come as news to school-based practitioners, research from the past 25 years of special education service delivery suggests that educators continue to struggle with adequately linking assessment data to IEP goals and services.

General Considerations

The primary aim of the PLOP section is to provide a concise summary of student data that clearly specifies the student's present level of performance with respect to the skills, knowledge, behaviors, or other areas that are to be addressed by the educational goals and objectives in the IEP. Information summarized in the PLOP should be *current* (based on recent data), *relevant* (related to how the student's disability affects his or her education), *specific* (described as precisely as possible), *objective* (unbiased and from a variety of sources, including observation, work samples, parent input, and formal/informal assessments), and *measurable* (quantifiable data from assessments or ongoing progress monitoring). Summarizing student needs in such a clear fashion not only leads to strong educational programs but also provides a baseline picture of the student's functioning that can be used to evaluate student progress at the end of the IEP's annual cycle. Table 8.1 provides examples of PLOP statements that incorporate the aforementioned principles.

> **Summarizing student needs in such a clear fashion not only leads to strong education programs but also provides a baseline picture of the student's functioning that can be used to evaluate student progress at the end of the IEP's annual cycle.**

Information from evaluations or classroom assessments should be narrowed down from broad characterizations of student functioning (e.g., standardized scores of intelligence, behavior, and achievement) to specific skills that need to be increased in order to improve the student's overall functioning. It can be helpful to think of the PLOP statement as the operational definition of a student's learning and/or behavior problems. From a problem-solving perspective, a "problem" is defined as the gap between what is occurring and what is expected. As such, the definition of student learning and behavior problems in the PLOP

TABLE 8.1. Sample PLOP Statements

Original	Rewrite
Joey needs to continue to improve in the area of written expression.	Joey's writing samples consistently show good use of semantics and conventions, but weak organization. In ninth grade, Joey's Word Use and Conventions (grammar, punctuation, capitalization) were rated at or above a "competent" level on the six Traits of Writing rubric on four of the five 5-paragraph essays assigned throughout the year. Joey's lowest-rated writing trait is Organization. None of the five 5-paragraph essays in ninth grade demonstrated a "competent" level of Organization (e.g., clear beginning, details in logical order, clear conclusion) on the six Traits of Writing rubric. By comparison, Joey's classmates demonstrated a "competent" level of Organization on an average of three out of five 5-paragraph essays assigned throughout the ninth-grade year.
Beth has trouble talking to others.	Beth demonstrates both strengths and weaknesses in the area of social skills. She approaches peers and adults to initiate conversations and interactions independently and with ease; however, she struggles to maintain conversations that are not on topics of her choosing. She presently participates in reciprocal conversation on an unfamiliar topic for 3 minutes in only 30% of opportunities during social skills group. Observation of typically developing peers in Beth's grade level indicates that they can participate in reciprocal conversation on an unfamiliar topic for at least 3 minutes in 90% of opportunities.

section should focus on those areas in which the student deviates significantly from peers and in which that difference in performance significantly affects educational functioning. Defining a problem in reference to peer comparison data is useful for two reasons. First, IEP teams are more likely to agree on areas of need and can easily tell when these needs have been sufficiently addressed (i.e., student catches up to same-age peers). Second, comparing the target student's performance with that of same-age peers on a specific, measurable skill clarifies the magnitude of the problem (i.e., how large the gap is between target student and peer), which helps IEP teams prioritize areas of need.

Finally, to provide a truly comprehensive description of student functioning, the PLOP section should include information about the child's strengths and mastered skills, as well as areas of educational need. Students' strengths and preferences are often overlooked in the IEP process, but they can help direct educators to materials or situations that can enable student learning. This is especially true for students with HFA/AS, who typically have very intense interests or hobbies. Incorporating students' interests into instruction can increase motivation for learning and task completion. In addition, summarizing areas of student strength is an important reminder to the IEP team to focus on the whole child, not just on the problems and challenges he or she faces.

Specific Considerations

The most recent reauthorization of IDEA (2004) clarifies expectations about the specific content on which teams should focus when developing a PLOP statement. Previously, the chief aim of the PLOP was to provide the IEP team with basic information concerning the student's specific levels of "educational performance" at the time of the IEP's development and to delineate "how the child's disability affects the child's involvement and progress in the general curriculum" (20 U.S.C. § 614(d)(1)(A)(i)(I)). IDEA (2004), however, changes the term "educational performance" to *academic achievement and functional performance* and "progress in the general curriculum" to "progress in the general *education* curriculum." Although these changes may seem mostly semantic in nature, such revisions are intended to both underscore the academic focus of curriculum present in the No Child Left Behind Act of 2001 (NCLB; 2001) and to clarify that the focus of the individual student's educational program should include functional performance (e.g., behavior, social-emotional functioning, daily living skills), as well as academic achievement (Gartin & Murdick, 2005).

Present Levels of Academic Achievement

"Present levels of academic achievement" refers to statements regarding the student's progress within the general education curriculum, including reading, writing, and mathematics skills. This section should include statements about the child's progress in the general education curriculum, regardless of where the child receives services currently. The President's Commission report (2002) unequivocally states that "children placed in special education are general education children first. . . . General education and special education share responsibilities for children with disabilities. They are not separable at any level" (p. 7). Even when the severity of a student's disability warrants significant curriculum or instructional modifications, accommodations, and support services, IDEA (2004) obligates the IEP team to determine ways for the child to access, be involved in, and make progress in the general education curriculum. In fact, under the 2004 reauthorization of IDEA, the development of a child's IEP is no longer the exclusive responsibility of the special educator, and the concentration has shifted to the development of the IEP for the student's success and implementation within the regular classroom (Lee-Tarver, 2006). As such, the PLOP statement must include information regarding how the child's disability affects his or her involvement and progress in the general education curriculum. For preschool children, the IEP team should consider how the disability affects the child's participation in age-appropriate activities.

> **Even when the severity of a student's disability warrants significant curriculum or instructional modifications, accommodations, and support services, IDEA (2004) obligates the IEP team to determine ways for the child to access, be involved in, and make progress in the general education curriculum.**

In keeping with the problem-solving model, this section should include data that summarize how the child is progressing in the general education curriculum in relation to local and national norms, as well as state-approved grade-level standards. The section on present level of academic achievement also can include descriptions of permanent products (i.e., work samples) or provide data on the student's work completion behaviors. It is particularly important that educators report any classroom strategies, interventions, additional or alternative instructional materials, instructional time, or personnel used to address academic needs and briefly summarize their efficacy in improving student academic performance. These data should be clear enough to demonstrate the need for the continuation or elimination of the goal statement, as information in this section will drive the development of the supports and services in the IEP.

Present Levels of Functional Performance

Beyond the child's academic skills, the IEP team also must consider the child's functioning in a broader context, including information regarding classroom performance and the results of any functional assessments that have been administered. Current functional levels and strengths and needs that may be developmental also should be included. The term *functional performance* encompasses activities of daily living such as hygiene, dressing, basic consumer skills, or community-based instruction, as well as social-emotional learning skills, behavioral difficulties, and the extent to which the student exhibits socially appropriate behavior. The added emphasis on functional performance is particularly important for students with HFA/AS, who sometimes demonstrate average to above-average academic skills but significant social skill deficits.

As with other problem definition statements, information included in this section should include performance data and current skill levels, not just a description of academic and behavioral deficits. Peer comparison data are particularly necessary for functional educational planning, because content standards and benchmarks typically are not available for social skills. It also is important to note that information on functional performance does not have to be indicative of a deficit. For example, the IEP team could write, "The child's functional performance in all areas is age appropriate."

STEP 2: PROBLEM ANALYSIS— CLARIFYING AREAS OF EDUCATIONAL NEED

In most problem-solving processes, problem definition and problem analysis stages are two distinct phases. The purpose of problem definition is to objectively state and define the problem to be solved, whereas problem analysis activities serve to uncover the root causes of the problem and to focus on key areas in greatest need of intervention. Within the context

> **Within the context of the IEP, however, educators often focus primarily on the problem definition, delineating a student's weaknesses at length without careful consideration of the source of these problems.**

of the IEP, however, educators often focus primarily on the problem definition, delineating a student's weaknesses at length without careful consideration of the source of these problems. In part, the reason may be that current and previous reauthorizations of IDEA do not expressly require a section attending to the analysis of student problems. However, without consideration of the underlying causes of educational weaknesses, IEP teams may find themselves treating mere symptoms rather than the true underlying problem.

Of primary importance is determining *why* a student demonstrates a particular skill weakness. On discovering that a student is engaging in a desired skill less often than other children his or her age, the team must determine whether this weakness is a skill deficit (i.e., a "can't do" problem) versus a performance deficit (i.e., a "won't do" problem; Bellini, 2006; VanDerHeyden, 2008). Clearly, the approach to addressing a "can't do" problem is significantly different from that used for a "won't do" problem, with the former focusing on providing instruction in the area of weakness and the latter focusing on reinforcement or self-monitoring. Skill versus performance deficits often are discussed with respect to academic problems but may be applicable to behavioral difficulties as well. When a skill deficit is clearly at hand, the IEP team must ensure that they have determined the point at which the student's skills begin to break down, so that foundational skills are supported and mastered before moving on to more advanced areas of learning. One such approach for analysis is the keystone method (Nelson & Hayes, 1986). The team conducts an analysis of relevant subskills related to a student's area of weakness (e.g., reading) to determine precisely where the student's skills begin to break down. From here, the team targets a specific ("keystone") skill or behavior that, if changed, would significantly improve the student's ability to perform or function in a broader sense (e.g., phonics skills). Consider the example of Jackson, a second-grade student whose DIBELS scores are suggestive of oral reading fluency weakness. Although his IEP team could have recommended interventions and supports aimed at increasing the rate and frequency with which he reads (e.g., repeated readings) immediately, they instead opted to conduct further assessment and learned that his phonics skills are significantly weaker than those of other children in his class. Had the team proceeded with fluency-focused interventions, Jackson's weak phonics skills may have gone unaddressed, and it is likely that his fluency would have remained below benchmark levels.

When challenging behaviors are the focus of the IEP team's attentions, a FBA should be used to determine the potential benefit a child obtains from engaging in those behaviors (e.g., to attract attention, to escape an unpreferred setting or situation, to access a tangible object, or to engage in sensory stimulation). O'Neill et al. (1997), in their seminal work on FBAs, state, "Functional assessment is not like a medical diagnosis. . . . Functional assessment is a process of redesigning environments so they 'work' for people with communication and behavioral disabilities. It is an intimate process" (p. 2). Conducting a FBA turns the IEP team's attention to the ecological aspects of a student's behavior, investigating the extent to which interactions with peers or adults, environmental conditions (e.g., noise levels, lighting, etc.), task demands, and other variables affect the child's behavior (see Chapter 4 for information on conducting FBAs). Furthermore, developing an understanding of the reasons for which a student engages in challenging behavior is essential in teaching a more socially appropriate way to cope with frustrating situations.

Although typically associated with beginning stages of problem solving, problem analysis activities also have an important place in progress monitoring. In particular, problem analysis is warranted when a student has failed to meet a particular goal (i.e., if a gap persists between student's current performance and expected achievement levels, *why* does that gap persist?). Perhaps the student failed to reach his or her goal due to a poor understanding of the problem's real cause (e.g., attributing poor performance to a skill deficit when it may have been a performance deficit). Other possible causes for failure to meet IEP goals include inadequate instructional methods, materials, intervention integrity, and others. It is important for educators to investigate a variety of variables about why goals were not met in order to revise IEP goals in a meaningful way. A good rule of thumb is that if a student has not made meaningful progress on a goal by the third quarter of an annual IEP cycle, the IEP chair should begin this analysis to prepare for the next IEP revision.

STEP 3: INTERVENTION/INSTRUCTIONAL PLANNING— GOALS, SERVICES, AND PLACEMENT

After sufficiently defining and analyzing the educational needs of students with HFA/AS, the next obvious step is to devise a plan of action to meet those needs and to promote additional learning. The IEP, as defined by IDEA (2004), delineates several required components for creating such a plan: (1) annual goals the child can reasonably accomplish in a year; (2) a list of special education and related services the child will receive, including any supplementary services or accommodations; (3) a statement regarding the extent to which the student will participate with children without disabilities in the general education setting and other school activities; (4) a statement regarding what, if any, accommodations or modifications are needed for the student to participate in state- and district-wide assessments. The first three of these components are addressed in the sections that follow; testing accommodations are not discussed because they should mirror those provided in the classroom on a regular basis.

Goals and Objectives

> Goals and objectives are often considered to be the "heart and soul" of IEPs. When derived from assessment and present-level information, goals and objectives create a truly individualized action plan that serves as a clear road map for the coming year.

Goals and objectives are often considered to be the "heart and soul" of IEPs. When derived from assessment and present-level information, goals and objectives create a truly individualized action plan that serves as a clear road map for the coming year. IEP goals are designed to meet the child's needs that result from the child's disability, thereby enabling the child to be involved in and make progress in the general education curriculum. Previous reauthorizations of IDEA required that IEPs include "specific, measurable annual goals and accompanying short-term objectives" for each area of need described in the PLOP (Gartin & Murdick, 2005).

Unfortunately, the distinction between goals and objectives has been a source of confusion for educators (Twachtman-Cullen & Twachtman-Reilly, 2002). Seigel (2001) describes IEP goals as the statement of broad educational aims for students, whereas objectives are provided to indicate the skills the child must attain in order to reach that goal. However, defining goals as "broad aims" may be ill-advised, as it may give license to use vague, unmeasurable terminology (e.g., *Anthony will improve his social skills*). Additionally, the presence of both goals and objectives often creates questions regarding measurement. In particular, which is measured for progress reporting purposes? The 2004 reauthorization of IDEA clarified the goals–objectives section by removing the requirement that all IEPs include short-term objectives or benchmarks for each annual goal (Gartin & Murdick, 2005). They continue to be required for students who will take alternative assessment and may still be used on standard IEPs if the team feels that they are necessary. In either case, the goal statement itself must be measurable without the presences of the objectives.

Consider the following fine-motor skills goal and objectives:

GOAL (Fine-Motor Skills): Kenya will independently write her name so it is recognizable to others in 80% of opportunities.

- *Objective 1: By the end of the third quarter (2008–2009 school year), Kenya will trace the letters in her name so they are recognizable to others in 80% of opportunities.*
- *Objective 2: By the end of the fourth quarter (2008–2009 school year), Kenya will copy the letters in her name from a model so they are recognizable to others in 80% of opportunities.*

- *Objective 3: By the end of the first quarter (2009–2010 school year), Kenya will write the individual letters in her name independently so they are recognizable to others in 80% of opportunities.*
- *Objective 4: By the end of the second quarter (2009–2010 school year), Kenya will independently write her name, with letters in the correct order and all letters recognizable to others, in 80% of opportunities.*

When written in this way, the goal is viable on its own, but the objectives lend clarity to the short-term steps the student will need to complete in order to meet this long-term goal.

Because goals (and objectives, if used) are the cornerstone of the IEP and are essential to its implementation and monitoring, educators must attend to the verbiage and details they include when writing them. IEP goals not only must be measurable but also must clearly specify precisely what skills or behaviors the student is expected to demonstrate, the conditions under which the student is expected to use these skills or behaviors, and the length of time in which they are expected to master these goals. Wright and Wright (2006) describe goals written in this way as "SMART IEP goals," using the mnemonic SMART to summarize the desired characteristics of a high-quality IEP goal: Specific, Measurable, Action words, Realistic and Relevant, and Time. In a review of the history of the SMART mnemonic, Morrison (2008) notes that it is *not* a formula or an order in which components of a goal should be written. Rather, SMART functions as a test to be applied to a goal or objective after it is written. Each of the SMART characteristics are reviewed in the section that follows. "Specific" and "action words" sections are discussed together, due to their similarity. Additionally, it should be noted that, although these characteristics are discussed in reference to the writing of goals, SMART is equally applicable to the writing of objectives, should the IEP team opt to utilize them.

Specific and Action Oriented

Writing a specific, objective statement of the behavior/skill to be modified ensures that the IEP team is in total agreement about what they are working toward. Here, the word *objective* is used to connote a goal that is written in clear, unambiguous terminology, such that all team members can recognize the behavior or skill when it is being observed. Without such objectivity, the individuals responsible for supporting the child may interpret a particular IEP goal in different ways and thus may have differing expectations. Consider the following example: *Jim will increase his self-confidence in social interactions with peers.* What does "self-confidence" look like? Would members of the IEP team know instantly when they have witnessed an instance of "self-confidence"? For this goal, IEP team members likely will need to use some degree of personal interpretation to draw conclusions about what "self-confidence" will look like for Jim, and these interpretations are likely to vary substantially, making data collection a tremendous, if not impossible, challenge. Furthermore, this goal has failed to identify clearly the specific social skills weaknesses that are contributing to Jim's lacking "self-confidence." Without this information, educators will be hard pressed to develop adequate instruction and/or environmental supports.

Sometimes, goals appear to be written using objective ter-minology that all IEP team members can identify and record, yet they fail to be truly specific. For example: *Art will respond to a peer on three of five opportunities.* This goal fails to identify the specific peer behaviors to which Art is expected to respond (e.g., conversation initiations, requests for materials, teasing remarks)? Although the IEP team may wish to see Art increase *all* prosocial responses to his peers throughout the course of the school year, this would be a challenging goal to instruct and progress monitor. Instead, a specific goal would delineate the precise conditions, situations, or behaviors to which the student will respond: *Art will respond to a peer's request for materials during independent seatwork periods. . . .* In addition, the use of the verb *respond* without additional qualification opens up many possibilities. In what way does the team expect Art to respond to a peer's request for materials? If Art turns his back when a peer asks for a pair of scissors, that behavior could be considered a "response," but it is unlikely that this is what Art's IEP team wants him to do. Clarifying the exact response desired from Art could enhance this objective: *Art will respond to a peer's request for materials by providing the requested item.*

Finally, when developing a statement of student behavior or skill, educators may be tempted to use familiar but unspecific terms, such as *inappropriate, difficulty, weak, unmotivated, limited, defiant, irresponsible, uncooperative,* and so on. These words are labels, not behaviors, and therefore are subjective in nature and difficult to measure. Using the observed actions that lead to these labels (e.g., "needs at least five prompts to follow directions") will help the IEP team key in on the specific problem that needs to be addressed and measure it consistently.

Measurable

Making IEP goals measurable is of utmost importance. Besides being required specifically by IDEA (2004), measurability affords IEP teams the ability to monitor progress and ultimately determine whether the goal has been achieved. Writing a specific goal, as discussed in the previous section, is an excellent first start, but it does not guarantee that the goal is truly measurable. Measurable IEP goals include three key components:

1. Objective, action-based statement of the behavior or skill to be modified (refer to the preceding section for more information).
2. Direction of the behavior (Will it increase? Decrease? Be maintained for a specific amount of time?).
3. Level of attainment or success criterion (i.e., degree of accuracy, frequency, or independence the student must demonstrate in order for the team to agree that the goal has been met; Wright & Wright, 2006).

Stating the direction of the behavior should be relatively easy if thorough assessment has been conducted prior to writing the goal. Generally, educators should aim to write goals that seek to increase the frequency or duration of desired behaviors or to improve the accuracy of skills, rather than aiming to decrease undesired behaviors. When writing academic goals, this concept is intuitive; educators strive to see their students make positive gains in the acquisition of skills. However, when it comes to behavior, it is often tempting to write goals such as *Maribel will decrease her call-outs during large-group instruction. . . .* By focusing on the undesired behavior, the IEP team has potentially overlooked two important considerations: (1) Why is Maribel calling out (i.e., making comments without raising her hand to be called on?), and (2) What does the team *want* Maribel to do during large-group instruction, instead of calling out (i.e., a replacement behavior, such as raising her hand or writing her question down)? The former question should have been addressed through the problem-identification and problem-analysis stages so the team is able to develop a viable answer to the latter question. Placing emphasis on an appropriate replacement behavior will ensure that Maribel's participation in large-group instruction is maximized.

If Maribel's IEP team revised the preceding goal to reflect emphasis on a replacement behavior (e.g., *Maribel will raise her hand and wait to be called on before making a comment during large-group instruction*), would the goal be sufficiently measurable? At first glance, this goal is written specifically and objectively, and it would be easy to observe Maribel and record instances of hand raising. Yet, without stating the criteria for evaluating Maribel's performance, the IEP team will have difficulty stating whether she has mastered this goal. If Maribel raises her hand once during large-group instruction but calls out three more times, has she made progress? By clarifying their expectations for Maribel's behavior (e.g., *Maribel will raise her hand and wait to be called on before making a comment in at least four of five opportunities during large-group instruction*), the IEP team has now written a measurable and achievable goal.

A caution with regard to writing success criteria: although it is important to specify the frequency, quality, or independence of a behavior in order to evaluate whether a goal has been attained, many IEPs use criteria that are unrealistic from a measurement perspective. Educators are often tempted to add "80% of the time" to the end of each goal to specify a reasonable rate of success. However, this criterion can be problematic from a data collection perspective. When developing a success criterion, it is essential that educators clarify the "whole part" before specifying the percentage that constitutes success (Bar-Lev, 2008). This refers to duration of

> **Educators are often tempted to add "80% of the time" to the end of each goal to specify a reasonable rate of success. However, this criterion can be problematic from a data collection perspective.**

time over which the student will be observed, in order to establish whether he or she has met the 80% criterion. If a goal simply states "80% of the time" without further clarification of the whole part, one could infer that IEP team is planning to observe the student 24 hours a day, 7 days a week! Similarly, "four of five opportunities" suggests that an IEP team member will be able to observe and measure all opportunities for a behavior. For many behaviors, there are so many opportunities that it would be impossible to observe and quantify them all (e.g., answering a question, maintaining personal space). Instead, consider modifying success criteria to specify the time frame or activity during which educators will look for the target behavior (e.g., "8 or more minutes during a 10-minute observation," or "80% of opportunities during a 45-minute lesson").

Realistic and Relevant

Specific, measurable goals are essential to the delivery of a high-quality IEP. However, if the team has developed goals and expectations that are not realistic, they are unlikely to be attained. As previously discussed, IEP teams often use "80% of the time" as a success criterion because it represents a reasonably high degree of success in a goal area. Yet, if Isabella's PLOP statement indicates that she currently does not correctly use pronouns at all, is it realistic to expect that she will use them correctly at least 80% of the time by the end of the year? Similarly, if Mateo stops working and puts away his materials only after five or more verbal prompts, is it realistic to expect him to do so independently (no verbal prompts) by the end of the year? Unfortunately, there are no clear-cut answers to questions such as these. Developing an adequate IEP goal requires a thorough understanding of each student's present level of functioning in the goal areas, his or her previous success with skill acquisition, the intended method(s) of instruction for each goal, and the intensity of the instructional methods or services. Most important, IEP teams must be careful not to fall into the habit of routinely assigning an 80% success criterion without careful consideration of whether this is a realistic expectation for the student in question.

Realistic goals not only are referenced to the student's present levels of functioning but also take into consideration local norms and average rates of skills/behaviors in same-age peers. IEP teams may wish to see a student master a particular skill at 100% accuracy when, in fact, other children his or her age do not regularly demonstrate the skill at that level of proficiency. Recall the example of Maribel: *Maribel will raise her hand and wait to be called on before making a comment during large-group instruction.* Success criteria should be developed in reference to developmental, social-emotional, and academic expectations for typically developing peers. In Maribel's case, expecting her to raise her hand 100% of the time is not realistic if her classmates only raise their hands 80% of the time. Instead, Maribel's team could determine the frequency of hand raising for an average classroom peer or take an average across all students during a given instructional period to develop a success criterion that is both attainable and age appropriate.

Additionally, IEP teams are tasked with developing *relevant* goals that address the student's educational needs caused by his or her disability. Due to the pervasive nature of social, communication, and behavioral difficulties associated with an ASD diagnosis, nearly all areas of development or education may require an IEP goal at some point in time, depending on individual student need. What is important for IEP teams to remember, however, is that IEP goals should address areas of *educational need* in which the student's difficulty prevents him or her from accessing or making progress in the general education curriculum. When a kindergarten student with HFA/AS presents with difficulty sustaining attention to large-group instruction for more than 20 minutes, is this an area of educational need that necessitates an IEP goal? Generally, most kindergarten-age children would demonstrate difficulty sustaining attention to large-group instruction for more than 20 minutes, so this is not a goal requiring the individualized attention and specialized instruction that an IEP affords. When a student demonstrates skills or behaviors consistent with their same-age peers in a given area, IEP goals are not relevant or necessary because they are not a result of the child's disability.

Time

Finally, SMART IEP goals consider the time needed to achieve a goal. Most IEPs are written annually, so goals are generally written to reflect a year's progress on a given skill or behavior. Again, IEP teams must consider the student's baseline levels of academic and functional performance in order to develop realistic goals that can be attained in a year's time. Educators also may consider utilizing benchmarks or objectives to mark the progress a student should make over smaller intervals of time within that year.

Consider Tyrone, a third-grade student with HFA who presently reads 20 words per minute. A goal for Tyrone might be written as follows: *By June 2010, Tyrone will increase his reading fluency by reading at least 90 words per minute with three or fewer errors.* Although this goal is indeed specific, action oriented, measurable, and realistic, it may be helpful for the team to break this goal down into substeps or objectives in order to better monitor Tyrone's progress toward this goal. For an annual goal, it may be appropriate to break the goal down into quarterly benchmarks. In Tyrone's case, this would represent a gain of 17–18 words per minute each quarter:

- Objective 1: *By October 2009, Tyrone will increase his reading fluency by reading at least 37 words per minute with three or fewer errors.*
- Objective 2: *By January 2010, Tyrone will increase his reading fluency by reading at least 54 words per minute with three or fewer errors.*
- Objective 3: *By March 2010, Tyrone will increase his reading fluency by reading at least 71 words per minute with three or fewer errors.*
- Objective 4: *By June 2010, Tyrone will increase his reading fluency by reading at least 90 words per minute with three or fewer errors.*

Table 8.2 provides a sample IEP goal analyzed using all of the SMART IEP goal characteristics.

Service Delivery

Clearly, well-written goals are necessary but not sufficient for the child with HFA/AS who is eligible for special education services to make educational gains. With only a road map but no vehicle, one would make little progress toward one's destination. In 1982, in *Board of Education of the Hendrick Hudson School District v. Rowley* (henceforth referred to as *Rowley*), the U.S. Supreme Court affirmed that all special education students had a right to FAPE and that mere access to public school programming is insufficient to guarantee FAPE. IDEA (2004) requires that specialized instruction and accommodations or modifica-

TABLE 8.2. Evaluating Goals and Objectives Using SMART Characteristics

Sample goal	Is the goal . . .	Analysis	Rewrite
Joey will master written expression skills at the tenth-grade level as measured by passing grades in his English class.	. . . Specific and action oriented?	Joey is expected to master *all* written expression skills at his grade level; this would entail a lot of data collection. Furthermore, it may not be clear to the uninformed reader what actions will be required of Joey in order to demonstrate mastery of tenth-grade writing curriculum.	*By June 15, given a graphic organizer prewriting activity and feedback after writing assignments, Joey will write a five-paragraph essay with "competent" or better use of the Organization trait, as measured by a rating of 4 or higher on the Organization rubric from six Traits of Writing.*
	. . . Measurable?	Is Joey's grade in English an adequate measure of his written expression skills? Put another way, if Joey gets a passing grade in English (D or better), can we guarantee that he has mastered all written expression skills? Grades are often indicative of both academic proficiency *and* work completion.	
	. . . Realistic and relevant?	Is it realistic to expect Joey to master written expressions at his grade level, given his disability and areas of need? Is this the most important goal for him, in light of his overall needs and levels of functioning? Alternatively, if Joey is a tenth-grader, this goal is not relevant because it is consistent with curriculum goals for all students his age.	
	. . . Time-oriented?	By what date will Joey demonstrate writing mastery: at the end of the first semester? By the end of the school year? What steps will he take to get there?	

tions to curriculum and/or instruction be provided to address each of the student's areas of educational need in order for that same student:

(aa) to advance appropriately toward attaining the annual goals;

(bb) to be involved in and make progress in the general education curriculum . . . and to participate in extracurricular and other nonacademic activities; and

(cc) to be educated and participate with other children with disabilities and children without disabilities in the regular class. (20 U.S.C. § 614(d)(1)(A)(i)(IV))

Related services (e.g., speech–language therapy, occupational therapy, or assistive technology supports, such as the use of Picture Exchange Communication System [PECS] or communication boards) also may be necessary to support specialized instruction and ensure the appropriateness of the child's educational program.

The U.S. Supreme Court in *Rowley* (1982) held that local education agencies, in collaboration with parents, hold the primary responsibility for choosing the educational methodology that will be used to educate students in special education. Furthermore, the Supreme Court asserted a laissez-faire stance to issues of methodology in special education by stating that, because courts lack the training and expertise to address questions of methodology, the specifics of service delivery would be left to the school district to decide as long as it can demonstrate that the requirements of IDEA have been met. Yet, within the past decade, the service delivery aspect of special education has received renewed scrutiny from policy experts and legislators. After an extensive review of the special education system, the President's Commission on Excellence in Special Education (2002) reported that the ever-increasing incidence of litigation and conflict within special education has created a "culture of compliance," in which districts tend to be more concerned with meeting the procedural requirements of IDEA than with realizing their true mission of educating all children (p. 8). The Commission (2002) further concluded that the educational system in general uses a "wait to fail" approach, characterized by insufficient efforts to prevent or remediate learning problems in the general education setting and a reluctance to embrace evidence-based strategies once they are established in the literature. As a result, new language in IDEA (2004) brings special education service delivery into alignment with the President's Commission's recommendations and NCLB's requirements for "evidence-based practices" by requiring that special education and related services must be "based on peer-reviewed research to the extent practicable" (20 U.S.C. § 614(d)(1)(A)(i)(IV)).

With respect to special education services for students with HFA/AS, Yell et al.'s (2003) review of recent litigation revealed that school districts are found in violation of the FAPE provision when they fail to provide services to the student despite evidence that such services are needed to provide FAPE (e.g., extended school year services, speech–language services, behavioral programming) and provide programming that does not result in student progress. Moreover, failure to ensure that school personnel (e.g., teachers, speech–language therapists) are trained appropriately for evaluating, teaching, or providing therapies to students with HFA/AS was found to be a common procedural violation of IDEA.

According to Yell et al. (2003), "a district violates IDEA . . . when it fails to employ faculty members who are knowledgeable about ASD to work with these students. The faculty members who implement the IEP must have the experience and training to do so" (p. 187). The extremely variable and individual nature of the autism spectrum of disorders requires that educators be highly knowledgeable so that they can select appropriate methodology that meets the educational needs of each student (Twachtman-Cullen & Twachtman-Reilly, 2002). Thus school districts must have a dual focus in their service delivery for students with HFA/AS, with equal emphasis on the provision of evidence-based services for students with HFA/AS in the here and now *and* on the availability of ongoing professional development that ensures the continuation of empirically supported instruction in the future.

> **School districts must have a dual focus in their service delivery for students with HFA/AS, with equal emphasis on the provision of evidence-based services for students with HFA/AS in the here and now *and* on the availability of ongoing professional development that ensures the continuation of empirically supported instruction in the future.**

Accommodations and Modifications

In addition to specifying the services and supports that will be used to help the student make progress, the IEP also must state all accommodations or modifications necessary to ensure the student's access to the general education environment. In general, accommodations and modifications are any changes made to the *teaching environment* (e.g., use of visuals or social stories to supplement verbal directions, physical arrangement of the room, behavioral management supports), to *instructional delivery* (e.g., individual front-loading of vocabulary, reteaching, breaking lessons down into smaller chunks, breaks between activities, organizational strategies and supports), or to *students' responses to instruction* (e.g., extended time to complete tasks, breaking down assignments into smaller chunks, word banks, test-taking accommodations). Furthermore, the IEP must not only state the accommodations to be used regularly in the classroom setting but also must specify which accommodations will be necessary for the student to access state- and district-wide assessments. Students should not be afforded accommodations on high-stakes tests that are not utilized in their everyday instruction or assessment context. For example, if Meghan does not demonstrate a need for shortened assignments, extended time on assignments or assessments, or more frequent breaks during long activities throughout the school year, then she should not need these accommodations during high-stakes assessment.

Educational Placement

In developing provisions for special education, legislators consistently have underscored the importance of educating students with disabilities in general education and alongside typically developing peers to the greatest extent possible. In keeping with previous iterations of special education legislation, the 2004 reauthorization of IDEA continues to require that to the maximum extent appropriate, children with disabilities, including children in public or private institutions or other care facilities, are educated with children who are not disabled, and that special classes, separate schooling, or other removal of children with disabilities from the regular educational environment occurs only when the nature or severity of the disability is such that education in regular classes with the use of supplementary aids and services cannot be achieved satisfactorily. (IDEA, 20 U.S.C. 1412 (5)(B))

This requirement, known as the least restrictive environment (LRE) mandate, has become one of the most controversial aspects of IDEA and is at the center of frequent legal disputes (Yell et al., 2003). Whereas the assessment, service delivery, and progress monitoring requirements of IDEA have faded into the background of the special education consciousness, the LRE provision of IDEA increasingly has been placed in a "front and center" position with each passing year (Twachtman-Cullen & Twachtman-Reilly, 2002, p. 92). Often, the term *least restrictive environment* is interpreted as being synonymous with *general education environment*, when this is not in fact the case. Rather, LRE is defined on a case-by-case basis, as it represents the setting and instructional format in which the student is able to do his or her best learning and is most likely to attain the goals set forth in that student's IEP. The previously cited section of IDEA (2004) sets forth a clear expectation that students with disabilities are educated with children who are not disabled to the greatest extent possible. Yet the legislation also leaves the door open for the possibility that student needs may, at times, necessitate a more restrictive, segregated placement (i.e., in a separate classroom or school setting) in order to provide an adequate degree of support. However, these decisions may not be made merely on the basis of a student's educational service category (e.g., autism, Other Health Impairment), of availability of resources or funding, or on any other single factor. It is only after comprehensive data have been gathered, synthesized into a PLOP statement, translated into high-quality (i.e., SMART) educational goals, and linked to evidence-based instructional services that an IEP team is finally in a position to make a determination about the student's most appropriate educational environment.

In some cases, when an IEP team reaches this point in the placement decision-making process, it becomes evident that the general education environment setting may be a *more* restrictive environment than a setting such as a self-contained classroom (Crockett & Kauffman, 1999). Consider the following case example:

Hope, a ninth-grade student diagnosed with AS, has had a difficult transition from middle school to high school. Although Hope has many strong intellectual and academic skills that are an asset for her educationally, she struggles significantly with transitioning from one environment to the next (which was not required in her middle school setting). At the beginning of her ninth-grade year, she refused to walk through the hallway during passing periods because of the loud noises and frequent physical contact with students walking beside her. The IEP team suggested that she leave her classes 5 minutes early to avoid the bustling hallway during passing periods. However, without adult supervision during transition times, Hope consistently went to the cafeteria to purchase her favorite snack rather than walking to her next class. After a functional behavioral assessment and sensory evaluation, a 9-week positive behavior plan rewarding Hope for on-time arrival to her classes (earning her favorite snacks for free) and teaching her coping strategies for dealing with sensory overload met with minimal success. When an adult aide was assigned to walk with her during transitions, Hope hit the aide and refused to walk with her by stating, "I'm not a baby." By the end of the second quarter, Hope often refused to attend her classes altogether to avoid the presence of the aide. Upon arriving at school, Hope often sat in the guidance office lobby and read her favorite books rather than going to class. Teachers' and administrators' attempts to verbally encourage Hope to join her peers in class usually ended with Hope swearing loudly and/or hitting adult staff members. By the end of the third quarter, Hope's mother reported that she was having trouble getting her on the bus because Hope "didn't want to go to that stupid place." At their fifth problem-solving meeting of the year, the IEP team estimated that the combined impact of Hope's late arrivals to class, refusal to join classes by staying in the lobby, eventual refusal to attend school at all, and suspensions for hitting staff members had caused her to miss a cumulative total of 34 school days by the end of the third quarter. She was in danger of failing five of her six courses.

This case study illustrates a district's good-faith efforts to maintain Hope's general education placement as long as possible by utilizing a problem-solving process to offer a variety of accommodations, assessments, positive interventions, and supplementary aids. Ultimately, however, the academic impact of Hope's lost instructional time was too much to ignore. The IEP team, including Hope's parents, agreed that a placement in the general educational setting was not Hope's LRE. The team chose to provide Hope's IEP services in a self-contained classroom for students with severe social-emotional and behavioral support needs, where she could remain throughout the school day with a consistent peer group.

The preceding case study represents only a single instance of a complicated placement decision-making process and illustrates a situation in which the educational team members and parents were in agreement. However, the extant literature and court cases in this area suggest that educators and parents often do not see eye to eye, which further complicates placement decision making. In a recent qualitative study investigating educators' and parents' attitudes, beliefs, and decision-making strategies regarding inclusive placements for students with ASD, educators and parents shared relatively similar definitions and attitudes of what "inclusive education" should look like yet failed to see each other as collaborative partners in placement decision making (J. M. Sansosti, 2008). Educators generally characterized parents as having "too much say" in the placement decision making process and suggested that many parents who push for their children with ASD to be in the general education setting are "in denial" about the extent of their children's needs. Meanwhile, parents of students with ASD reported feeling significantly excluded from placement decision making and viewed the decision-making process as being controlled by educators with limited knowledge about ASD. Both legal mandates and scholarly literature insist that parent involvement is essential in supporting students with ASD and other disabilities, and both general education and special education literature support the academic and behavioral benefits of home–school collaboration. Yet the aforementioned data and the preponderance of litigation suggest that placement continues to be a highly contentious issue in special education, needing significant improvement in many school districts.

Transition Planning

As students progress through the educational curriculum and near the time when they will leave the school system, IDEA (2004) requires that the IEP team help students access information, resources, and experiences that will facilitate their transition from school to postschool activities such as postsecondary or vocational schools, employment settings (with or without support), independent living, and community participation. Transition services are particularly important for students with HFA/AS, as research indicates that they are disproportionately likely to demonstrate poor outcomes after exiting K–12 education. For example, studies examining long-term outcomes have demonstrated that individuals with HFA/AS develop serious mental

> **Transition services are particularly important for students with HFA/AS, as research indicates that they are disproportionately likely to demonstrate poor outcomes after exiting K–12 education.**

health conditions, fail to establish long-term relationships, and may encounter problems with the legal system (Barnhill, 2007; Engstrom, Ekstrom, & Emilsson, 2003; Howlin, 2000; Howlin, Goode, Hutton, & Rutter, 2004). Moreover, and most dishearteningly, only 12% of individuals with HFA/AS are employed as adults (Barnard et al., 2001).

In addition to IEP goals and services described earlier, the IEP team must develop a statement of the transition service needs for students who are age 14 or older, indicating how the student's course of study (i.e., current course load) helps prepare him or her for post-secondary settings. After age 16, transition planning becomes significantly more involved. Age-appropriate transition assessment related to postsecondary education and training, employment, and (if necessary) independent living skills is used to provide a clear profile of the student's transition service needs. The IEP team then writes measurable postsecondary goals to ensure the student's progress in these areas. Goals are written to reflect completion after the student graduates from high school (e.g., *Upon graduation, Bill will attend Acme Vocational Academy and take course work in the landscaping program*). Because this goal is postsecondary, the school district is not responsible for ensuring that Bill does, in fact, attend vocational school. Rather, they must demonstrate a good-faith effort to provide Bill with any necessary course work, information, or other supports in the high school setting so that he is able to pursue and attain this goal after graduation. Any additional transition services needed to attain these goals are listed in this section. Because a detailed survey of transition planning considerations is beyond the scope of this chapter, the interested reader is referred to the work of deFur (2003) for a more comprehensive discussion of this topic.

STEP 4: PROGRESS MONITORING— EVALUATING IEP OUTCOMES

The final step of the problem-solving process involves gathering data to ensure that the goals of the plan are being achieved and, if they are not, revising the plan for better outcomes. Progress monitoring is an essential aspect of IEP service delivery. The 1997 reauthorization of IDEA added several elements designed to underscore the importance of improving educational outcomes for students with disabilities, including the requirement that IEP goals be measurable and that students' progress regularly be reported to parents (Yell et al., 2003). Most critically, IDEA 1997 made it clear that IEP teams must revise a student's plan if progress monitoring data indicate that a student is failing to make progress toward his or her IEP goal, rather than allowing the student to continue to struggle. IDEA 2004 maintains this emphasis on data-based decision making, with only minor modifications to the location or specific wording of progress reporting requirements (Gartin & Murdick, 2006).

Methods for measuring progress monitoring are determined by the IEP team and should be linked to day-to-day instructional and assessment processes. In order to accurately evaluate whether a student has made progress in an area of educational weakness, data should be gathered to answer three key questions:

1. *What progress has the student made toward mastering the IEP goal, as defined by success criteria set forth by the IEP team (e.g., "80% of the time," "for at least 5 minutes," etc.)?* This question can be answered by comparing the student's present rate or level of performance to his or her baseline level described in the IEP, using an aim line and trend line to demonstrate progress toward individualized goals.

2. *What progress has the student made toward reducing educational need?* At times, the answers to this question may be one and the same, when IEP goals aim for the student to perform at levels consistent with those of peers in one year's time. However, in other situations, the IEP team may wish to set a more reasonable goal that does not yet reach the level of peer attainment. In this case, progress monitoring data should be referenced not only to the student's success criterion but also to peer levels of behavior.

3. *Has the student demonstrated any skill regressions, and, if so, how long does it take the student to recoup those skills to their prebreak levels?* This question is particularly relevant for students with HFA/AS, who may find school breaks particularly disruptive to their sense of routine. In order for a child to be eligible for extended school year (ESY) services through IDEA (2004), the IEP team must provide evidence of regression and demonstrate diminished capacity for recoupment. Specifically, does the child revert to a lower level of functioning following an interruption in educational programming (e.g., winter or spring break) and, upon returning to school, does the child have the ability to recover the skills to levels demonstrated prior to the interruption in a reasonable amount of time? When a child's difficulties with regression and recoupment make it unlikely that the child will be able to maintain the skills and behaviors targeted in the IEP, he or she is a good candidate for ESY services. Educators should not need to gather additional data for ESY purposes if they already are engaging in frequent classroom-based assessments of skills as a part of gen-

eral IEP progress monitoring. Rather, the team should be prepared to have data from time periods involving school breaks available at a periodic review meeting to be able to answer questions regarding ESY.

Goals can be measured through formal or informal formative assessment tools, such as curriculum-based assessments, portfolios, observations, anecdotal records, performance assessments, checklists, work samples, inventories, and rubrics. It is important to note that forms of summative evaluation, such as standardized assessments or statewide testing conducted on an annual basis, are *not* recommended as progress monitoring tools. Although information from a formal 3-year reevaluation can be useful for providing the IEP team with updated information on the student's functioning across a variety of domains, several problems exist when trying to use summative evaluation data to document IEP goal progress: (1) content assessed on standardized measures may not match the specific skills or behaviors targeted in the student's IEP goals exactly; (2) scores from summative evaluations are typically norm- or criterion-referenced and do not provide a clear rate, frequency, or consistency with which the student can perform the desired behavior; and (3) summative evaluations are not conducted with enough frequency to be sensitive to small changes in student functioning, nor to allow the IEP to make changes in course midway through the IEP cycle if needed. Rather, the triennial reevaluation offers the IEP team the opportunity to cast a wider net and to determine whether there are other areas of need arising—especially if previous educational needs have been successfully addressed.

Although this step is the fourth and final step in a basic problem-solving model, it is truly an integral part of all other steps, particularly Steps 1 (problem identification) and 2 (problem analysis). Data should be referenced back to the original problem definition in order to draw conclusions about the extent to which the student has demonstrated progress in an area of need. Consider the example of Joe, previously presented in Table 8.1, whose writing weaknesses were documented by his ratings on a writing evaluation rubric called "the Six Traits of Writing." Because these data were marshaled initially to

> Data should be referenced back to the original problem definition in order to draw conclusions about the extent to which the student has demonstrated progress in the area of need, ... but also should be incorporated into the PLOP statement of the student's next IEP.

demonstrate the existence of a problem (i.e., no ratings at the "competent" level in the area of Organization), these same data need to be gathered throughout the term of the intervention or services to evaluate whether Joey has made progress on his writing goal. Progress monitoring data not only determine whether current goals have been met but also should be incorporated into the PLOP statement of the student's next IEP.

At least once a year, the IEP team must convene to review the child's progress and determine whether the child is achieving his or her annual goals. Although IDEA (2004) requires IEPs to be reviewed at least once a year, in fact the team may review and revise the IEP more frequently if necessary. Both parent and educator members of the IEP team can convene the team at any time to address concerns (of minimal progress) or of more rapid progress than expected (i.e., the child has met most or all of the goals in the IEP well in advance of the annual review; U.S. Department of Education Office of Special Education and Rehabilitation Services, 2000). In either case, the IEP team would meet to revise the student's plan. When completing an annual review of a student's IEP and writing new IEP goals, the team should first review previous goals and progress monitoring data as a part of the new IEP's PLOP. The previous year's goals and data should link directly to the coming year's goals, objectives, and service plans, and this link should be documented clearly in the IEP for all team members to see.

Despite the clear emphasis on the need for data-based decision making in special education law, Yell et al.'s (2003) review of ASD-specific IEP litigation reveals that failure to monitor IEP goals adequately is a common violation of IDEA's FAPE provision. Their judicial review found at least 11 cases of "procedural violations" related to progress monitoring, including failure to collect data to determine whether students were progressing in the special education program, to demonstrate that students were making progress in the school's special education program, or to alter programs when the students did not progress (Yell et al., 2003). These data highlight the essential nature of progress monitoring as a part of the IEP process and the legal vulnerabilities districts may face if they fail to meet IDEA's requirements in this regard.

TOOLS FOR ENHANCING THE QUALITY AND FUNCTIONALITY OF IEPS

Federal, state, and local requirements for writing IEPs have become increasingly cumbersome since the initial passage of special education litigation in 1975. Furthermore, general education and related services personnel have become important members of the IEP team who are involved actively in the development of IEPs at all levels. To coordinate the efforts of numerous team members across such a vast range of IEP compliance standards is a challenging endeavor that requires a common framework against which all team members can judge the quality of the plans they develop. Form 8.1 in the Appendix provides a rubric developed by Rosas, Winterman, Kroeger, and Jones (2009) that may be a useful way to remind IEP team members of required components when developing an IEP or to evaluate whether existing IEP documents are in compliance with the updated requirements of IDEA (2004).

> To coordinate the efforts of numerous team members across such a vast range of IEP compliance standards is a challenging endeavor that requires a common framework against which all team members can judge the quality of the plans they develop.

Once an IEP is written, the work of improving student outcomes is nowhere near complete. The IEP team must ensure that the student's instructional program provides specialized supports aimed at increasing functioning in areas of need. An IEP program-planning matrix, illustrated in Figure 8.2, provides a mechanism for ensuring that opportunities for targeting areas of need are embedded throughout the school day (Janney & Snell, 2011). Janney and Snell suggest that an IEP program-planning matrix is particularly useful when

Student Name: Henry P.	Grade: 3	Date: 8/25/2009

Team Members: Mr. Block (GE), Mrs. Gregory (SE), Mrs. Schwartz (SLP), Mrs. Holland (Title I tutor), Ms. Swank (PE), Mrs. Peabody (Art), Ms. Day (Library), Mr. Wendell (Music), Mrs. Corianno (SE Associate)

Abbreviated IEP Objectives	Daily Schedule/Activities										
	Arrival	Journal	Lang. Arts	Break	Spelling	Math	Lunch/Recess	Shared Rdg.	Specials	Sci./Social Stu.	Dismissal
Content Area: Reading											
Read high-frequency sight words from Gr. 2 Dolch list		X				X				X	
Determine the meaning of unknown words using a variety of context clues		X								X	
Read passages aloud at a rate of at least 100 words per minute (<3 errors)		X									
Content Area: Writing											
Use the upper-case/lower-case letters appropriately within a word		X	X		X					X	
Write letters using the guidelines for height on paper		X	X		X					X	
Provide uniform spacing between words		X	X		X					X	
Content Area: Functional Skills/Communication											
Use active listening strategies, such as making eye contact and asking for clarification/explanation	X	X	X	X	X	X	X	X	X	X	X
Follow two- and three-step oral directions.	X	X	X	X	X	X	X	X	X	X	X
Content Area: Social Skills											
Maintain topic within a 3-min. conversation with peers and/or adults	X			X			X	X	X		X
Identify elements of nonverbal communication (e.g., facial expressions, tone of voice, personal space)	X		X	X			X	X	X		X

FIGURE 8.2. Sample IEP program-planning matrix. Adapted from Janney and Snell (2011). Copyright 2011 by Pearson Education, Inc. Adapted by permission of Pearson Education, Inc.

planning instruction for students who need a more functional curriculum to assist teams in identifying ways in which general education instruction can be accommodated or modified to address altered curriculum objectives. For students with HFA/AS, however, the matrix serves as a document that alerts all members of the IEP team to their responsibilities to address IEP goals during their particular instructional period. See Form 8.2 in the Appendix for a reproducible version.

Each adult working directly with a student, including classroom, special area (e.g., P.E., art) and special education teachers, related services personnel, tutors, and associates should receive a copy of the student's matrix. Once team members are aware of the student's goals and objectives in their particular area of instruction, they are more empowered to provide direct support in those areas, to monitor progress, and to make adjustments to instruction as needed. Of course, the IEP program matrix cannot and should not be used as a substitute for the student's entire IEP. The matrix is intended to be a brief reiteration of the students' IEP objectives plotted alongside their daily schedules, while the full IEP is rich in details regarding the student's background, success criterion for achieving annual goals, and expectations for progress monitoring. Nevertheless, for teams working to provide cohesive, consistent support for students with HFA/AS across a variety of settings, educators, and service providers, the IEP program-planning matrix offers an essential communication tool for coordinating their efforts.

CONCLUSION

The highly enigmatic and unpredictable nature of HFA/AS requires that educators develop individualized, assessment-driven plans of instructional support for children with HFA/AS. Yet, in the increasingly litigious climate of special education, IEPs tend to be overly focused on legal protection and compliance rather than on individualized educational services. When school districts attempt to protect themselves from potential litigation by becoming consumed with procedural compliance, they may neglect to ensure that students are provided high-quality, research-based programming that results in measurable student progress. This chapter has reviewed the contents of the IEP through the lens of the problem-solving model. By infusing into the IEP the scientific thinking, data-based decision making, and evidence-based practices of problem-solving processes, educational teams are better poised to develop IEPs that meet both procedural and substantive requirements of IDEA and to provide the truly "special" education that some students with HFA/AS need to overcome the limitations of their disability.

CHAPTER 9

Collecting Data, Evaluating Outcomes, and Ensuring Success

with JULIE E. GOLDYN

OVERVIEW

Too often, many educators consider *data* a dirty "four-letter word"! Within education, a world already replete with excessive paperwork, the mere thought of collecting data several times a week frequently is viewed as an intrusive, time-consuming task that interferes with teaching (especially within the context of general education). Such thoughts and opinions are only magnified when data is collected from multiple students within the same classroom. Despite these feelings, which very often are grounded in the reality of school-based practice, educators work in an educational environment that is now dominated by accountability and outcomes-based reform. Within today's schools and classrooms, the proof of learning resides in positive results rather than correct procedures. Therefore, a lack of outcome data puts educators at risk for criticism from administrators and parents, at best, and due process hearings and/or litigation, at worst. With this in mind, it is essential that educators become familiar with procedures for collecting data and evaluating the effectiveness of prevention and intervention strategies for students with HFA/AS. This chapter provides specific information not only on how to collect and use data within educational contexts but also on how to ensure that students continue to demonstrate success.

Julie E. Goldyn, MEd, is a doctoral candidate in the School Psychology Program at Kent State University. She is employed as a school psychologist by Partners for Success and Innovation (PSI) and serves Cleveland city schools. Ms. Goldyn has experience working with individuals with ASD in both home and school settings, providing consultative services to teachers in Northeast Ohio, and presenting at local and national venues on utilizing naturalistic interventions to enhance communication and social skills in individuals with autism.

THE IMPORTANCE OF DATA COLLECTION (WHY COLLECT DATA?)

Of the steps involved in the assessment of and intervention for academic, behavioral, and social difficulties in individuals with HFA/AS, data collection is the one step that mostly likely is ignored or performed irregularly. However, there are several excellent reasons for frequently collecting data as a critical part of prevention and intervention efforts within schools. First, through data collection, it is possible to determine the effects of a particular strategy or intervention (Alberto & Troutman, 2008). Without data, educators may not be able to notice a student's improvements from his or her initial and to current behavior. This is likely the result of a student's making progress but still performing outside the range of what is expected. Data gathered regularly not only serve to illustrate a student's, sometimes minor, improvement but also encourages educators to keep up their efforts (Crone & Horner, 2003).

Second, systematic data collection allows formative evaluation. That is, data collected while a strategy or an intervention is being implemented allow educators to identify problems early on in the process and make changes during the course of the intervention rather than waiting to see whether it was successful after several weeks or months (Alberto & Troutman, 2008). For example, Michael's team wanted to increase his ability to join in activities appropriately. To accomplish this task, the team created an intervention that consisted of video-modeled Social Stories™. Data collection demonstrated initial success for the first several days of the intervention, followed immediately by a regression in skills and, in some instances, aggression towards his peers (see Sansosti & Powell-Smith, 2008, for a full review of this example). Over the course of a week, Michael engaged in arguments with his peers with greater intensity than prior to the implementation of the video-modeled Social Stories. As could be expected, Michael's teachers were ready to eliminate this strategy, thinking it was a failure. However, Michael's team reviewed the data, made hypotheses as to why he was not using the skills appropriately, and conducted several qualitative observations on the playground. This examination revealed that Michael, in fact, was using his skills appropriately. It was his peers who were not providing Michael with opportunities to practice his skills. In fact, during one observation, Michael was observed standing on top of a jungle gym screaming, "Why won't anybody play with me? I saw it on my videotape, and, I'm doing it right!" Based on this knowledge, Michael's team made a few adjustments to the intervention to include prompts and child confederates. These minor modifications resulted in an abrupt improvement in Michael's behavior that maintained modestly after the intervention was terminated. From this example, it is fair to presume that Michael's team would have completely abandoned the intervention, thinking that their efforts did not make a difference, had it not been for the careful analysis of the data collected.

Finally, collecting data is the ultimate tool for accountability. Because educators now work within an environment of outcomes, it is essential that data be gathered on *all* aspects of intervention and instruction. In this era of evidence-based accountability, schools, districts, educators, and students are responsible for results and educational planning. Data are used not only to demonstrate that various stakeholders have met performance-based standards, whether for an entire school or as an individual goal on an IEP, but also to provide support for educational decision making. For example, frequent data collection should be used as the foundation for determining whether or not a student with HFA/AS qualifies for extended school year (ESY). To qualify for this service on the IEP, the educational team *must*

> Data are used not only to demonstrate that various stakeholders have met performance-based standards, whether for an entire school or as an individual goal on an IEP, but also to provide support for educational decision making.

demonstrate that the child loses significant progress on a skill or skills over a school break (e.g., winter or spring break). In order to do so, the team *must* have data to support their determination. That is, data need to demonstrate that access to school over the summer months is a need, not a want!

DATA COLLECTION PROCESS

Step 1: Identify a Target Behavior

The identification of a target behavior often is not a difficult task. Educators and parents frequently report dozens of difficulties that individuals with HFA/AS experience within school and home settings, respectively. Identifying the goal of instruction based on information shared is often obvious and straightforward, because the need for the behavior is widely accepted and the consequences for not engaging in the behavior are undesired (Kazdin, 1994). However, it is not realistic to identify all of the behaviors or academic and social skills difficulties that a student (or students) with HFA/AS may display. It is more important to focus prevention and intervention efforts on clearly defined target behaviors that take into consideration the situation or context in which the behavior occurs.

Step 2: Define the Target Behavior

After a target behavior has been identified, it needs to be defined in terms that are specific, observable, and measurable (Alberto & Troutman, 2008). The behavioral definition should provide a clear and objective picture of exactly what the behavior looks like when it is occurring. With a solid definition, multiple observers should be able to agree on the occurrence and nonoccurrence of the target behavior. For example, Ms. Campana is interested in increasing Charley's in-seat behavior. She defined in-seat behavior as Charley sitting in his chair. Ms. Campana and the classroom aide, Ms. Mazze, began to take

> The behavioral definition should provide a clear and objective picture of exactly what the behavior looks like when it is occurring. With a solid definition, multiple observers should be able to agree on the occurrence and nonoccurrence of the target behavior.

data on the number of times the student was in his seat during first period. After a week of collecting data, they realize that their recordings were discrepant. After discussing their observations of the target behavior, they realize that the behavioral definition established was ambiguous and vague. That is, the behavioral definition meant different things to each of them. Specifically, Ms. Campana perceived Charley to be in his seat when he was facing the front of the classroom and sitting on his bottom with both feet on the floor, whereas Ms. Mazze felt that Charley was in his seat as long as the majority of his body was on the chair, even if he was kneeling in his seat and facing the back of the classroom. After this revelation, the teacher and the aide revised the behavioral definition to reduce its ambiguity. Now, in-seat behavior was defined as occurring when Charley's bottom was touching the seat of the chair, body positioned upright, both feet on the floor, and legs and body facing the front of the classroom. The previous example provides a snapshot of a relatively common occurrence within educational contexts. In order to ensure that a target behavior is defined explicitly and includes descriptions of actions that are directly observable, educators should share their definitions with members of the team and allow them to ask questions. Such questions may include, "Tell me what the student currently does," "What is the sequence of actions we are looking for?" or "What do we want the student to do?"

Step 3: Determine How to Collect Data

Once a target behavior has been defined, the next step is to determine how to collect data. Educators and support teams must ask themselves several questions when deciding how to measure the target behavior, including, "Am I (are we) concerned with how often the target behavior occurs?", "Am I (are we) concerned with the length of time a behavior lasts or takes to get started?" or "Am I (are we) interested in the function of a behavior?" Answers to these questions will assist in the determination of what data collection system to use. Specific

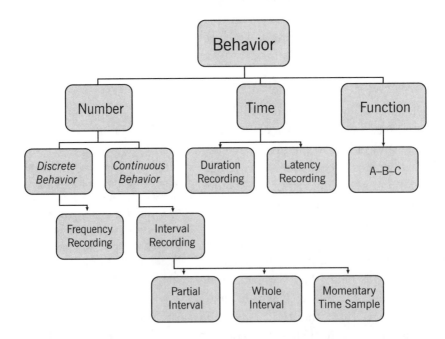

FIGURE 9.1. Decision tree for determining what data collection method to use.

information regarding each data collection system is given in the following paragraphs, and Figure 9.1 provides a decision tree regarding how to select the appropriate data collection system.

Number

FREQUENCY RECORDING

When one is interested in the number of times a behavior occurs, a frequency recording system often is used. Frequency recording is used with behaviors that are discrete—those behaviors that have a clear beginning and end. Only when a target behavior is determined to be discrete can separate instances of the response be counted. Frequency recording requires merely noting the instances in which the behavior occurs by tallying marks on a sheet of paper or using a hand counter. For example, Mrs. Ackerman used a golf stroke counter to track the number of times Dena initiated interactions with her peers during recess. The obvious advantage of frequency counts is that it is relatively easy to gather data. Moreover, educators often are creative in the manner in which they gather frequency data. For example, a former teacher used to collect data regarding the number of times a student "called out" in class by moving a bingo chip from her left pocket to her right. Another teacher simply moved rubber bands from her right hand to her left when recording the number of times a student with HFA/AS did not have the materials for a particular assignment. Figure 9.2 provides a sample frequency recording data sheet. See Form 9.1 in the Appendix for a reproducible version.

The information in a frequency recording system is graphed according to one of two broad methods. If data are taken for the same length of time across sessions (e.g., always 20 minutes), or if the number of opportunities to perform the target behavior is the same across sessions, then the data are reported simply as a frequency count (the number of times the behavior occurred). However, there often are times within educational contexts that the behavior of a student is observed for 30 minutes one day and 20 minutes on another day. Because the time does not remain constant, the frequencies of the behaviors are not comparable. When time is not constant, a *rate of response* can be determined by dividing the frequency of the behavior by the number of minutes the student was observed. A rate of response calculation allows for comparison of different durations of observations.

INTERVAL RECORDING

An interval recording system also can be used when we are interested in recording the number of times a behavior occurs. However, this particular system is used with behaviors that are continuous. With continuous behaviors, it is difficult to count each individual occurrence because there is not a clear beginning or end of the behavior. This may be due to the nature of the target behavior (e.g., behaviors that occur for long periods of time) or behaviors that occur at a high frequency (e.g., hand flapping). Interval recording systems provide an approximation of the actual occurrence of the target behavior (Alberto & Troutman,

Student: Bobbi B.	Time of Day: 10:20–10:40 (typically)
Observer: Hank	Activity: Large-Group Math Instruction
Target Behavior: Blurting/calling out answers without raising hand	

DIRECTIONS: This chart is a quick, nonintrusive way for classroom teachers to record the frequency with which a student displays a particular behavior.

1. Choose an OBSERVATIONAL PERIOD most appropriate to the target behavior. Use the same observation period each day. A minimum of 5 days of charting should be conducted before any intervention is implemented in order to establish baseline information.
2. RECORD: Work upward from the bottom of the column for each day, marking a number each time the target behavior occurs during the evaluation period.
3. CONNECT the highest numbers marked across the columns to graph progress.

Date	9/8	9/9	9/10	9/11	9/12	9/15	9/16	9/17	9/18	9/19	9/22				
	25	25	25	25	25	25	25	25	25	25	25	25	25	25	25
	24	24	24	24	24	24	24	24	24	24	24	24	24	24	24
	23	23	23	23	23	23	23	23	23	23	23	23	23	23	23
	22	22	22	22	22	22	22	22	22	22	22	22	22	22	22
	21	21	21	21	21	21	21	21	21	21	21	21	21	21	21
	20	20	20	20	20	20	20	20	20	20	20	20	20	20	20
	19	19	19	19	19	19	19	19	19	19	19	19	19	19	19
	18	18	18	18	18	18	18	18	18	18	18	18	18	18	18
	17	17	17	17	17	17	17	17	17	17	17	17	17	17	17
	16	16	16	16	16	16	16	16	16	16	16	16	16	16	16
	15	15	15	15	15	15	15	15	15	15	15	15	15	15	15
	14	14	14	14	14	14	14	14	14	14	14	14	14	14	14
	13	13	13	13	13	13	13	13	13	13	13	13	13	13	13
	12	12	12	12	12	12	12	12	12	12	12	12	12	12	12
	11	11	11	11	11	11	11	11	11	11	11	11	11	11	11
	10	10	10	10	10	10	10	10	10	10	10	10	10	10	10
	9	9	9	9	9	9	9	9	9	9	9	9	9	9	9
	8	8	8	8	8	8	8	8	8	8	8	8	8	8	8
	7	7	7	7	7	7	7	7	7	7	7	7	7	7	7
	6	6	6	6	6	6	6	6	6	6	6	6	6	6	6
	5	5	5	5	5	5	5	5	5	5	5	5	5	5	5
	4	4	4	4	4	4	4	4	4	4	4	4	4	4	4
	3	3	3	3	3	3	3	3	3	3	3	3	3	3	3
	2	2	2	2	2	2	2	2	2	2	2	2	2	2	2
	1	1	1	1	1	1	1	1	1	1	1	1	1	1	1
	← Baseline →					← Intervention Phase →									

(Left vertical axis label: FREQUENCY OF BEHAVIOR)

FIGURE 9.2. Sample frequency recording data sheet.

2008). To determine the intervals, the observation period is divided into equal segments or intervals. Typically, the intervals are 15 seconds long, but they can range anywhere from 5 seconds to 1 minute. For example, if the observation time is 20 minutes and the intervals are set at 15 seconds, then there will be 80 intervals. For each interval, the occurrence of a target behavior is recorded with a tally or plus sign (see Figure 9.3).

Within an interval recording system, data can be recorded using a partial interval, a whole interval, or a momentary time-sample procedure (see Alberto & Troutman, 2008, for detailed information regarding data collection procedures). When using a partial-interval recording system, the occurrence of the target behavior is recorded if it occurs *at any time during the interval*. This means that each interval has only one notation regardless of the number of times the behavior occurred. Partial-interval recording methods are often the best choice for behaviors that do not last for a long period of time (e.g., praising others, making a particular comment). The sample data sheet provided in Figure 9.4 provides an example of how a partial-interval recording procedure was used to gather data regarding the occurrence of sportsmanship behaviors during a 20-minute period (divided into 2-minute intervals). During the first 10 minutes of the observation period, the target behavior occurred during three intervals; the first, fourth, and fifth. Over the entire 20-minute period, the target behavior occurred during six, or 30%, of the intervals.

In a whole-interval recording system, the occurrence of the target behavior is recorded only if the behavior occurs *the entire time during the interval*. Whole-interval recording allows educators to record data for ongoing behaviors that may continue for several intervals (Alberto & Troutman, 2008). This method of recording requires that the behavior be present throughout the entire interval if it is to be considered an occurrence. Examples of behaviors that lend themselves to whole-interval recording include writing, reading, working on an assignment, and/or occurrences of social engagement. Figure 9.5 provides an example of a whole-interval recording procedure. Within this example, Dennis was observed to maintain conversations in 8 of the 30 intervals (or 27% of the intervals).

Finally, in momentary time sampling, the observer records whether the behavior occurred or did not occur *at the end of each interval*. For example, at every 30 seconds, the observer will record whether or not the target behavior occurred. Momentary time sampling is concerned with recording the presence or absence of behaviors *within* specified time intervals, whereas interval recording procedures (both partial and whole) are concerned with recording behaviors *during* specified time intervals. Momentary time sampling tends to produce the most accurate estimation of the occurrence of the target behavior. In addition, momentary recording systems tend to be the easiest for educators to implement. In Figure 9.6, a sample data sheet demonstrates the use of momentary time sampling to

Intervals

1	2	3	4	5	6	7	8	9	10
+	+		+			+	+		+

+ = *behavior occurred during interval*

FIGURE 9.3. Example of interval scoring sheet for one individual.

Student: Georgio A.	Date: 9/25/2008
Observer: Marcus	Time Started: 9:30 AM
Setting: Recess	Time Ended: 9:50 AM

Target Behavior: Sportsmanship

Behavior Definition: Following the rules of a game, helping a player up off the ground, offering positive encouragement ("way to go," "good job," "good luck," "maybe next time"), taking turns, etc.

Key: + = Occurrence − = Nonoccurrence

Each interval = 1 minute(s)

1	2	3	4	5	6	7	8	9	10
+	−	−	+	+	−	−	−	−	−
−	−	−	+	−	+	−	+	−	−

Number (Percent) of Intervals of Occurrence:	#: 6 Intervals	%: 30% of Intervals
Number (Percent) of Intervals of Nonoccurrence:	#: 14 Intervals	%: 70% of Intervals

FIGURE 9.4. Sample partial-interval recording data sheet.

Student: Dennis B.	Date: 8/7/2008
Observer: Mr. Butler	Time Started: 12:10 PM
Setting: Lunch	Time Ended: 12:40 PM

Target Behavior: Maintaining conversations

Behavior Definition: Engaging in "small talk," listening to an ongoing conversation and showing approval (e.g., nodding), talking about information heard from a peer in the conversation, engaging in reciprocal conversation

Key: + = Occurrence − = Nonoccurrence

Each interval = 1 minute(s)

1	2	3	4	5	6	7	8	9	10
−	−	−	−	+	−	−	+	+	−
+	+	−	−	−	−	−	−	−	−
−	−	−	−	−	+	+	+	−	−

Number (Percent) of Intervals of Occurrence:	#: 8 Intervals	%: 27% of Intervals
Number (Percent) of Intervals of Nonoccurrence:	#: 22 Intervals	%: 73% of Intervals

FIGURE 9.5. Sample whole-interval recording data sheet.

Student: D. Lux	Date: 6/25/2008
Observer: Rebecca	Time Started: 9:10 AM
Setting: Morning Play Routine	Time Ended: 10:10 AM
Target Behavior: Cooperative play	
Behavior Definition: Sharing toys, developing a plan to build with blocks and/or Legos, engaging in reciprocal interactions while playing with dolls, trucks, puppets, etc.	

Key: + = Occurrence – = Nonoccurrence

Each interval = __10__ minute(s)

*** RECORD AT THE END OF EACH INTERVAL ***

1	2	3	4	5	6	7	8	9	10
+	–	–	+	–	–	–	–	–	–

Number (Percent) of Intervals of Occurrence:	#: 2 Intervals	%: 20% of Intervals
Number (Percent) of Intervals of Nonoccurrence:	#: 8 Intervals	%: 80% of Intervals

FIGURE 9.6. Sample momentary time-sampling recording data sheet.

measure the occurrences of cooperative play of a child with HFA/AS within a summer treatment camp. Over the entire 60-minute period, the target behavior occurred during 2, or 20%, of the intervals. (See Form 9.2 in the Appendix for a reproducible data sheet.)

Time

DURATION RECORDING

A duration recording system is used when educators are interested in the length of time, or *how long*, that a behavior occurs (Alberto & Troutman, 2008). This method is useful for ongoing responses that are continuous rather than discrete and that occur at high rates. For example, Michael, a student with AS, often approaches peers during free play to interact socially but quickly runs away from his classmates. As a result of this behavior, his teacher, Ms. Stevens, is interested in increasing the amount of time that Michael interacts with his peers during free play. Once Michael initiates an interaction with a peer, Ms. Stevens begins timing how long the interaction lasts. She records the duration of the target behavior with a stopwatch or, in some instances, her wristwatch (a clock can also be used).

When one is reporting information obtained from duration recording systems, two procedures can be used: total duration recording or average duration recording. *Total-duration recording* measures the *total amount of time* that a student engages in a targeted behavior during a specified period of observation. Typically, total-duration data are gathered when the number of opportunities to perform the target behavior is the same across sessions. For example, Ms. Stevens may observe Michael's social interactions during recess, an activity that typically lasts for 15 minutes. During one of the observations, Michael was interacting appropriately from 11:30 to 11:35 (5 minutes), from 11:37 to 11:38 (1 minute), and from 11:40 to 11:42 (2 minutes). Such observations established that Michael was socially engaged three times for a total duration of 8 minutes during the observation.

In contrast, *average-duration recording* measures the *average amount of time* that a student engages in a targeted behavior during a period of observation. Typically, the average-duration method is used when the behavior occurs regularly but for extended periods of time. As an example, Mr. McNeil, a sixth-grade social studies teacher, is concerned about Paulo's out-of-seat behavior. Because out-of-seat behavior is a discrete behavior, event recording could be used (i.e., simply tallying the number of times Paulo is out of his seat). However, Mr. McNeil notes that Paulo gets out of his seat only a few times each period but spends much time walking around the room. For this reason, average-duration recording was selected because it permitted the collection of data on how long Paulo was out of his seat in Mr. McNeil's class. On Wednesday, Mr. McNeil began recording the number of minutes Paulo was out of his seat. In that one period, Paulo was out of his seat three times, for 11, 9, and 3 minutes, respectively. If he continued to collect data in this manner for the rest of the week, Mr. McNeil would be able to calculate Paulo's average duration of out-of-seat behavior for the week.

LATENCY RECORDING

A latency recording system is used when educators are interested in measuring the amount of time it takes a student to initiate a requested behavior (Alberto & Troutman, 2008). Specifically, latency recording begins after a direction has been given by the teacher (this is called an antecedent stimulus) and ends when the student engages in the behavior (this is called response initiation). For example, Mr. Willard is concerned with the amount of time it takes Stuart to begin in-class assignments. He decides to use latency recording to gather data on the amount of time it takes Stuart to get out his books and begin assignments (response) once he gives the class directions (antecedent stimulus). Just like duration, latency is measured with the use of a timer, clock, or wristwatch. With latency recording, data are reported as the actual amount of time in seconds, minutes, or hours.

Gathering data for duration or latency is relatively simple. For both, a timing device, such as a stopwatch, wristwatch, or clock, and a simple data collection sheet is all that is needed. A duration recording data sheet should note: (1) the time the student began the target behavior, (2) the time the student ended the target behavior, and (3) the duration of the behavior (see Figure 9.7 for an example, and Form 9.3 in the Appendix for a reproducible version). Similarly, a latency recording sheet should note (1) the time a command or cue was provided to the student (antecedent stimulus), (2) the time the student actually began to respond in the targeted/desired behavior, and (3) the calculated latency of the behavior (see Figure 9.8 for an example, and Form 9.4 in the Appendix for a reproducible version). In addition to these formats, Figures 9.9 and 9.10 provide alternative examples of how duration

Student: Michael C.			Date: 10/6/2008
Observer: George			Time Started: 11:30 AM
Setting: Recess			Time Ended: 11:45 AM
Target Behavior: Social Interaction/Engagement			
Behavior Definition: Instances when child initiates or participates in some play activity or conversation with one or more children; instances when child actively contributed to a reciprocal conversation or attended to a topic of conversation			

Episode	Behavior Started	Behavior Ended	Duration
1	11:30	11:35	5
2	11:37	11:38	1
3	11:40	11:42	2

Total Duration of Target Behavior	8 minutes
Percent of Time Target Behavior Displayed (Duration/Total Time)	53.33%

FIGURE 9.7. Sample duration recording data sheet.

and latency recording procedures can be made into simple data collection sheets based on 20-second intervals (or whatever interval is needed to measure the target behavior). (See Forms 9.5 and 9.6 in the Appendix for reproducible versions.)

Function

A–B–C RECORDING

A–B–C recording is an extremely useful method to help educators identify the function of a behavior. Specifically, A–B–C recording is the process of not only noting a target behavior but also indicating the environmental events that occur immediately before and immediately after the occurrence of the behavior (Alberto & Troutman, 2008). The "A" stands for the antecedent variable that occurred right before the student demonstrated the behavior ("B"). Subsequently, the "C" stands for the consequence that immediately followed the problematic behavior. The purpose of A–B–C recording is to help educators identify response patterns that may set off a behavior and/or maintain its occurrence. Figures 9.11 and 9.12 provide two examples of using A–B–C cards to determine the function of behavior. In the first example, a narrative A–B–C card is used to demonstrate that the student, Brenda, throws tantrums in order to escape a task that she does not want to complete. In the second example, a checklist style A–B–C card that is used to conclude that Vincenzo makes inappropriate comments when a nonpreferred task is introduced in order to get attention from his peers. (See Forms 9.7 and 9.8 in the Appendix for reproducible versions.) Alternative

Student: Jeremy	Date: 10/6/2008
Observer: Lane	Time Started: 1:15 PM
Setting: Social Studies Class	Time Ended: 2:05 PM
Target Behavior: Out-of-Seat	
Behavior Definition: Instances when child is physically out of his seat and walking around the classroom. Out-of-Seat only is recorded if the child is not working on the assigned activities.	
Behavioral Initiation: Child sits in his seat with at least one foot on the floor (sitting on one leg is permitted)	

Episode	Command/Cue	Response	Latency
1	1:23	1:34	11
2	1:37	1:46	9
3	1:50	1:53	3
4	2:00	2:05	5

Total Latency of Target Behavior	28 minutes
Percent of Time Target Behavior Displayed (Latency/Total Time)	56%

FIGURE 9.8. Sample latency recording data sheet.

formats of A–B–C data collection sheets can be found in Alberto & Troutman, 2008; Fad, Patton, & Polloway, 2000; and O'Neill et al., 1997).

Other Useful Data Sources

ANECDOTAL REPORTS

An anecdotal report simply is a complete description of a student's behavior in a particular setting or during instruction (Alberto & Troutman, 2008). Typically, an anecdotal report is written to describe an occurrence within a classroom to report to a principal or parent. For example, it may be reported that "Marcus constantly blurts out answers and does not raise his hand in class," or "Denny cannot seem to get himself under control after he sees the janitor walk by the classroom with a vacuum cleaner," or "Sean constantly is talking about dinosaurs throughout the day and is getting picked on by other students because of it." The use of such reports does not provide objective information regarding the frequency, duration, or function of a student's behavior, but they can be used as a method of analysis when making important educational decisions. That is, anecdotal reports often provide a high degree of qualitative information that can be used by educators when investigating the reasons that an intervention is not working to the degree expected. Very often, anecdotal reports will provide fodder for developing and testing hypotheses aimed at improving the effectiveness of instruction or intervention(s).

Student: Vincenzo	Time of Day: 1:10–1:30
Observer: Billy	Activity: Independent Seat Work
Target Behavior: Singing, humming, and drumming during work time	

DIRECTIONS: This chart is a quick, nonintrusive way for classroom teachers to record how long (duration) a student displays a particular behavior. Each of the numbers represents TIME IN SECONDS.

1. Choose an OBSERVATIONAL PERIOD most appropriate to the target behavior. Use the same observation period each day. A minimum of 5 days of charting should be conducted before any intervention is implemented in order to establish baseline information.
2. RECORD: Work upward from the bottom of the column for each day, marking the time the target behavior occurs during the evaluation period.
3. CONNECT the highest numbers marked across the columns to graph progress.

Date	9/15	9/16	9/17	9/18	9/19	9/22	9/23	9/24	9/25	9/26	9/29				
	10:00	10:00	10:00	10:00	10:00	10:00	10:00	10:00	10:00	10:00	10:00	10:00	10:00	10:00	10:00
	40	40	40	40	40	40	40	40	40	40	40	40	40	40	40
	20	20	20	20	20	20	20	20	20	20	20	20	20	20	20
	9:00	9:00	9:00	9:00	9:00	9:00	9:00	9:00	9:00	9:00	9:00	9:00	9:00	9:00	9:00
	40	40	40	40	40	40	40	40	40	40	40	40	40	40	40
	20	20	20	20	20	20	20	20	20	20	20	20	20	20	20
	8:00	8:00	8:00	8:00	8:00	8:00	8:00	8:00	8:00	8:00	8:00	8:00	8:00	8:00	8:00
	40	40	40	40	40	40	40	40	40	40	40	40	40	40	40
	20	20	20	20	20	20	20	20	20	20	20	20	20	20	20
	7:00	7:00	7:00	(7:00)	7:00	7:00	7:00	7:00	7:00	7:00	7:00	7:00	7:00	7:00	7:00
	40	40	40	40	(40)	40	40	40	40	40	40	40	40	40	40
	20	(20)	20	20	20	20	20	20	20	20	20	20	20	20	20
	6:00	6:00	(6:00)	6:00	6:00	(6:00)	6:00	6:00	6:00	6:00	6:00	6:00	6:00	6:00	6:00
	(40)	40	40	40	40	40	40	40	40	40	40	40	40	40	40
	20	20	20	20	20	20	20	20	20	20	20	20	20	20	20
	5:00	5:00	5:00	5:00	5:00	5:00	5:00	5:00	5:00	5:00	5:00	5:00	5:00	5:00	5:00
	40	40	40	40	40	40	40	(40)	40	40	40	40	40	40	40
	20	20	20	20	20	20	20	20	20	20	20	20	20	20	20
	4:00	4:00	4:00	4:00	4:00	4:00	4:00	4:00	4:00	4:00	4:00	4:00	4:00	4:00	4:00
	40	40	40	40	40	40	(40)	40	40	40	40	40	40	40	40
	20	20	20	20	20	20	20	20	20	(20)	20	20	20	20	20
	3:00	3:00	3:00	3:00	3:00	3:00	3:00	3:00	3:00	3:00	3:00	3:00	3:00	3:00	3:00
	40	40	40	40	40	40	40	40	40	40	(40)	40	40	40	40
	20	20	20	20	20	20	20	20	20	20	20	20	20	20	20
	2:00	2:00	2:00	2:00	2:00	2:00	2:00	2:00	2:00	2:00	2:00	2:00	2:00	2:00	2:00
	40	40	40	40	40	40	40	40	40	40	40	40	40	40	40
	20	20	20	20	20	20	20	20	20	20	20	20	20	20	20
	1:00	1:00	1:00	1:00	1:00	1:00	1:00	1:00	1:00	1:00	1:00	1:00	1:00	1:00	1:00
	40	40	40	40	40	40	40	40	40	40	40	40	40	40	40
	20	20	20	20	20	20	20	20	20	20	20	20	20	20	20
	← Baseline →					← Intervention Phase →									

(Vertical axis label: DURATION OF BEHAVIOR)

FIGURE 9.9. Sample duration recording data sheet.

Student: Rosario	**Time of Day:** 8:35–8:45
Observer: Mrs. C	**Activity:** Transition from bus
Target Behavior: Following verbal commands (backpack, lunch box)	

DIRECTIONS: This chart is a quick, nonintrusive way for classroom teachers to record how long (duration) a student displays a particular behavior. Each of the numbers represents TIME IN SECONDS.

1. Choose an OBSERVATIONAL PERIOD most appropriate to the target behavior. Use the same observation period each day. A minimum of 5 days of charting should be conducted before any intervention is implemented in order to establish baseline information.
2. RECORD: Work upward from the bottom of the column for each day, marking the time the target behavior occurs during the evaluation period.
3. CONNECT the highest numbers marked across the columns to graph progress.

Date	1/6	1/7	1/8	1/9	1/10	1/13	1/14	1/15	1/16	1/17	1/20	1/21	1/22	1/23	
	10:00	10:00	10:00	10:00	10:00	10:00	10:00	10:00	10:00	10:00	10:00	10:00	10:00	10:00	10:00
	40	40	40	40	40	40	40	40	40	40	40	40	40	40	40
	20	20	20	20	20	20	20	20	20	20	20	20	20	20	20
	9:00	9:00	9:00	9:00	9:00	9:00	9:00	9:00	9:00	9:00	9:00	9:00	9:00	9:00	9:00
	40	40	40	40	40	40	40	40	40	40	40	40	40	40	40
	20	20	20	20	20	20	20	20	20	20	20	20	20	20	20
	8:00	8:00	8:00	8:00	8:00	8:00	8:00	8:00	8:00	8:00	8:00	8:00	8:00	8:00	8:00
	40	40	40	40	40	40	40	40	40	40	40	40	40	40	40
	20	20	20	20	20	20	20	20	20	20	20	20	20	20	20
	7:00	7:00	7:00	7:00	7:00	7:00	7:00	7:00	7:00	7:00	7:00	7:00	7:00	7:00	7:00
	40	40	40	40	40	40	40	40	40	40	40	40	40	40	40
	20	20	20	20	20	20	20	20	20	20	20	20	20	20	20
	6:00	6:00	6:00	6:00	6:00	6:00	6:00	6:00	6:00	6:00	6:00	6:00	6:00	6:00	6:00
	40	40	40	40	40	40	40	40	40	40	40	40	40	40	40
	20	20	20	20	20	20	20	20	20	20	20	20	20	20	20
	5:00	5:00	5:00	5:00	5:00	5:00	5:00	5:00	5:00	5:00	5:00	5:00	5:00	5:00	5:00
	40	40	40	40	40	40	40	40	40	40	40	40	40	40	40
	20	20	20	20	20	20	20	20	20	20	20	20	20	20	20
	4:00	4:00	4:00	4:00	4:00	4:00	4:00	4:00	4:00	4:00	4:00	4:00	4:00	4:00	4:00
	40	40	40	40	40	40	40	40	40	40	40	40	40	40	40
	20	20	20	20	20	20	20	20	20	20	20	20	20	20	20
	3:00	3:00	3:00	3:00	3:00	3:00	3:00	3:00	3:00	3:00	3:00	3:00	3:00	3:00	3:00
	40	40	40	40	40	40	40	40	40	40	40	40	40	40	40
	20	20	20	20	20	20	20	20	20	20	20	20	20	20	20
	2:00	2:00	2:00	2:00	2:00	2:00	2:00	2:00	2:00	2:00	2:00	2:00	2:00	2:00	2:00
	40	40	40	40	40	40	40	40	40	40	40	40	40	40	40
	20	20	20	20	20	20	20	20	20	20	20	20	20	20	20
	1:00	1:00	1:00	1:00	1:00	1:00	1:00	1:00	1:00	1:00	1:00	1:00	1:00	1:00	1:00
	40	40	40	40	40	40	40	40	40	40	40	40	40	40	40
	20	20	20	20	20	20	20	20	20	20	20	20	20	20	20
	← Baseline →					← Intervention Phase →								

LATENCY OF BEHAVIOR (vertical label, left side)

FIGURE 9.10. Sample latency recording data sheet.

Student: Brenda Z.	Teacher: P. Leone	Date: 10/30/2008
Location: Classroom	Activity: Transition	Time of Incident: 9:25

A (Antecedent)	B (Behavior)	C (Consequence)
Teacher asks student to clean up.	Stomps feet and cries	Teacher ignores tantrum and sends student to time-out. Once calm, the student goes to next activity.
Teacher tells student that it is time to move to the second activity.	Screams and refuses to look at the teacher	Teacher allows student five more minutes to complete her task.
The teacher told the class to switch centers.	Student throws her toys down and begins crying.	The tantrum is ignored and the student plays with her toys for a few minutes until told again to switch centers.

FIGURE 9.11. Sample A–B–C card (narrative format).

RUBRICS/CHECKLISTS

Additional observational data can be collected using checklists designed to capture the frequency of specific skills. Many forms of checklists can be created that provide a simple way for educators simply to check off whether or not a behavior occurred. For example, the Observation of Apptopriate Social Interaction Skills (OASIS; see Figure 9.13 for an example, and Form 9.9 in the Appendix for a reproducible version), a social skills checklist designed by F. J. Sansosti, can be used to gather additional information regarding the frequency of desired social interaction skills (e.g., eye contact, body basics, conversational skills). The OASIS and other similar checklists are completed by placing a check or tally mark in the appropriate column when one of the stated behaviors occurs. Throughout an intervention, the totals and ratios of yes/no responses can be calculated for each observation or aggregated to compare changes across baseline and intervention phases. Regardless of how the data are used, educators often prefer checklists because they require minimal time to complete. The use of checklists can augment other behavior recording methods and provide valuable information regarding those skills that are not directly targeted for observation.

Step 4: Develop an Action Plan

Once a data collection system is selected, it is important to develop a plan for collecting the data consistently and frequently (this likely will ensure accountability). The plan should address when data will be

> It is important to develop a plan for collecting the data consistently and frequently (this likely will ensure accountability).

Student: Vincenzo P.　　　　**Teacher:** Mrs. Herr　　　　**Date:** 8/28/2008　　**Time of Incident:** 11:40 AM

Behavior: Makes inappropriate comments or swears so the entire class can hear

What Happened Before?	What Happened After?	Activity/Setting
☐ Demand / Request	☐ Behavior Ignored	☐ Structured Activity
☐ Denial	☐ Reprimand / Warning	☐ Unstructured Activity
☐ Difficult Task Introduced	☐ Verbal Redirection	☑ Small-Group Instruction
☑ Nonpreferred Task Introduced	☐ Physical Redirection	☐ Large-Group Instruction
☐ Consequences Imposed	☐ Loss of Privileges	☐ Other (specify): _____
☐ Denied Access to Activity / Object	☐ Removal of Activity / Materials	
☐ Provoked by Another Student	☑ Peer Attention / Laughter	**Additional Comments**
☐ Interruption of Routine / Activity	☐ Adult Attention / Assistance	
☐ Transition Time (Tasks)	☐ Time-Out in Class	**Related Issues:** Illnesses, conflict, fight, fatigue, eating routine, weather, things obtained or avoided . . . .
☐ Transition Setting (Halls, etc.)	☐ Time-Out in Another Class	
☐ Attention Given to Others	☐ Removal from Setting	
☐ No Direct Adult Attention	☐ Office Referral	
☐ Presence of Specific Adult, Peer, or	☐ Suspension: ISS OSS	
☐ Sensory Events (e.g., lights, noise)	☐ Physical Restraint	
☐ Other: _____	☐ Home Note / Parent Conference	
	☐ Other (specify): _____	

FIGURE 9.12. Sample A–B–C card (checklist format).

Student: Clint			Date: 2/24/2007
Observer: H. Davidson			Time Started: 1:15 PM
Setting: Recess Playground			Time Ended: 2:05 PM

Directions. Carefully read each item. Ask yourself if the child can do what the items say. Check either *Yes* or *No* by each item. If you are uncertain or doubt that the child can do what the item says, check *No*.

Check *Yes* for those items that the child can do right now or is beginning to do.

Check *No* if the child cannot do what the item says. Remember, if you have not heard it or seen it, mark *No*.

Yes	No		Items
X		1	Smiles at a familiar person
	X	2	Calls peers by their names
	X	3	Ask questions using words such as "who," "what," and "where"
	X	4	Starts a conversation with his or her peers
X		5	Refers to himself or herself by name
X		6	Makes eye contact with peers close to him or her for at least 5 seconds
	X	7	Uses age-appropriate language to talk to peers
X		8	Responds to other peers verbally, physically, or gesturally
	X	9	Engages in reciprocal conversations with peers
	X	10	Hands something to or receives something from peers
	X	11	Invites others to join in activities
	X	12	Gives compliments to peers
	X	13	Cooperates with peers without prompting
	X	14	Joins ongoing activity or group without being told to do so
	X	15	Accepts peers' ideas for group activities

Total Appropriate Skills: 4   Percentage Appropriate Skills: 27%

FIGURE 9.13. Sample OASIS checklist. From Sansosti (2003). Reprinted with permission of the author.

collected, who will be responsible for collecting data, and where data will be collected within and/or across school, home, and community environments. In addition, this plan should include information on the length of time during which data will be gathered (e.g., 2 weeks), as well as, a suggested date for educators to meet as a team to review data and determine whether the instruction/intervention was effective. Action plans are essential to ensure accountability because they (1) keep educational teams focused on the goals and/or objectives for students, (2) keep educational teams moving toward demonstrable outcomes, and (3) provide educational teams with a record (defensible data) of how much progress has been made (Crone & Horner, 2003).

HOW MUCH DATA SHOULD BE COLLECTED?

Baseline Data Considerations

It is necessary to collect at least three to five data points during the baseline phase of data collection. This will allow educators to describe accurately the student's present level of performance and to predict how the student likely will perform in the future if no intervention is provided (Kazdin, 1994). Aside from gathering sufficient data points, it is vital to determine whether baseline data are stable or whether the trend of the data is going in the opposite direction from what is desired. Stable (defined by Barlow and Hersen, 1984, as three successive data points in the same direction) or countertherapeutic data trends signal to educators that an intervention is needed to improve the student's performance and, more important, provide a unit of comparison for determining success or failure of instruction.

Within school-based settings, it may be difficult to establish pure stability within baseline data. In fact, most educational data likely will demonstrate daily fluctuations (variability) in student performance. Moreover, educational settings frequently lack the resources and time necessary to eliminate such variability (Sidman, 1960). How, then, can educators determine whether baseline data are stable enough to proceed with an intervention and later conclude that there is a causal link (functional relationship) between the student's improved outcomes and the intervention? The key is to decide what level of fluctuation in student performance (variability) is acceptable. For educational settings, a more lenient parameter of 50% variability has been established (Barlow & Hersen, 1984). Figure 9.14 illustrates a procedure for computing the stability of baseline data using this criterion.

Intervention Phase

The answer to how much data should be collected during an intervention phase depends on several factors. First, enough time must pass to ensure that the intervention has had sufficient time to take effect. Although some behavioral changes may be observed within days, others may require weeks. Remember, many of the behavioral and social skills diffi-

Session	Data Value
1	14
2	23
3	16
4	19
5	26

Calculated Mean of Baseline Data	=	(14 + 23 + 16 + 19 + 26)/5= 98/5 = 19.6 = 20
50% of Mean	=	10
Acceptable Range of Baseline Data	=	20 +/− 10 (10 to 30)
Are the Baseline Data Stable?		Yes, because none of the data values vary more than 50% from the mean

FIGURE 9.14. Calculating stability of baseline data.

culties displayed by individuals with HFA/AS are difficult to change quickly and likely will require a significant period of intervention implementation. Although there is no standard for educators to adhere to, interventions for individuals with HFA/AS should be implemented for a minimum of 2 weeks and a maximum of 12 weeks in order to reliably predict that change has occurred. Second, the amount of data collected during an intervention period will depend on specific trends displayed in student performance. For example, trends that signal that an

> **Although there is no standard for educators to adhere to, interventions for individuals with HFA/AS should be implemented for a minimum of 2 weeks and a maximum of 12 weeks in order to reliably predict that change has occurred.**

intervention is effective and results in a rapid change in behavior likely will require less implementation time. Conversely, trends that indicate that behavior is slow to change or require a significant "closing of the gap" between the student's level of performance and that of his or her peers may necessitate additional weeks of intervention. Either way, data trends during the intervention phase will dictate for how long a period interventions should be implemented, as well as provide guidance in determining whether to continue, modify, or discard an intervention(s).

FACTORS THAT INFLUENCE DATA COLLECTION

Four factors may influence the accuracy of data collection: reactivity, simplicity, observer drift, and expectancy (Alberto & Troutman, 2008; Kazdin, 1977, 1994). *Reactivity* refers to changes in a student's behavior when he or she knows that he or she is being watched. Fortunately, reactivity is temporary, if it even occurs at all. Educators can minimize reactivity by taking data from a distance or glancing around the room at other students so that a particular student does not feel that he or she is being watched. Over time, students will become used to being monitored, and their behavior most likely will return to normal. *Simplicity* refers to the ease of the data collection system. Basically, the easier the data collection system is to implement, the more likely the observer will be able to record accurate data. Although some data systems may give more information on the target behavior, educators should use what is feasible within the classroom. Examples of easy-to-use data sheets have been presented throughout this chapter, and educators are encouraged to copy these forms as they appear at the end of the chapter. The third factor, *observer drift*, refers to the tendency of observers to depart from the original definition of the target behavior (Kazdin, 1994). That is, the observer may record behaviors that do not conform to the original definition (Alberto & Troutman, 2008). A retraining session and feedback regarding the definition(s) of behavior can help minimize observer drift and ensure that observers are recording student behavior(s) accurately. Finally, *expectancy* refers to an observer's recording what he or she wants to see from a target student rather than what he or she actually saw. In essence, expectancy is a form of observer bias that results from the sharing of information. Biases can occur due to a student's race, gender, and/or appearance. More often, expectancy bias occurs because parents, teachers, and/or administrators describe positive comments about the student's behavior (e.g., "You should have seen how well Josh did in his group today!" "We are so proud that Suzy is meeting her behavioral goals"). Such comments may cause educators to expect change, and they may make a concentrated effort to find it. Of course, the reverse is also true, and any negative information that is shared can have the same effect on observers (e.g., *Nothing can be done with this student; why even try?*"). AAlthough stringent standards for ensuring that these four factors do not affect data collection most likely are part of research studies, educators should be aware of how the data they collect can be potentially biased.

GRAPHING DATA

So far, this chapter has discussed a variety of methods for gathering performance data using an assortment of formats as an effort to demonstrate increased student outcomes and educator accountability. (*AUTHOR'S WARNING: Collecting data using these methods may result in a significant pile of data sheets!*) However, the mere act of collecting data is meaningless unless the data are used to make important educational decisions. Too often in education, untold amounts of data are collected and then stored away in a filing cabinet or buried on a computer's hard drive, inanimately waiting to be used. To be helpful, data gathered must be presented in a manner that permits various stakeholders to assess that the skill level of a student (or students) with HFA/AS

> **The mere act of collecting data is meaningless unless the data are used to make important educational decisions. Too often in education, untold amounts of data are collected and then stored away in a filing cabinet or buried on a computer's hard drive, inanimately waiting to be used.**

improved across the time of instruction or intervention. The best method for doing so is to use a graph. Graphs not only provide educators with an ongoing analysis (formative evaluation) of the effectiveness of an intervention but also serve as a method of organizing and communicating countless bits of data to other educators, parents, and, perhaps, the child in a quick, interpretable fashion (Alberto & Troutman, 2008). It is far easier to display a picture of the student's progress than it is to thumb through piles of data sheets in an IEP meeting—not to mention, more accountable!

Creating graphs need not be an intimidating task. With the continual advancement of technology, creating graphs on a computer is a relatively easy task (although the execution of patience and some practice is required). Those who are technically savvy can use Microsoft Excel (or Numbers—part of Apple's iWork productivity suite) to organize data and create very appealing graphs. Although presenting step-by-step procedures for creating a graph via these programs is beyond the scope of this chapter, access to easy-to-understand materials is available. Interested readers are encouraged to enter "using Excel to make a graph" into any online search engine to retrieve countless step-by-step tutorials; or search for recent manuals such as *Excel for Dummies* that are available at low costs (go to *www.dummies.com* for product listings). In addition, educators may want to consult with the media personnel within their respective schools or districts. Such individuals may be able to provide resources, assistance, or maybe training in graphing procedures. For those who want to create accurate graphs but do not have the time (or patience!) and resources to do so, use of an online graphing program is recommended. For example, interested readers can use ChartDog 2.0 and The Behavior Reporter, both available at *www.interventioncentral. org.*

METHODS FOR EVALUATING DATA

For the most part, a visual inspection of a graph will indicate whether or not the desired treatment effects were obtained. However, a variety of methods can be used to ensure that changes in behavior from baseline to intervention occurred reliably. Methods of visual analysis such as calculating trend, change in mean level, percent of nonoverlapping data, and effect size are used for evaluating the reliability of change from baseline.

Visual Analysis

Calculating Trends

Trend lines indicate whether the student's performance on the target behavior is increasing, decreasing, or unchanging. When the direction of the data depicted in the graph is obvious, trend lines can be determined simply by visual inspection. However, there may be times when the trend of the data is not so clear and requires more systematic calculation. To calculate a trend within any phase, the quarter-intersect method (see White & Liberty, 1976, for a detailed explanation) can be used (see Figure 9.15)

Obviously, trends that are going in the intended direction indicate that the intervention is effective, whereas trends in the opposite direction, or trend lines that indicate no change, suggest that the intervention is not effective in producing the desired change. If the trend of a student's target behavior is going in the desired direction during baseline and continues into the treatment phase, then educators may conclude that the intervention did not produce the desired change, but rather another variable.

Change in Mean Level

A change in the mean level indicates that a change in the average rate of performance from the baseline to the intervention phase occurred (Alberto & Troutman, 2008). In each phase, the mean is determined by taking the sum of the data and dividing the sum by the total number of data points. The mean of the data for each phase may be indicated on the graph by drawing a dashed horizontal line corresponding to the appropriate level (see Figure 9.16 for an example). Educators should examine the degree of the mean change and whether the change occurred in the appropriate direction.

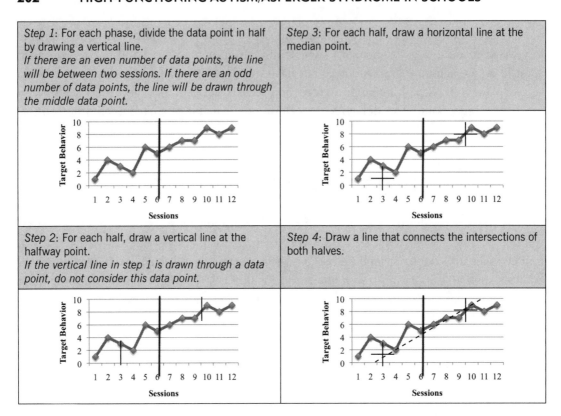

Step 1: For each phase, divide the data point in half by drawing a vertical line. *If there are an even number of data points, the line will be between two sessions. If there are an odd number of data points, the line will be drawn through the middle data point.*	*Step 3*: For each half, draw a horizontal line at the median point.

Step 2: For each half, draw a vertical line at the halfway point. *If the vertical line in step 1 is drawn through a data point, do not consider this data point.*	*Step 4*: Draw a line that connects the intersections of both halves.

FIGURE 9.15. Steps for calculating trends.

Percentage of Nonoverlapping Data

The percentage of nonoverlapping data (PND) provides an indication of the impact of an intervention on the target behavior (Alberto & Troutman, 2008). This is calculated by determining the range of data points in the baseline condition, counting the number of data points in the treatment condition that do not fall within the range of the baseline data points, dividing the number of data points in the treatment condition that do not fall within the range of the baseline data points by the total number of data points in the treatment con-

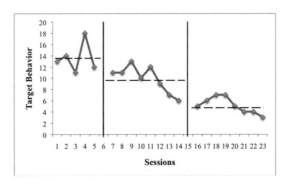

FIGURE 9.16. Example of mean change.

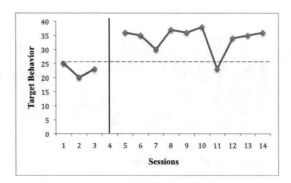

FIGURE 9.17. Sample percentage nonoverlapping data calculation. Within this example, all but the sixth intervention data point are above the highest baseline data point. Therefore, 9 of the 10 intervention data points do not overlap with the baseline—the PND = 90%.

dition, and then multiplying this number by 100 (to calculate a percentage). The higher the percentage obtained, the stronger the intervention effectiveness. Specifically, PND scores above 85% indicate that the intervention was highly effective. Scores between 65% and 85% show moderate intervention effects. PND scores of 65% or below suggest that the effects of the intervention were weak. See Figure 9.17 for an example of PND calculation.

Calculating PND allows educators to determine the extent of fluctuation (variability) of students' skills from day to day. Naturally, the more stable the data are, the easier it is to predict future behavior and draw conclusions about the impact of the intervention. Within applied settings, data that fall within 50% of the mean are commonly considered stable (Alberto & Troutman, 2008). As was demonstrated earlier with regard to baseline stability, the percentage of variability is determined by the following three steps (1) determine the mean, (2) divide the mean by two, and (3) add and subtract the quotient determined in the previous step to and from the mean. Data points that fall within the boundaries are determined to be within 50% of the mean and are considered stable. If a data point falls on or outside the boundary line, then the student's performance is considered to be highly variable.

Effect Size

Typically, the effectiveness of an intervention in single-subject research or evaluation is determined by visual inspection of graphical data. Through visual inspection, a large effect is indicated by a stark contrast in the levels of data between the baseline and intervention phase(s). However, when a visual effect is not large, a reliable method of quantification is needed to detect treatment effects. Effect size measures the magnitude of the effect that the intervention had on the target behavior. Typically, effect size is calculated by determining the mean of each phase, subtracting the mean of the treatment phase from the mean of the baseline phase, and dividing the answer obtained in step 2 by the standard deviation of the baseline phase (Busk & Serlin, 1992). As was true with PND, the higher the effect size, the stronger the intervention effectiveness. Specifically, an effect size of 0.80

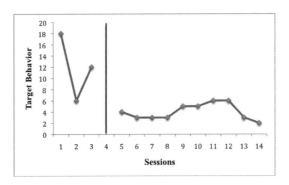

FIGURE 9.18. Sample effect size calculation. *Step 1*: Calculate the mean of the baseline data points. In the example above, the mean of the three baseline data points (18, 6, 12) is 12.0. *Step 2*: Calculate the mean of the intervention data points. In the example above, the mean of the 10 intervention data points (4, 3, 3, 3, 5, 5, 6, 6, 3, 2) is 4.0. *Step 3*: Calculate the standard deviation of the baseline data points. In the example above, the standard deviation of the three baseline data points (18, 6, 12) is 6.0. *Step 4*: Calculate the difference between the mean of the intervention data and the mean of the baseline data and divide that by the standard deviation of the baseline data. ES = (Mean of intervention data − Mean baseline data)/Standard deviation of baseline data. ES = (4.0 − 12.0)/6.0 = 1.33.

or greater is considered large, an effect size of 0.50–0.79 is considered moderate, and an effect size of 0.20–0.49 is considered small (Cohen, 1988). Figure 9.18 provides directions for calculating effect size. Once the effect size is calculated, interpretation simply refers to the contrast of baseline and intervention levels of performance. When included in reports or discussions, effect sizes allow practitioners to develop a sense of relative strength of the intervention.

Social Validity

The best way to understand social validity is to think of the more familiar concept of consumer satisfaction (Bellini, 2008; Wolf, 1978). In the case of students with HFA/AS, the consumers are parents, teachers, community members, and the child. Specifically, social validity refers to the level of satisfaction, appropriateness, and effectiveness of intervention goals, procedures, and outcomes (Gresham & Lambros, 1998; Wolf, 1978). Methods of social validation typically involve having teachers, parents, and other stakeholders complete rating scales. Several commercially available rating scales measure social validity, such as the Behavioral Intervention Rating Scale (BIRS; Von Brock & Elliott, 1987), the Intervention Rating Profile (IRP-15; Witt & Elliott, 1985), or the Treatment Evaluation Inventory (TEI; Kazdin, 1980). Each of these social validity measures assesses teacher and/or parent perceptions of treatment acceptability and effectiveness of instruction/intervention. The Children's Intervention Rating Profile (CIRP; Witt & Elliott, 1985) is a brief scale for assessing child perceptions of acceptability. In addition to these commercially available measures, educators can create their own tools to assess social validity. For example, educators implementing a Social Story intervention may create an easy-to-complete scale that asks teachers and parents to rate their perceptions regarding the acceptability and effectiveness of using a Social Story, as well as their willingness to continue using such an intervention in the future.

ENSURING SUCCESS: MAINTENANCE AND GENERALIZATION

Programming for Maintenance

Maintenance refers to changes in a target behavior that are maintained at the appropriate level over time and occur without the presence of the intervention. It is essential that strategies be employed for increasing the ability of an individual with HFA/AS to maintain the skill taught through instruction or intervention. There are several simple methods that educators can utilize that have proven effectiveness. First, educators will need to make a decision about when to gradually fade out components of the intervention

> **It is essential that strategies be employed for increasing the ability of an individual with HFA/AS to maintain the skill taught through instruction or intervention.**

and/or decrease the intensity in which the intervention is applied. Second, it is essential that the use of tangible reinforcers, such as edibles, stickers, and tokens, be paired with more naturalistic reinforcers such as play activities, praise, and social engagement. Once the student begins to demonstrate the appropriate target behavior consistently, artificial reinforcers can be faded and replaced by more naturally occurring forms of reinforcement. In addition, educators will want to vary the frequency with which they provide reinforcement. Specifically, educators should move from immediate reinforcement to a more intermittent schedule.

Programming for Generalization

When designing interventions, it is important to program for generalization. Generalization refers to changes in behavior that are maintained over time and occur across settings and related behaviors (Baer, Wolf, & Risley, 1968). In the classroom, educators often design interventions that rely on a "train and hope" approach (Stokes & Baer, 1977). With this approach, educators train students to increase target behaviors under specific conditions and hope that the learned skills will occur when students are in other situations and interacting with different individuals. Children with HFA/AS tend to have difficulty generalizing learned skills, and they have even greater difficulty under this approach. Due to their difficulties with generalization, educators must design interventions that incorporate strategies to facilitate skill generalization.

> **Due to their difficulties with generalization, educators must design interventions that incorporate strategies to facilitate skill generalization.**

Stimulus Generalization

During initial acquisition stages, learning trials often involve educators repeatedly present-ing the same stimulus to a child until he or she masters the skill. For example, Ms. Stevens has a student, Carmen, who has difficulty responding appropriately when people greet him. In order to increase his ability to appropriately answer greetings, Ms. Stevens arranged for the principal to greet this student every day by saying, *"Good morning, Carmen, how is your day?"* Ms. Stevens has worked with Carmen on how to appropriately respond only to this common conversation starter. However, once a skill is mastered, students with HFA/AS may have difficulty demonstrating the learned skill when presented with a different stimulus. For example, Carmen may not know how to appropriately respond if the principal greeted him by saying, *"Hi, Johnny, how are things going?"* In order to facilitate general-ization across various stimuli, teach the target behavior across a variety of exemplars. For instance, Ms. Stevens may want to expose Carmen to a variety of different greetings right away and teach him how his response would be appropriate for each greeting. With this approach, skill acquisition may take longer because the student will need to learn a larger subset of items, but generalization to a novel stimulus may be more likely.

Generalization across Settings

At times, students with HFA/AS may have difficulty functioning in various environments because of their sensitivity to various stimuli (e.g., noise). Due to these distractions, some students with HFA/AS may demonstrate target behaviors in one setting but not another. For example, a student may be able to work well one-on-one with the teacher in the corner of the classroom but may not be able to perform the same target behavior when asked by the teacher in a small-group setting. In order to facilitate generalization across settings, educators need to provide skill training to students in a variety of environments, such as a classroom, the home, and/or a play setting. For students who have a difficult time focusing or shifting attention, educators may want to begin by providing the intervention in a highly structured setting with minimal distractions. Once a student begins to acquire the skill, educators may then gradually expose the child to more naturalistic settings.

Generalization across Persons

Inevitably, some children with HFA/AS fail to demonstrate their target behaviors when interacting with people other than the primary person responsible for implementing the intervention. In order to facilitate generalization across people, educators should keep in mind the roles that a variety of people can play in the implementation of the intervention. The intervention should be designed so that various people can implement the procedures, including teachers, parents, and other educational personnel (e.g., lunchroom monitor, para-professional). Although there may be a primary person responsible for the implementation, the intervention should be provided by other individuals who come into frequent contact with the individual with HFA/AS. For example, educational personnel can increase the number of opportunities that an individual with HFA/AS has to practice his or her skills by training a small group of peers. In addition, additional student services personnel (e.g., speech–language pathologist) who are working with the student should be informed of the intervention protocol and encouraged to incorporate aspects of interventions into their routines. When they do so, opportunities to practice target skills with a variety of individuals are increased.

CONCLUSION

As the educational environment continues to focus on accountability and positive student outcomes, it is imperative that practitioners within schools embrace a model of data-based decision making. Without data, it becomes next to impossible to judge whether or not an individual with HFA/AS has benefited from instruction. Moreover, frequent data collection provides important information on how to modify programming to best meet the needs of a child. As was mentioned throughout this chapter, data collection can be performed through the use of observations, interviews, and rating scales. Typically, most data collection methods for working with individuals with HFA/AS will include observation recording systems such as frequency, duration, latency, and time-sampling procedures. Interviews and rating scales also can be used to reflect educator and/or parent perceptions of progress, as well as the success of the intervention implementation (social validity). Although collecting data is essential to practice, a stack of data sheets reflecting student progress is meaningless without interpretation. Therefore, data must be organized into graphs to demonstrate that instruction has worked or is working and to communicate the impact of instruction to various stakeholders in a quick, interpretable fashion. Data collection need not be a daunting task. Rather, data collection should be thought of as a part of a much larger system of intervention development and implementation. Without the use of data to make important educational decisions, it is likely that administrators and, especially, families of children with HFA/AS will scrutinize practices in schools. Practitioners owe it to themselves and, most important, to the individuals they work with to prove the impact of their services. To do so means frequent and ongoing data collection that demonstrates accountability.

Reproducible Forms

CHAPTER 4

FORM 4.1 Parent Interview of Social Functioning   211

FORM 4.2 Teacher Interview of Social Functioning   213

FORM 4.3 Child Interview of Social Functioning   215

CHAPTER 7

FORM 7.1 Peer Buddies Sociometric Form   217

CHAPTER 8

FORM 8.1 Rubric for Evaluating IEPs Using Criteria from IDEA (2004)   218

FORM 8.2 IEP Program Planning Matrix   220

CHAPTER 9

FORM 9.1 Frequency Recording Data Sheet   221

FORM 9.2 Interval/Momentary Time-Sampling Recording Data Sheet   222

FORM 9.3 Duration Recording Data Sheet (Table Format)   223

FORM 9.4 Latency Recording Data Sheet (Table Format)   224

FORM 9.5 Duration Recording Data Sheet (Graph Format)   225

FORM 9.6 Latency Recording Data Sheet (Graph Format)   226

FORM 9.7 Narrative Antecedent–Behavior–Consequence (A–B–C) Form   227

FORM 9.8 Antecedent–Behavior–Consequence (A–B–C) Checklist   228

FORM 9.9 Observation of Appropriate Social Interaction Skills (OASIS) Checklist   229

Parent Interview of Social Functioning

Social Functioning

1. How many friends does your child have? If none, does he/she express an interest in having friends? Has he/she ever had friends?

   a. How many close friends?

   b. Describe their relationship.

   c. Does he/she prefer playing with younger children rather than same-age peers?

   d. Does he/she appear more comfortable interacting with adults rather than peers?

2. How does your child play with other children?

   a. Does he/she join in games with other children?

   b. Does he/she ask others to join him/her?

   c. Does he/she have trouble taking turns?

3. How does your child typically display his/her emotions?

   a. Are they appropriate to the situation?

   b. Does your child exhibit fear or distress regarding social interactions?

   c. Does he/she avoid social situations?

4. Describe his/her eye contact during social interactions. Does he/she maintain eye contact? If not, what does he/she look at?

5. Does your child appear argumentative when disagreeing with others?

6. Does he/she often say things that are "taken the wrong way" by others?

Social Communication

1. Does your child ask many questions?

   a. To request something (tangible item)?

   b. To request assistance?

   c. To request information about a topic?

   d. To request information about a person?

(cont.)

2. How would you describe the tone of your child's voice?

   a. Different from those of other children?

3. How would you describe your child's ability to engage in conversations?

   a. Are they one-sided or do they involve give and take?
   b. Does he/she have difficulty shifting topics in conversations?
   c. Does he/she initiate interactions? What do these interactions look like?

Interests

1. What are your child's interests? How often does he/she talk about or engage in these activities?

2. Does your child have difficulty transitioning from one activity to another?

   a. Difficulty starting a task?
   b. Difficulty finishing?

3. Does your child have any play behaviors that are different from those of other children his/her age? Describe.

4. Does your child have any sensory sensitivities that interfere with social interactions (sounds, visual, tactile, smells, taste)?

Other Important Questions

1. What are your child's strengths?

2. What are your goals (short and long term) for your child?

3. What do you see as the biggest obstacle to your child's establishing social relationships?

Teacher Interview of Social Functioning

Social Functioning

1. Please describe the student's social relationships with peers.

   a. How many close friends?

   b. Describe their relationship.

   c. What types of children does he/she prefer to play with?

   d. Does he/she appear more comfortable interacting with adults than with peers?

   e. How do other children treat him/her?

2. What does the student typically do at recess?

   a. Does he/she mostly play alone or with other children?

   b. Does he/she join in games with other children?

   c. Does he/she ask others to join him/her?

   d. Does he/she have trouble taking turns?

3. How does the student typically display his/her emotions?

   a. Are they appropriate to the situation?

   b. Does the child exhibit fear or distress regarding social interactions?

   c. How would you describe his/her ability to regulate his/her emotions?

   d. Does he/she avoid social situations?

4. Describe his/her eye contact during social interactions.

   a. Does he/she maintain eye contact?

   b. If not, what does he/she look at?

5. Does the student appear argumentative when disagreeing with others?

6. Does he/she often say things that are "taken the wrong way" by others?

7. Compare the student's social skills to those of students in his/her class.

(cont.)

Communication

1. Describe the student's language ability compared to that of other children in the class. Does the student ask many questions?
   a. To request something (tangible item)?
   b. To request assistance?
   c. To request information about a topic?
   d. To request information about a person?

2. How would your describe the tone of the student's voice?
   a. Different from other children?

3. How would you describe his/her conversational ability?
   a. Are the conversations one-sided or do they involve give and take?
   b. Do the conversations seem planned, or do they appear random and poorly planned?
   c. Does he/she initiate interactions?
   d. How would you describe the quality of his/her interactions?
   e. Does the child have difficulty shifting from one topic to another?

Interests

1. What are the student's interests? How often does he/she talk about or engage in these interests?

2. Does the child have any peculiar play behaviors? Describe.

3. Does the child have any repetitive behaviors (hand flapping, rocking, spinning, etc.)?

4. Does the child have any sensory sensitivities (sounds, visual, tactile, smells, taste) that may hinder social participation?

Other Important Questions

1. What are your major social concerns for the student?

2. What do you feel is a major obstacle to his or her establishing social relationships?

3. What are the student's strengths?

4. What are the goals (short and long term) for the student?

214

Child Interview of Social Functioning

Social

1. How many friends do you have? (If child responds that he/she does not have friends, go to Question 5.)

2. What are their names? What grades are they in? How old are they?

3. Please describe them.

4. What kind of things do you do with your friends? (If the child responds that he/she does not have friends, skip to Question 5.)

5. Would you like to have friends?

6. What is a friend?

7. How are you (or how would you be) a good friend?

8. Do you ever get teased or bullied? Why? What do you do when you are teased or bullied?

9. Do people ever do things that bother you? What?

10. Do you ever do things that bother or upset others? What?

Emotional

1. What kinds of things make you feel happy?

2. What kinds of things make you scared? What makes you nervous? Can you describe what scared feels like? Nervous? (Provide examples if necessary; for instance, "do your hands shake?") What do you do when you feel nervous? Does it help?

3. What kinds of things make you angry? What do you do when you feel angry? Does it help?

4. What kinds of things make you sad? What do you do when you feel sad? Does it help?

5. Do you ever feel lonely? When? What do you do when you feel lonely? Does it help?

6. How do you know when someone else is (sad, happy, scared, angry, etc.)?

(cont.)

Interests/Routines and Stereotypical Behaviors

1. What kind of things do you like to do?

2. How much time do you spend on these interests?

3. Does it bother you when you are asked to switch from one activity to another?

4. Do any sounds bother you?

5. Does it bother you to be in a noisy, crowded room? Where do you work best?

6. What makes you different from other people? The same? (If the child engages in any stereotypical behaviors such as hand flapping, use this answer to assess whether he/she is aware of the behavior and if he/she perceives it as problematic.)

Additional Questions

1. What is your best quality? What do you like most about yourself?

2. What is your worst quality? What do you like least about yourself?

3. If you could change one thing about yourself or your life, what would it be?

Peer Buddies Sociometric Form

On the lines below, you will be asked to name some students in your class. The reason you are being asked to do this is to learn more about children's friendships. Please do not put your name on this paper. Your answers will not be known by anyone. Please do not tell anyone how you answered, and do not talk about this activity with other students in your class once you are done.

1. List the names of three classmates with whom you like to play:

_____

_____

_____

2. List the names of three classmates with whom you do not like to play:

_____

_____

_____

3. List the names of three classmates whom you would invite to your birthday party:

_____

_____

_____

4. List the names of three classmates whom you would not invite to a birthday party:

_____

_____

_____

Rubric for Evaluating IEPs Using Criteria from IDEA (2004)

Key area	Requirement	Yes	No
Student's present levels of academic achievement and functional performance	Statement that explains the effect of a student's disability on his or her educational performance, as well as involvement and progress in the general education curriculum	☐	☐
	Statement that clearly indicates actual performance in academic and functional areas (e.g., behavioral, communication) using measurable data.	☐	☐
	Statement of child's strengths and needs (present levels of academic achievement and functional performance). Details on level of functioning are sufficient to develop goals.	☐	☐
Goals	Statement of measurable annual goals that include goals in academic and/or functional areas.	☐	☐
	Goals are written using specific, observable, and measurable terms.	☐	☐
	Goals describe skills that can realistically be achieved within 1 year.	☐	☐
	Goals are clearly connected to the statement(s) on the student's present levels of academic achievement and functional performance.	☐	☐
Benchmarks and short-term objectives for students who take alternate assessments	Alternate assessments are included in the IEP.	☐	☐
	At least two objectives written for each goal.	☐	☐
	Each objective includes a condition and measurable behavior.	☐	☐
	Specific criteria that match the skills being measured are written for each objective.	☐	☐
	Objectives are clearly connected to the present levels of academic achievement, functional performance and goals, addressing student abilities and needs.	☐	☐
Measure and report progress	Statement of how a student's progress toward meeting his or her annual goals will be measured.	☐	☐
	Statement on when and how periodic reports will be provided to the student's parents.	☐	☐
	Statement lets the reader know that the reports are issued as frequently as students in general education receive their report cards.	☐	☐

From Rosas, Winterman, Kroeger, and Jones (2009). Copyright 2009 by the *International Journal of Applied Educational Studies*. Reprinted with permission in Frank J. Sansosti, Kelly A. Powell-Smith, and Richard J. Cowan (Guilford Press, 2010). Permission to photocopy this form is granted to purchasers of this book for personal use only (see copyright page for details).

Key area	Requirement	Yes	No
Services to achieve goals	Statement of the special education and related services and supplementary aids and services to be provided to the student.	☐	☐
	Statement of the program modifications or supports for school personnel that will enable the student to advance appropriately toward attaining his or her annual goals.	☐	☐
	Statement of the program modifications or supports for school personnel that will enable the student to be involved in and make progress in the general education curriculum.	☐	☐
	Special education and related services and supplementary aids and services are based on peer-reviewed research to the extent practicable.	☐	☐
	Statement that students have access to the general curriculum.	☐	☐
		☐	☐
Least restrictive environment (LRE)	Explain rationale for a child's not participating in general education curriculum.	☐	☐
Accommodations	Accommodations match the services delivered in the classroom on a regular basis.	☐	☐
	Accommodations derived from student needs (present levels of academic achievement and functional performance).	☐	☐
	The accommodations adhere to local and federal guidelines.	☐	☐
		☐	☐
Transition services (beginning at age 16)	Statement of quality-of-life goals: results oriented, focused on improving academic and functional achievement, facilitate movement from school to postschool activities, including postsecondary education, vocational education, integrated employment (including supported employment), continuing and adult education, adult services, independent living, or community participation.	☐	☐
	Vision: based on the child's needs, taking into account the child's strengths, preferences, and interests.	☐	☐
	Resources and interagency collaboration: description of the course of study needed to reach stated goals, including instruction, related services, community experiences, development of employment and other postschool adult living objectives, and, when appropriate, acquisition of daily living skills and functional vocational evaluation.	☐	☐
	Stakeholders: Parents of a child transitioning from Part C services (early childhood) to part B services (school age) can request that an invitation to the initial IEP meeting be sent to representatives of the Part C system to assist with a smooth transition of services.	☐	☐
Technical	Signatures and dates	☐	☐
	Frequency of review	☐	☐
	Location where services will take place	☐	☐
	Duration of services and modifications	☐	☐

IEP Program Planning Matrix

Student Name:		Grade:	Date:
Team Members:			

Abbreviated IEP Objectives	Daily Schedule/Activities											
Content Area: _____												
Content Area: _____												
Content Area: _____												

Frequency Recording Data Sheet

Student:	Time of Day:
Observer:	Activity:
Target Behavior:	

DIRECTIONS: This chart is a quick, nonintrusive way for classroom teachers to record the frequency with which a student displays a particular behavior.

1. Choose an OBSERVATIONAL PERIOD most appropriate to the target behavior. Use the same observation period each day. A minimum of 5 days of charting should be conducted before any intervention is implemented in order to establish baseline information.
2. RECORD: Work upward from the bottom of the column for each day, marking a number each time the target behavior occurs during the evaluation period.
3. CONNECT the highest numbers marked across the columns to graph progress.

Date															
	25	25	25	25	25	25	25	25	25	25	25	25	25	25	25
	24	24	24	24	24	24	24	24	24	24	24	24	24	24	24
	23	23	23	23	23	23	23	23	23	23	23	23	23	23	23
	22	22	22	22	22	22	22	22	22	22	22	22	22	22	22
	21	21	21	21	21	21	21	21	21	21	21	21	21	21	21
	20	20	20	20	20	20	20	20	20	20	20	20	20	20	20
	19	19	19	19	19	19	19	19	19	19	19	19	19	19	19
	18	18	18	18	18	18	18	18	18	18	18	18	18	18	18
	17	17	17	17	17	17	17	17	17	17	17	17	17	17	17
	16	16	16	16	16	16	16	16	16	16	16	16	16	16	16
	15	15	15	15	15	15	15	15	15	15	15	15	15	15	15
	14	14	14	14	14	14	14	14	14	14	14	14	14	14	14
	13	13	13	13	13	13	13	13	13	13	13	13	13	13	13
	12	12	12	12	12	12	12	12	12	12	12	12	12	12	12
	11	11	11	11	11	11	11	11	11	11	11	11	11	11	11
	10	10	10	10	10	10	10	10	10	10	10	10	10	10	10
	9	9	9	9	9	9	9	9	9	9	9	9	9	9	9
	8	8	8	8	8	8	8	8	8	8	8	8	8	8	8
	7	7	7	7	7	7	7	7	7	7	7	7	7	7	7
	6	6	6	6	6	6	6	6	6	6	6	6	6	6	6
	5	5	5	5	5	5	5	5	5	5	5	5	5	5	5
	4	4	4	4	4	4	4	4	4	4	4	4	4	4	4
	3	3	3	3	3	3	3	3	3	3	3	3	3	3	3
	2	2	2	2	2	2	2	2	2	2	2	2	2	2	2
	1	1	1	1	1	1	1	1	1	1	1	1	1	1	1
	← Baseline →					← Intervention Phase →									

(Left vertical axis label: FREQUENCY OF BEHAVIOR)

Interval/Momentary Time-Sampling Recording Data Sheet

Student:	Date:
Observer:	Time Started:
Setting:	Time Ended:
Target Behavior:	
Behavior Definition:	

Key: + = Occurrence − = Nonoccurrence

Each interval = _____ minute(s)

Measurement Format Used:

☐ Whole-Interval Measurement (behavior occurred throughout entire interval)

☐ Partial-Interval Measurement (behavior occurred at some point during interval)

☐ Momentary Time Sampling (behavior occurred at the end of each interval)

1	2	3	4	5	6	7	8	9	10

Number (Percent) of Intervals of Occurrence:	#:	%:
Number (Percent) of Intervals of Nonoccurrence:	#:	%:

Duration Recording Data Sheet (Table Format)

Student:	Date:
Observer:	Time Started:
Setting:	Time Ended:
Target Behavior:	
Behavior Definition:	

Episode	Behavior Started	Behavior Ended	Duration

Total Duration of Target Behavior	
Percent of Time Target Behavior Displayed (Duration/Total Time)	

Latency Recording Data Sheet (Table Format)

Student:	Date:
Observer:	Time Started:
Setting:	Time Ended:
Target Behavior:	
Behavior Definition:	
Behavioral Initiation:	

Episode	Command/Cue	Response	Latency

Total Latency of Target Behavior	
Percent of Time Target Behavior Displayed (Latency/Total Time)	

FORM 9.5

Duration Recording Data Sheet (Graph Format)

Student:	Time of Day:
Observer:	Activity:
Target Behavior:	

DIRECTIONS: This chart is a quick, nonintrusive way for classroom teachers to record how long (duration) a student displays a particular behavior. Each of the numbers represents TIME IN SECONDS.

1. Choose an OBSERVATIONAL PERIOD most appropriate to the target behavior. Use the same observation period each day. A minimum of 5 days of charting should be conducted before any intervention is implemented in order to establish baseline information.
2. RECORD: Work upward from the bottom of the column for each day, marking the time the target behavior occurs during the evaluation period.
3. CONNECT the highest numbers marked across the columns to graph progress.

Date															
DURATION OF BEHAVIOR	10:00	10:00	10:00	10:00	10:00	10:00	10:00	10:00	10:00	10:00	10:00	10:00	10:00	10:00	10:00
	40	40	40	40	40	40	40	40	40	40	40	40	40	40	40
	20	20	20	20	20	20	20	20	20	20	20	20	20	20	20
	9:00	9:00	9:00	9:00	9:00	9:00	9:00	9:00	9:00	9:00	9:00	9:00	9:00	9:00	9:00
	40	40	40	40	40	40	40	40	40	40	40	40	40	40	40
	20	20	20	20	20	20	20	20	20	20	20	20	20	20	20
	8:00	8:00	8:00	8:00	8:00	8:00	8:00	8:00	8:00	8:00	8:00	8:00	8:00	8:00	8:00
	40	40	40	40	40	40	40	40	40	40	40	40	40	40	40
	20	20	20	20	20	20	20	20	20	20	20	20	20	20	20
	7:00	7:00	7:00	7:00	7:00	7:00	7:00	7:00	7:00	7:00	7:00	7:00	7:00	7:00	7:00
	40	40	40	40	40	40	40	40	40	40	40	40	40	40	40
	20	20	20	20	20	20	20	20	20	20	20	20	20	20	20
	6:00	6:00	6:00	6:00	6:00	6:00	6:00	6:00	6:00	6:00	6:00	6:00	6:00	6:00	6:00
	40	40	40	40	40	40	40	40	40	40	40	40	40	40	40
	20	20	20	20	20	20	20	20	20	20	20	20	20	20	20
	5:00	5:00	5:00	5:00	5:00	5:00	5:00	5:00	5:00	5:00	5:00	5:00	5:00	5:00	5:00
	40	40	40	40	40	40	40	40	40	40	40	40	40	40	40
	20	20	20	20	20	20	20	20	20	20	20	20	20	20	20
	4:00	4:00	4:00	4:00	4:00	4:00	4:00	4:00	4:00	4:00	4:00	4:00	4:00	4:00	4:00
	40	40	40	40	40	40	40	40	40	40	40	40	40	40	40
	20	20	20	20	20	20	20	20	20	20	20	20	20	20	20
	3:00	3:00	3:00	3:00	3:00	3:00	3:00	3:00	3:00	3:00	3:00	3:00	3:00	3:00	3:00
	40	40	40	40	40	40	40	40	40	40	40	40	40	40	40
	20	20	20	20	20	20	20	20	20	20	20	20	20	20	20
	2:00	2:00	2:00	2:00	2:00	2:00	2:00	2:00	2:00	2:00	2:00	2:00	2:00	2:00	2:00
	40	40	40	40	40	40	40	40	40	40	40	40	40	40	40
	20	20	20	20	20	20	20	20	20	20	20	20	20	20	20
	1:00	1:00	1:00	1:00	1:00	1:00	1:00	1:00	1:00	1:00	1:00	1:00	1:00	1:00	1:00
	40	40	40	40	40	40	40	40	40	40	40	40	40	40	40
	20	20	20	20	20	20	20	20	20	20	20	20	20	20	20
	← Baseline →					← Intervention Phase →									

Latency Recording Data Sheet (Graph Format)

Student:	Time of Day:
Observer:	Activity:
Target Behavior:	

DIRECTIONS: This chart is a quick, nonintrusive way for classroom teachers to record how long (duration) a student displays a particular behavior. Each of the numbers represents TIME IN SECONDS.

1. Choose an OBSERVATIONAL PERIOD most appropriate to the target behavior. Use the same observation period each day. A minimum of 5 days of charting should be conducted before any intervention is implemented in order to establish baseline information.
2. RECORD: Work upward from the bottom of the column for each day, marking the time the target behavior occurs during the evaluation period.
3. CONNECT the highest numbers marked across the columns to graph progress.

Date															
	10:00	10:00	10:00	10:00	10:00	10:00	10:00	10:00	10:00	10:00	10:00	10:00	10:00	10:00	10:00
	40	40	40	40	40	40	40	40	40	40	40	40	40	40	40
	20	20	20	20	20	20	20	20	20	20	20	20	20	20	20
	9:00	9:00	9:00	9:00	9:00	9:00	9:00	9:00	9:00	9:00	9:00	9:00	9:00	9:00	9:00
	40	40	40	40	40	40	40	40	40	40	40	40	40	40	40
	20	20	20	20	20	20	20	20	20	20	20	20	20	20	20
	8:00	8:00	8:00	8:00	8:00	8:00	8:00	8:00	8:00	8:00	8:00	8:00	8:00	8:00	8:00
	40	40	40	40	40	40	40	40	40	40	40	40	40	40	40
	20	20	20	20	20	20	20	20	20	20	20	20	20	20	20
	7:00	7:00	7:00	7:00	7:00	7:00	7:00	7:00	7:00	7:00	7:00	7:00	7:00	7:00	7:00
	40	40	40	40	40	40	40	40	40	40	40	40	40	40	40
	20	20	20	20	20	20	20	20	20	20	20	20	20	20	20
	6:00	6:00	6:00	6:00	6:00	6:00	6:00	6:00	6:00	6:00	6:00	6:00	6:00	6:00	6:00
	40	40	40	40	40	40	40	40	40	40	40	40	40	40	40
	20	20	20	20	20	20	20	20	20	20	20	20	20	20	20
	5:00	5:00	5:00	5:00	5:00	5:00	5:00	5:00	5:00	5:00	5:00	5:00	5:00	5:00	5:00
	40	40	40	40	40	40	40	40	40	40	40	40	40	40	40
	20	20	20	20	20	20	20	20	20	20	20	20	20	20	20
	4:00	4:00	4:00	4:00	4:00	4:00	4:00	4:00	4:00	4:00	4:00	4:00	4:00	4:00	4:00
	40	40	40	40	40	40	40	40	40	40	40	40	40	40	40
	20	20	20	20	20	20	20	20	20	20	20	20	20	20	20
	3:00	3:00	3:00	3:00	3:00	3:00	3:00	3:00	3:00	3:00	3:00	3:00	3:00	3:00	3:00
	40	40	40	40	40	40	40	40	40	40	40	40	40	40	40
	20	20	20	20	20	20	20	20	20	20	20	20	20	20	20
	2:00	2:00	2:00	2:00	2:00	2:00	2:00	2:00	2:00	2:00	2:00	2:00	2:00	2:00	2:00
	40	40	40	40	40	40	40	40	40	40	40	40	40	40	40
	20	20	20	20	20	20	20	20	20	20	20	20	20	20	20
	1:00	1:00	1:00	1:00	1:00	1:00	1:00	1:00	1:00	1:00	1:00	1:00	1:00	1:00	1:00
	40	40	40	40	40	40	40	40	40	40	40	40	40	40	40
	20	20	20	20	20	20	20	20	20	20	20	20	20	20	20
	← Baseline →					← Intervention Phase →									

LATENCY OF BEHAVIOR

Narrative Antecedent–Behavior–Consequence (A–B–C) Form

Student:	Teacher:	Date:
Location:	Activity:	Time of Incident:

A (Antecedent)	B (Behavior)	C (Consequence)

Antecedent–Behavior–Consequence (A–B–C) Checklist

Student:	Teacher:	Date:	Time of Incident:

Behavior:

Activity/Setting

- ☐ Structured Activity
- ☐ Unstructured Activity
- ☐ Small-Group Instruction
- ☐ Large-Group Instruction
- ☐ Other (specify): _____

What Happened Before?

- ☐ Demand / Request
- ☐ Denial
- ☐ Difficult Task Introduced
- ☐ Nonpreferred Task Introduced
- ☐ Consequences Imposed
- ☐ Denied Access to Activity / Object
- ☐ Provoked by Another Student
- ☐ Interruption of Routine / Activity
- ☐ Transition Time (Tasks)
- ☐ Transition Setting (Halls, etc.)
- ☐ Attention Given to Others
- ☐ No Direct Adult Attention
- ☐ Presence of Specific Adult, Peer, or Sensory Events (e.g., lights, noise)
- ☐ Other: _____

What Happened After?

- ☐ Behavior Ignored
- ☐ Reprimand / Warning
- ☐ Verbal Redirection
- ☐ Physical Redirection
- ☐ Loss of Privileges
- ☐ Removal of Activity / Materials
- ☐ Peer Attention / Laughter
- ☐ Adult Attention / Assistance
- ☐ Time-Out in Class
- ☐ Time-Out in Another Class
- ☐ Removal from Setting
- ☐ Office Referral
- ☐ Suspension: ISS OSS
- ☐ Physical Restraint
- ☐ Home Note / Parent Conference
- ☐ Other (specify): _____

Additional Comments

Related Issues: Illnesses, conflict, fight, fatigue, eating routine, weather, things obtained or avoided . . . .

_____
_____
_____
_____
_____
_____
_____

FORM 9.9

Observation of Appropriate Social Interaction Skills (OASIS) Checklist

Student:	Date:
Observer:	Time Started:
Setting:	Time Ended:

Directions. Carefully read each item. Ask yourself if the child can do what the items say. Check either *Yes* or *No* by each item. If you are uncertain or doubt that the child can do what the item says, check *No*.

Check *Yes* for those items that the child can do right now or is beginning to do.

Check *No* if the child cannot do what the item says. Remember, if you have not heard it or seen it, mark *No*.

Yes	No		Items
		1	Smiles at a familiar person
		2	Calls peers by their names
		3	Ask questions using words such as "who," "what," and "where"
		4	Starts a conversation with his or her peers
		5	Refers to himself or herself by name
		6	Makes eye contact with peers close to him or her for at least 5 seconds
		7	Uses age-appropriate language to talk to peers
		8	Responds to other peers verbally, physically, or gesturally
		9	Engages in reciprocal conversations with peers
		10	Hands something to or receives something from peers
		11	Invites others to join in activities
		12	Gives compliments to peers
		13	Cooperates with peers without prompting
		14	Joins ongoing activity or group without being told to do so
		15	Accepts peers' ideas for group activities

Total Appropriate Skills: _____   Percentage Appropriate Skills: _____

References

Alberto, P. A., & Troutman, A. C. (2008). *Applied behavioral analysis for teachers* (8th ed.). Upper Saddle River, NJ: Merrill Prentice Hall.

Allik, H., Larsson, J. O., & Smedje, H. (2006). Sleep patterns of school-age children with Asperger syndrome or high-functioning autism. *Journal of Autism and Developmental Disorders, 36,* 585–595.

American Psychiatric Association. (2000). *Diagnostic and statistical manual of mental disorders* (4th ed., text rev.). Washington, DC: Author.

Apple, A . L., Billingsley, F., & Schwartz, I. S. (2005). Effects of video modeling alone and with self-management on compliment-giving behaviors of children with high-functioning ASD. *Journal of Positive Behavior Interventions, 7,* 33–46.

Aspy, R., & Grossman, B. G. (2007). *The ziggurat model: A framework for designing comprehensive interventions for individuals with high-functioning autism and Asperger syndrome.* Shawnee Mission, KS: Autism Asperger Publishing.

Attwood, T. (1998). *Asperger's syndrome: A guide for parents and professionals.* London: Kingsley.

Attwood, T. (2000). Strategies for improving the social integration of children with Asperger syndrome. *Autism, 4,* 85–100.

Attwood, T. (2007). *The complete guide to Asperger's syndrome.* London: Kingsley.

Bacon, A. L., Fein, D., Morris, R., Waterhouse, L., & Allen, D. (1998). The responses of autistic children to the distress of others. *Journal of Autism and Developmental Disorders, 28,* 129–142.

Baer, D. M., Wolf, M. M., & Risley, T. R. (1968). Some current dimensions of applied behavior analysis. *Journal of Applied Behavior Analysis, 1,* 91–97.

Baker, J. E. (2003). *Social skills training for children and adolescents with Asperger syndrome and social communication problems.* Shawnee Mission, KS: Autism Asperger Publishing.

Bandura, A. (1977). *Social learning theory.* Englewood Cliffs, NJ: Prentice Hall.

Bandura. A. (1986). *Social foundations of thought and action: A social cognitive theory.* Englewood Cliffs, NJ: Prentice Hall.

Bar-Lev, N. B. (2008). *Memorandum: Examples and tips of making IEP annual goals measurable.* Retrieved September 27, 2008, from *www.fetaweb.com/03/iep.goals.revise.measurable2.htm.*

Barnard, J., Harvey, J., Prior, A., & Potter, D. (2001). *Ignored or ineligible?: The reality for adults with autism spectrum disorders.* London: National Autistic Society.

Barnhill, G. P. (2007). Outcomes of adults with

Asperger syndrome. *Focus on Autism and Other Developmental Disabilities, 22,* 116–126.

Barnhill, G. P., Hagiwara, T., Myles, B. S., Simpson, R. L., Brick, M. L, & Griswold, D. E. (2000). Parent, teacher, and self-report of problem and adaptive behaviors in children and adolescents with Asperger syndrome. *Diagnostique, 25,* 147–167.

Barlow, D. H., & Hersen, M. (1984). *Single case experimental designs: Strategies for studying behavior change* (2nd ed.). New York: Pergamon Press.

Baron-Cohen, S. (2002). The extreme male brain theory of autism. *Trends in Cognitive Sciences, 6,* 248–254.

Baron-Cohen, S., & Swettenham, J. (1997). Theory of mind in autism: Its relationship to executive function and central coherence. In D. Cohen & F. Volkmar (Eds.), *Handbook of autism and pervasive developmental disorders* (2nd ed., pp. 880–893). New York: Wiley.

Barry, L., & Burlew, S. (2004). Using Social Stories to teach choice and play skills to children with autism. *Focus on Autism and Other Developmental Disabilities, 19,* 45–51.

Barton, M., & Volkmar, F. (1998). How commonly are known medical conditions associated with autism? *Journal of Autism and Developmental Disorders, 28,* 273–278.

Bass, J. D., & Mulick, J. A. (2007). Social play skill enhancement of children with autism using peers and siblings as therapists. *Psychology in the Schools, 44,* 727–735.

Batsche, G., Elliott, J., Graden, J., Grimes, J., Kovaleski, J., Prasse, D., et al. (2005). *Response to intervention: Policy considerations and implementation.* Alexandria, VA: National Association of State Directors of Special Education.

Bauer, S. (1996). *Asperger syndrome.* Retrieved April, 3, 20008, from *www.udel.edu/bkirby/asperger.*

Bauminger, N., Shulman, C., & Agam, G. (2003). Peer interaction and loneliness in high-functioning children with autism. *Journal of Autism and Developmental Disorders, 33,* 489–507.

Bellini, S. (2008). *Building social relationships: A systematic approach to teaching social in-* teraction skills to children and adolescents with autism spectrum disorders and other social difficulties. Shawnee Mission, KS: Autism Asperger Publishing.

Bellini, S. (in press). *Autism Social Skills Profile* (ASSP). Shawnee Mission, KS: Autism Asperger Publishing.

Bellini, S., & Akullian, J. (2007). A meta-analysis of video-modeling and video self-modeling interventions for children and adolescents with autism spectrum disorders. *Exceptional Children, 73,* 264–287.

Bellini, S., & Hopf, A. (2007). The development of the Autism Social Skills Profile: A preliminary analysis of psychometric properties. *Focus on Autism and Other Developmental Disabilities, 22,* 80–87.

Bennetto, L., Pennington, B. F., & Rogers, S. J. (1996). Intact and impaired memory functions in autism. *Child Development, 67,* 1816–1835.

Bergan, J. R., & Kratochwill, T. R. (1990). *Behavioral consultation and therapy.* New York: Plenum Press.

Berkowitz, M. W., & Bier, M. C. (2005). *What works in character education: A research-driven guide for educators.* Washington, DC: Character Education Partnership.

Berney, T. (2004). Asperger syndrome from childhood into adulthood. *Advances in Psychiatric Treatment, 10,* 341–351.

Bertrand, J., Mars, A., Boyle, C., Bove, F., Yeargin-Allsopp, M., & Decoufle, P. (2001). Prevalence of autism in a United States population: The Brick Township, New Jersey, investigation. *Pediatrics, 108,* 1155–1161.

Blankenship, C. S. (1985). Using curriculum-based assessment data to make instructional management decisions. *Exceptional Children, 42,* 233–238.

Board of Education of the Hendrick Hudson School District v. Rowley, 458 U.S. 176 (1982).

Bodfish, J. W. (2004). Training the core features of autism: Are we there yet? *Mental Retardation and Developmental Disabilities Research Reviews, 10,* 318–326.

Bowen, J., Jenson, W. R., & Clark, E. (2004). *School-based interventions for students with behavior problems.* New York: Kluwer Academic/Plenum.

Bracken, B. A., & McCullum, R. S. (1998). *The Universal Nonverbal Intelligence Test* (UNIT). Itasca, IL: Riverside.

Bramlett, R. K., & Murphy, J. J. (1998). School psychology perspectives on consultation: Key contributions in the field. *Journal of Educational and Psychological Consultation, 9,* 29–55.

Bromley, J., Hare, D. J., Davison, K., & Emerson, E. (2004). Mothers supporting a child with autistic spectrum disorders: Social support, mental health status and satisfaction with services. *Autism, 8,* 419–433.

Bronfenbrenner, U. (1979). *The ecology of human development.* Cambridge, MA: Harvard University Press.

Bronfenbrenner, U. (1986). Ecology of the family as a context for human development research perspectives. *Developmental Psychology, 22,* 723–742.

Brown, F., Nietupski, J., & Hamre-Nietupski, S. (1976). The criterion of ultimate functioning and public school services for severely handicapped children. In M. A. Thomas (Ed.), *Hey, don't forget about me: New directions for serving the severely handicapped* (pp. 2–15). Reston, VA: Council for Exceptional Children.

Bruininks, R. H., Woodcock, R. W., Weatherman, R. F., & Hill, B. K. (1984). *Scales of Independent Behavior—Revised (SIB-R).* Itasca, IL: Riverside.

Bryan, L. C., & Gast, D. L. (2000). Teaching on-task and on-schedule behaviors to high-functioning children with autism via picture activity schedules. *Journal of Autism and Developmental Disorders, 30,* 553–568.

Busk, P. L., & Serlin, R. C. (1992). Meta-analysis for single-case research. In T. R. Kratochwill & J. R. Levin (Eds.), *Single-case research design and analysis: New directions for psychology and education* (pp. 187–212). Hillsdale, NJ: Erlbaum.

Callahan, K., & Rademacher, J. A. (1999). Using self-management strategies to increase the on-task behavior of a student with autism. *Journal of Positive Behavior Interventions, 1,* 117–122.

Carr, E. G., & Durand, V. M. (1985). The social–communicative basis of severe behavior problems in children. In S. Reiss & R. R. Bootzin (Eds.), *Theoretical issues in behavior therapy* (pp. 219–254). New York: Academic Press.

Centers for Disease Control and Prevention. (2007). *Autism and developmental disabilities monitoring network.* Retrieved March 3, 2008, from *www.cdc.gov/ncbddd/autism/faq_prevalence.htm.*

Chakrabarti, S., & Fombonne, E. (2001). Pervasive developmental disorders in preschool children. *Journal of the American Medical Association, 285,* 3093–3099.

Chapman, L., & Trowbridge, M. (2000). Social Stories for reducing fear in the outdoors. *Horizons, 11,* 39–40.

Charlop-Christy, M. H., & Daneshvar, S. (2003). Using video modeling to teach perspective taking to children with autism. *Journal of Positive Behavior Interventions, 5,* 12–21.

Charlop-Christy, M. H., & Haymes, L. K. (1998). Using objects of obsession as token reinforcers for children with autism. *Journal of Autism and Developmental Disorders, 28,* 189–198.

Charlop-Christy, M. H., Le, L., & Freeman, K. A. (2000). A comparison of video modeling with in vivo modeling for teaching children with autism. *Journal of Autism and Developmental Disorders, 30,* 537–552.

Chiang, H., & Lin, Y. (2007). Mathematical ability of students with Asperger syndrome and high-functioning autism: A review of the literature. *Autism, 11*(6), 547–556.

Christenson, S. L., & Sheridan, S. M. (2001). *Schools and families: Creating essential connections for learning.* New York: Guilford Press.

Church, C., Alisanski, S., & Amanullah, S. (2000). The social, behavioral, and academic experiences of children with Asperger syndrome. *Focus on Autism and Other Developmental Disabilities, 15,* 12–20.

Cohen, I. L., & Sudhalter, V. (2005). *PDD Behavior Inventory (PDDBI).* Lutz, FL: Psychological Assessment Resources.

Cohen, J. (1988). *Statistical power analysis for the behavioral sciences* (2nd ed.). Hillsdale, NJ: Erlbaum.

Comer, J. P. (1984). Home–school relationships as they affect the academic success of children. *Education and Urban Society, 16,* 323–337.

Committee for Children. (1986). *Second step.* Seattle, WA: Author.

Connolly, A. J. (2008). *KeyMath—Third edition (KeyMath-3.* Circle Pines, MN: American Guidance Resources.

Consortium on the School-Based Promotion of Social Competence. (1996). The school-based promotion of social competence. In R. J. Haggerty, L. R. Sherrod, N. Garmezy, & M. Rutter (Eds.), *Stress, risk, and resilience in children and adolescence: Processes, mechanisms, and interventions* (pp. 268–316). New York: Cambridge University Press.

Constantino, J. N. (2002). *Social Responsiveness Scale (SRS).* Los Angeles: Western Psychological Services.

Constantino, J. N., Davis, S. A., Todd, R. D., Schindler, M. K., Gross, M. M., Brophy, S. L., et al. (2003). Validation of a brief quantitative measure of autistic traits: Comparison of the social responsiveness scale with the Autism Diagnostic Interview—Revised. *Journal of Autism and Developmental Disorders, 33,* 427–433.

Constantino, J. N., Gruber, C. P., Davis, S., Hayes, S., Passanante, N., & Przybeck, T. (2004). The factor structure of autistic traits. *Journal of Child Psychology and Psychiatry, 45,* 719–726.

Constantino, J. N., Przybeck, T., Friesen, D., & Todd, R. D. (2000). Reciprocal social behavior in children with and without pervasive developmental disorders. *Journal of Developmental and Behavioral Pediatrics, 21,* 2–11.

Cooper, J. O., Heron, T. E., & Heward, W. L. (1987). *Applied behavior analysis.* Columbus, OH: Merrill.

Coucouvanis, J. (2005). *Super skills: A social skills group program for children with Asperger syndrome, high-functioning autism, and related challenges.* Shawnee Mission, KS: Autism Asperger Publishing.

Courchesne, E., & Pierce, K. (2005). Brain overgrowth in autism during a critical time in development: Implications for frontal pyramidal neuron and interneuron development and connectivity. *International Journal of Developmental Neuroscience, 23,* 153–170.

Courchesne, E., Townsend, J. P., Akshoomoff, N. A., Yeung-Courchesne, R., Press, G. A., Murakami, J. W., et al. (1994). A new finding: Impairment in shifting attention in autistic and cerebellar patients. In H. Broman & J. Grafman (Eds.), *Atypical cognitive deficits in developmental disorders: Implications for brain function* (pp. 101–137). Hillsdale, NJ: Erlbaum.

Cowan, R., & Allen, K. D. (2007). Using naturalistic procedures to enhance learning in individuals with autism: A focus on generalized teaching within the school setting. *Psychology in the Schools, 44,* 701–716.

Cowan, R. J., & Sheridan, S. M. (2009). Evidence-based approaches to working with children with disruptive behavior. In T. Gutkin & C. Reynolds (Eds.), *The handbook of school psychology* (4th ed., pp. 569–590). New York: Wiley.

Cowan, R. J., Swearer, S. M., & Sheridan, S. M. (2004). Home–school collaboration. In C. Spielberger (Ed.), *Encyclopedia of applied psychology* (pp. 127–141). San Diego, CA: Academic Press.

Crockett, J. B., & Kauffman, J. M. (1999). *The least restrictive environment: Its origins and interpretations in special education.* Mahwah, NJ: Erlbaum.

Crone, D. A., & Horner, R. H. (2003). *Building positive behavior support systems in schools: Functional behavioral assessment.* New York: Guilford Press.

D'Ateno, P., Mangiapanello, K., & Taylor, B. A. (2003). Using video modeling to teach complex play sequences to a preschooler with autism. *Journal of Positive Behavior Interventions, 5,* 5–11.

Dawson, G., Meltzoff, A. N., Osterling, J., Rinaldi, J., & Brown, E. (1998). Children with autism fail to orient to naturally occurring social stimuli. *Journal of Autism and Developmental Disorders, 28,* 479–485.

deFur, S. H. (2003). IEP and transition planning: From compliance to quality. *Exceptionality, 11*(2), 115–128.

De Martini-Scully, D., Bray, M. A., & Kehle, T. J. (2000). A packaged intervention to reduce disruptive behaviors in general education students. *Psychology in the Schools, 37,* 149–156.

Delano, M. E. (2007a). Improving written language performance of adolescents with Asperger syndrome. *Journal of Applied Behavior Analysis, 40*, 345–351.

Delano, M. E. (2007b). Use of strategy instruction to improve the story writing skills of a student with Asperger syndrome. *Focus on Autism and Other Related Developmental Disabilities, 22*(4), 252–258.

Deno, S. L. (1985). Curriculum-based measurement: The emerging alternative. *Exceptional Children, 52*, 219–232.

Deno, S. L. (1987). Curriculum-based measurement. *Teaching Exceptional Children, 20*, 41.

Deno, S. L. (1990). Individual differences and individual difference: The essential difference of special education. *Journal of Special Education, 24*, 160–173.

Deno, S. L. (1995). School psychologist as problem solver. In A. Thomas & J. Grimes (Eds.), *Best practices in school psychology: III* (pp. 471–484). Washington, DC: National Association of School Psychologists.

Deno, S. L. (2002). Problem solving as best practice. In A. Thomas & J. Grimes (Eds.), *Best practices in school psychology: IV* (pp. 37–55). Bethesda, MD: National Association of School Psychologists.

Deno, S. L., Marston, D. B., & Mirkin, P. (1982). Valid measurement procedures for continuous evaluation of written expression. *Exceptional Children, 48*, 68–71.

Deno, S. L., & Mirkin, P. (1980). Data-based IEP development: An approach to substantive compliance. *Testing Exceptional Children, 12*, 92–97.

DeRosier, M. E., & Mercer, S. H. (2007). Improving student social behavior: The effectiveness of a storytelling-based character education program. *Journal of Research in Character Education, 5*, 131–148.

Donahue, M. L., & Foster, S. K. (2004). Social cognition, conversation, and reading comprehension: How to read a comedy of manners. In C. A. Stone, E. R. Silliman, B. J. Ehren, & K. Apel (Eds.), *Handbook of language and literacy: Development and disorders* (pp. 363–379). New York: Guilford Press.

Doyle, P. D., Jenson, W. R., Clark, E., & Gates, G. (1999). Free time and dots as negative reinforcement to improve academic completion and accuracy for mildly disabled students. *Proven Practice, 2*, 10–15.

Dunn, M. A. (2005). *S. O. S. social skills in our schools: A social skills program for verbal children with pervasive developmental disorders and their typical peers.* Shawnee Mission, KS: Autism Asperger Publishing.

Dunn, W., Saiter, J., & Rinner, L. (2002). Asperger syndrome and sensory processes: A conceptual model and guidance for intervention planning. *Focus on Autism and Other Developmental Disabilities, 17*(3), 172–185.

Edwards, D., Hunt, M. H., Meyers, J., Grogg, K. R., & Jarrett, O. (2005). Acceptability and student outcomes of a violence prevention curriculum. *Journal of Primary Prevention, 26*, 401–418.

Ehlers, S., & Gillberg, C. (1993). The epidemiology of Asperger syndrome: A total population study. *Journal of Child Psychology and Psychiatry and Allied Disciplines, 34*, 1327–1350.

Elliot, C. D. (2007). *Differential Ability Scales—Second Edition* (DAS-II). San Antonio, TX: Psychological Corporation.

Elliot, S., & Gresham, F. (1991). *Social skills intervention guide.* Circle Pines, MN: American Guidance.

Engstrom, I., Ekstrom, L., & Emilsson, B. (2003). Psychological functioning in a group of Swedish adults with Asperger syndrome or high-functioning autism. *Autism, 7*, 99–110.

Epstein, J. L., Sanders, M. G., Simon, B. S., Salinas, K. C., Jansorn, N. R., & Van Voorhis, F. L. (2002). *School, family, and community partnerships: Your handbook for action* (2nd ed.). Thousand Oaks, CA: Corwin.

Fad, K., Patton, J., & Polloway, E. (2000). *Behavioral intervention planning.* Austin, TX: Pro-Ed.

Fiedler, J. F., & Knight, R. R. (1986). Congruence between assessed needs and IEP goals of identified behaviorally disabled students. *Behavioral Disorders, 12*, 22–27.

Fighting Autism. (2008). *Graphing IDEA.* Retrieved March 3, 2008, from *www.fightingautism.org/idea/index.php.*

Fitzgerald, M., & Bellgrove, M. A. (2006). The overlap between alexithymia and Asperger's syndrome. *Journal of Autism and Developmental Disorders, 36*, 573–576.

Flanagan, D. P., & Harrison, P. L. (2005). *Contemporary intellectual assessment: Theories, tests, and issues.* New York: Guilford Press.

Fombonne, E., & Chakrabarti, S. (2001). No evidence for a new variant of measles–mumps–rubella-induced autism. *Pediatrics, 108*, 58.

Frederickson, N., & Turner, J. (2003). Utilizing the classroom peer group to address children's social needs: An evaluation of the Circle of Friends intervention approach. *Journal of Special Education, 36*, 234–245.

Frederickson, N., Warren, L., & Turner, N. (2005). "Circle of Friends": An exploration of impact over time. *Educational Psychology in Practice, 21*, 197–217.

Freeman, R., Eber, L., Anderson, C., Irvin, L., Horner, R., Bounds, M., et al. (2006). Building inclusive school culture using schoolwide positive behavior support: Designing effective individual support systems for students with significant disabilities. *Research and Practice for Persons with Severe Disabilities, 5*, 4–17.

Freitag, C. M., Kleser, C., Schneider, M., & von Gontard, A. (2007). Quantitative assessment of neuromotor function in adolescents with high-functioning autism and Asperger syndrome. *Journal of Autism and Developmental Disorders, 37*, 948–959.

Frey, K. S., Nolen, S. B., Edstrom, L. V., & Hirschstein, M. K. (2005). Effects of a school-based social–emotional competence program: Linking children's goals, attributions, and behavior. *Journal of Applied Developmental Psychology, 26*, 171–200.

Frith, U. (2003). *Autism: Explaining the enigma* (2nd ed.). Malden, MA: Blackwell.

Frith, U. (2004). Emmanuel Miller lecture: Confusions and controversies about Asperger syndrome. *Journal of Child Psychology and Psychiatry and Allied Disciplines, 45*, 672–686.

Fuchs, L. S., & Deno, S. L. (1994). Must instructionally useful performance assessment be based in the curriculum? *Exceptional Children, 61*, 15–24.

Fuchs, L. S., & Fuchs, D. (1986). Effects of systematic formative evaluation: A meta-analysis. *Exceptional Children, 53*, 199–208.

Fuchs, L. S., Fuchs, D., & Hamlett, C. L. (1995). *Monitoring basic skills progress (MBSP): Basic math computation and basic math concepts and applications.* Austin, TX: PRO-ED.

Gagnon, E. (2001). *The Power Card strategy: Using special interests to motivate children and youth with Asperger syndrome and autism.* Shawnee Mission, KS: Autism Asperger Publishing.

Gagnon, E., & Myles, B. S. (1999). *This is Asperger syndrome.* Shawnee Mission, KS: Autism Asperger Publishing.

Gartin, B. C., & Murdick, N. L. (2005). IDEA 2004: The IEP. *Remedial and Special Education, 26*, 327–331.

Gately, S. E. (2008). Facilitating reading comprehension for students on the autism spectrum. *Teaching Exceptional Children, 40*(3), 40–45.

Geir, D. A., & Geir, M. R. (2004). A comparative evaluation of the effects of MMR immunization and mercury doses from thimerosal-containing childhood vaccines on the population prevalence of autism. *Medical Science Monitor, 19*, 133–139.

Geurts, H. M., Verté, S., Oosterlaan, J., Roeyers, H., & Sergeant, J. A. (2004). How specific are executive functioning deficits in attention-deficit/hyperactivity disorder and autism? *Journal of Child Psychology and Psychiatry, 45*, 836–854.

Ghaziuddin, M., Ghaziuddin, N., & Greden, J. (2002). Depression in persons with autism: Implications for research and clinical care. *Journal of Autism and Developmental Disorders, 32*, 299–306.

Ghaziuddin, M., & Mountain-Kimchi, K. (2004). Defining the intellectual profile of Asperger syndrome: Comparison with high-functioning autism. *Journal of Autism and Developmental Disorders, 34*, 279–284.

Gickling, E., & Havertape, J. (1981). *Curriculum-based assessment.* Minneapolis, MN: National School Psychology Inservice Training Network.

Gickling, E. E., Shane, R. L., & Croskery, K. M. (1989). Developing math skills in low-achieving high school students through curriculum-based assessment. *School Psychology Review, 18*(3), 344–355.

Gillberg, C. (2002). *A guide to Asperger's syndrome.* Cambridge, UK: Cambridge University Press.

Gilliam, J. E. (2001). *Gilliam Asperger's Disorder Scale* (GADS). Austin, TX: PRO-ED.

Gilliam, J. E. (2006). *Gilliam Autism Rating Scale—Second Edition* (GARS-2). Austin, TX: PRO-ED.

Gold, D. (1994). "We don't call it a 'circle' ": The ethos of a support group. *Disability and Society, 9,* 435–452.

Goldberg, E. (2001). *The executive brain: Frontal lobes and the civilized mind.* New York: Oxford University Press.

Goldstein, S., Naglieri, J. A., & Ozonoff, S. (2009). *Assessment of autism spectrum disorders.* New York: Guilford Press.

Gould, K., & Pratt, C. (2008). Schoolwide discipline and individual supports for students with autism spectrum disorders. *Principal, 87,* 38–41.

Graham, S., & Harris, K. R. (2005). *Writing better: Effective strategies for teaching students with learning difficulties.* Baltimore: Brookes.

Graham, S., Harris, K. R., MacArthur, C., & Schwartz, S. (1991). Writing and writing instruction for students with learning disabilities: Review of a research program. *Learning Disability Quarterly, 14,* 89–114.

Gray, C. A (2000). *The new social story book.* Arlington, TX: Future Horizons.

Gray, C. A. (2003). *Social Stories 10. 0.* Arlington, TX: Future Horizons.

Gray, C. A., & Garand, J. D. (1993). Social Stories: Improving responses of students with autism with accurate social information. *Focus on Autistic Behavior, 8,* 1–10.

Gresham, F. M. (2002). Social skills assessment and instruction for students with emotional and behavioral disorders. In K. L. Lane, F. M. Gresham, & T. E. O'Shaughnessy (Eds.), *Interventions for children with or at risk for emotional and behavioral disorders* (pp. 242–258). Boston: Allyn & Bacon.

Gresham, F. M., & Elliott, S. N. (1990). *Social Skills Rating System* (SSRS). Circle Pines, MN: American Guidance Service.

Gresham, F. M., & Elliott, S. N. (2008). *Social Skills Improvement System* (SSIS). Minneapolis, MN: Pearson Assessments.

Gresham, F. M., & Lambros, K. M. (1998). Behavioral and functional assessment. In T. S. Watson & F. M. Gresham (Eds.), *Handbook of child behavior therapy* (pp. 3–22). New York: Plenum Press.

Gresham, F. M., Sugai, G., & Horner, R. H. (2001). Interpreting outcomes of social skills training for students with high-incidence disabilities. *Exceptional Children, 67,* 331–344.

Gresham, F. M., & Witt, J. C. (1997). Utility of intelligence tests for treatment planning, classification, and placement decisions: Recent empirical findings and future directions. *School Psychology Quarterly, 12,* 249–267.

Griswold, D. E., Barnhill, G. P., Myles, B. S., Hagiwara, T., & Simpson, R. L. (2002). Asperger syndrome and academic achievement. *Focus on Autism and Other Developmental Disabilities, 17,* 94–102.

Gueldner, B. A. (2006). *An investigation of the effectiveness of a social–emotional learning program with middle school students in a general education setting and the impact of consultation support using performance feedback.* Unpublished doctoral dissertation, University of Oregon, Eugene.

Gutkin, T. B. (1993). Moving from behavioral to ecobehavioral consultation: What's in a name? *Journal of Educational and Psychological Consultation, 4,* 95–99.

Gutkin, T. B. (1996). Core elements of consultation service delivery for special service personnel. *Remedial and Special Education, 17,* 333–340.

Gutkin, T. B., & Curtis, M. J. (1990). School-based consultation: Theory, techniques, and research. In T. B. Gutkin & C. R. Reynolds (Eds.), *The handbook of school psychology* (2nd ed., pp. 577–611). New York: Wiley.

Gutkin, T. B., & Curtis, M. J. (1999). School-based consultation theory and practice: The art and science of indirect service delivery. In T. B. Gutkin & C. R. Reynolds (Eds.), *The handbook of school psychology* (3rd ed., pp. 598–637). New York: Wiley.

Hagiwara, T., & Myles, B. S. (1999). A multimedia social story intervention: Teaching skills to children with autism. *Focus on Autism and Other Developmental Disabilities, 14,* 82–95.

Hammill, D. D., & Larsen, S. C. (2009). *Test of Written Language—Fourth Edition (TOWL-4).* Austin, TX: PRO-ED.

Happé, F. (1997). *Autism: Understanding the mind, fitting together the pieces.* Retrieved May 15, 2008, from *www.mindship.org/happe.htm.*

Happé, F. (1999). Understanding assets and deficits in autism: Why success is more interesting than failure. *Psychologist, 12,* 540–547.

Harlacher, J. E. (2008). *Social and emotional learning as a universal level of support: Evaluating the follow-up effect of Strong Kids on social and emotional outcomes.* Unpublished doctoral dissertation, University of Oregon, Eugene.

Harrington, N. G., Giles, S. M., Hoyle, R. H., Feeney, G. J., & Yungbluth, S. C. (2001). Evaluation of the All Stars character education and problem behavior prevention program: Effects on mediator and outcome variables for middle school students. *Health Education and Behavior, 28,* 533–546.

Harrison, P. L., & Oakland, T. (2003). *Adaptive Behavior Assessment System—Second Edition (ABAS-II).* San Antonio, TX: Psychological Corporation.

Hedley, D., & Young, R. (2006). Social comparison processes and depressive symptoms in children and adolescents with Asperger syndrome. *Autism, 10,* 139–153.

Heimann, M., Nelson, K. E., Tjus, T., & Gillberg, C. (1995). Increasing reading and communication skills in children with autism through an interactive multimedia program. *Journal of Autism and Developmental Disorders, 25,* 459–480.

Hill, E. L., & Frith, U. (2003). Understanding autism: Insights from mind and brain. In U. Frith & E. L. Hill (Eds.), *Autism: Mind and brain* (pp. 1–19). New York: Oxford University Press.

Hintze, J. M., Christ, T. J., & Methe, S. A. (2006). Curriculum-based assessment. *Psychology in the Schools, 43*(1), 45–56.

Honda, H., Shimizu, Y., & Rutter, M. (2005). No effect of MMR withdrawal on the incidence of autism: A total population study. *Journal of Child Psychology and Psychiatry, 46,* 572–579.

Horner, R. H., Sprague, J. R., & Flannery, K. B. (1993). Building functional curricula for students with severe disabilities and severe problem behavior. In R. Van Houton & S. Axelrod (Eds.), *Behavior analysis and treatment* (pp. 47–71). New York: Plenum Press.

Horner, R. H., Sugai, G., Todd, A. W., & Lewis-Palmer, L. (2005). Schoolwide positive behavior support. In L. M. Bambara & L. Kern (Eds.), *Individualized supports for students with problem behaviors* (pp. 359–390). New York: Guilford Press.

Hosp, M. K., & MacConnell, K. L. (2008). Best practices in curriculum-based evaluation in early reading. In A. Thomas & J. Grimes (Eds.), *Best practices in school psychology: V* (pp. 363–396). Bethesda, MD: National Association of School Psychologists.

Howell, K. W. (2008). Best practices in curriculum-based evaluation and advanced reading. In A. Thomas & J. Grimes (Eds.), *Best practices in school psychology: V* (pp. 397–418). Bethesda, MD: National Association of School Psychologists.

Howell, K. W., Hosp, J. L., & Kurns, S. (2008). Best practices in curriculum-based evaluation. In A. Thomas & J. Grimes (Eds.), *Best practices in school psychology: V* (pp. 349–362). Bethesda, MD: National Association of School Psychologists.

Howell, K. W., & Nolet, V. (2000). *Curriculum-based evaluation: Teaching and decision-making* (3rd ed.). Belmont, CA: Wadsworth/Thomson.

Howlin, P. (1998). *Children with autism and Asperger syndrome: A guide for practitioners and carers.* New York: Wiley.

Howlin, P. (2000). Outcome in adult life of more able individuals with Asperger syndrome. *Autism, 4,* 63–83.

Howlin, P., Goode, S., Hutton, J., & Rutter, M. (2004). Adult outcomes for children with autism. *Journal of Child Psychology and Psychiatry, 45,* 212–229.

Hughes, C., Russell, J., & Robbins, T. W. (1994). Evidence for executive dysfunction in autism. *Neuropsychologica, 32,* 477–492.

Hughes, C. A., Schumaker, J. B., Deshler, D. D., & Mercer, C. D. (2002). *Learning strategies curriculum: The test taking strategy* (6th ed.). Lawrence, KS: Edge Enterprise.

Hurlbutt, K., & Chalmers, L. (2004). Employment and adults with Asperger syndrome. *Focus on Autism and Other Developmental Disabilities, 19,* 215–222.

Hurth, J., Shaw, E., Izeman, S. G., Whaley, K., & Rogers, S. J. (1999). Areas of agreement about effective practices among programs serving young children with autism spectrum disorders. *Infants and Young Children, 12,* 17–26.

Hyman, S. L., Rodier, P. M., & Davidson, P. (2001). Pervasive developmental disorders in young children. *Journal of the American Medical Association, 285,* 3141–3142.

Individuals with Disabilities Education Improvement Act of 2004, 20 U.S.C. § 614 *et seq.*

Isava, D. M. (2004). *An investigation of the impact of a social–emotional learning curriculum on problem symptoms and knowledge gains among adolescents in a residential treatment center.* Unpublished doctoral dissertation, University of Oregon, Eugene.

Janney, R., & Snell, M. E. (2011). Planning and implementing instructional programs. In M. E. Snell & F. Brown (Eds.), *Instruction of students with severe disabilities* (7th ed.). Upper Saddle River, NJ: Merrill/Prentice Hall.

Joseph, R. M., Tager-Flusberg, H., & Lord, C. (2002). Cognitive profiles and social–communicative functioning in children with autism spectrum disorder. *Journal of Child Psychology and Psychiatry, 43,* 807–821.

Kalyva, E., & Avramidis, E. (2005). Improving communication between children with autism and their peers through the "Circle of Friends": A small-scale intervention study. *Journal of Applied Research in Intellectual Disabilities, 18,* 253–261.

Kaminski, R. A., Cummings, K. D., Powell-Smith, K. A., & Good, R. H., III. (2008). Best practices in using Dynamic Indicators of Basic Early Literacy Skills (DIBELS) for formative assessment and evaluation. In A. Thomas, & J. Grimes (Eds.), *Best practices in school psychology: V* (pp. 1181–1204). Bethesda, MD: National Association of School Psychologists.

Kaminski, R. A., & Good, R. H., III. (1996). Toward a technology of assessing basic early literacy skills. *School Psychology Review, 25,* 215–227.

Kaminski, R. A., & Good, R. H., III. (1998). Assessing early literacy skills in a problem-solving model: Dynamic Indicators of Basic Early Literacy Skills. In M. R. Shinn (Ed.), *Advanced applications of curriculum-based measurement* (pp. 113–142). New York: Guilford Press.

Kamphaus, R. W. (2001). *Clinical assessment of child and adolescent intelligence* (2nd ed.). Needham Heights, MA: Allyn and Bacon.

Kaufman, A. S., & Kaufman, N. L. (2004). *Kaufman Assessment Battery for Children—Second Edition (KABC-II).* Circle Pines, MN: American Guidance Service.

Kazdin, A. E. (1977). Artifact, bias, and complexity of assessment: The ABC's of reliability. *Journal of Applied Behavior Analysis, 10,* 141–150.

Kazdin, A. E. (1980). Acceptability of alternative treatments for deviant child behavior. *Journal of Applied Behavior Analysis, 13,* 259–273.

Kazdin, A. E. (1994). *Behavior modification in applied settings* (5th ed.). Pacific Grove, CA: Brooks/Cole.

Keeling, K., Myles, B. S., Gagnon, E., & Simpson, R. L. (2003). Using the Power Card strategy to teach sportsmanship skills to a child with autism. *Focus on Autism and Other Developmental Disabilities, 18,* 103–109.

Kehle, T. J., Bray, M. A., Theodore, L. A., Jenson, W. R., & Clark, E. (2000). A multicomponent intervention designed to reduce disruptive classroom behavior. *Psychology in the Schools, 37,* 475–481.

Kelley, B. (2008). Best practices in curriculum-based evaluation and math. In A. Thomas & J. Grimes (Eds.), *Best practices in school psychology: V* (pp. 419–438). Bethesda, MD: National Association of School Psychologists.

Kim, J. A., Szatmari, P., Bryson, S. E., Streiner, D. L., & Wilson, F. J. (2000). The prevalence of anxiety and mood problems among children with autism and Asperger syndrome. *Autism, 4,* 117–132.

Kincaid, D., Childs, K., Blase, K. A., & Wallace, F. (2007). Identifying barriers and facilitators in implementing schoolwide positive behavior support. *Journal of Positive Behavior Interventions, 9,* 174–184.

Kinney, E. M., Vedora, J., & Stromer, R. (2003). Computer-presented video models to teach generative spelling to a child with an autism spectrum disorder. *Journal of Positive Behavior Interventions, 5,* 22–29.

Klin, A., Jones, W., Schultz, R., Volkmar, F., & Cohen, D. (2002). Designing and quantifying the social phenotype in autism. *American Journal of Psychiatry, 159,* 895–908.

Klin, A., McPartland, J., & Volkmar, F. R. (2005). Asperger syndrome. In F. R. Volkmar, R. Paul, A. Klin, & D. J. Cohen (Eds.), *Handbook of autism and pervasive developmental disorders: Vol. 2. Assessment, interventions, and policy* (3rd ed., pp. 88–125). New York: Wiley.

Klin, A., Saulnier, C., Tsatsanis, K., & Volkmar, F. R. (2005). Clinical evaluation in autism spectrum disorders: Psychological assessment within a transdisciplinary framework. In F. R. Volkmar, R. Paul, A. Klin, & D. J. Cohen (Eds.), *Handbook of autism and pervasive developmental disorders: Vol. 2. Assessment, interventions, and policy* (3rd ed., pp. 772–798). New York: Wiley.

Klin, A., Sparrow, S. S., Marans, W. D., Carter, A., & Volkmar, F. R. (2000). Assessment issues in children and adolescents with Asperger syndrome: In A. Klin, F. R. Volkmar, & S. S. Sparrow (Eds.), *Asperger syndrome* (pp. 309–339). New York: Guilford Press.

Klin, A., Sparrow, S. S., Volkmar, F. R., Cicchetti, D. V., & Rourke, B. P. (1995). Asperger syndrome. In B. P. Rourke (Ed.), *Syndrome of nonverbal learning disabilities: Neurodevelopmental manifestations* (pp. 93–118). New York: Guilford Press.

Klin, A., & Volkmar, F. R. (1999). Autism and other pervasive developmental disorders. In S. Goldstein & C. R. Reynolds (Eds.), *Handbook of neurodevelopmental and genetic disorders in children* (pp. 247–274). New York: Guilford Press.

Klin, A., & Volkmar, F. R. (2000). Treatment and intervention guidelines for individuals with Asperger syndrome. In A. Klin, F. R. Volkmar,

& S. S. Sparrow (Eds.), *Asperger syndrome* (pp. 340–366). New York: Guilford Press.

Koegel, L. K., Koegel, R. L., Frea, W., & Green-Hopkins, I. (2003). Priming as a method of coordinating educational services for students with autism. *Language, Speech, and Hearing Services in Schools, 34,* 228–235.

Kolko, D. J., & Kazdin, A. E., (1993). Emotional/behavioral problems in clinic and nonclinic children: Correspondence among child, parent, and teacher reports. *Journal of Child Psychology and Psychiatry, 34,* 991–1006.

Korinek, L., & Popp, P. A. (1997). Integrating social skills with academic instruction. *Preventing School Failure, 4,* 148–152.

Kovacs, M. (1991). *The Children's Depression Inventory.* North Tonawanda, NY: Multi-Health Systems.

Kratochwill, T. R. (2008). Best practices in school-based problem-solving consultation: Applications in prevention and intervention systems. In A. Thomas & J. Grimes (Eds.), *Best practices in school psychology: V* (pp. 1673–1688). Bethesda, MD: National Association of School Psychologists.

Kratochwill, T. R., & Bergan, J. R. (1990). *Behavioral consultation in applied settings: An individual guide.* New York: Plenum.

Kratochwill, T. R., Elliott, S. N., & Busse, R. T. (1995). Behavioral consultation training: A five-year evaluation of consultant and client outcomes. *School Psychology Quarterly, 10,* 87–117.

Kratochwill, T. R., Elliott, S. N., & Callan-Stoiber, K. (2002). Problem-solving consultation. In A. Thomas & J. Grimes (Eds.), *Best practices in school psychology: IV* (pp. 583–608). Bethesda, MD: National Association of School Psychologists.

Kratochwill, T. R., & Stoiber, K. C. (2000). Empirically supported interventions and school psychology: Conceptual and practice issues: Part II. *School Psychology Quarterly, 15,* 233–253.

Krug, D. A., & Arick, J. R. (2003). *Krug Asperger's Disorder Index* (KDAI). Austin, TX: PRO-ED.

Kunce, L. J., & Mesibov, G. B. (1998). Educational approaches to high-functioning autism and Asperger's syndrome. In E. Schopler, G. B. Mesibov, & L. J. Kunce (Eds.), *Asperger syndrome or high functioning autism?* (pp. 227–261). New York: Plenum Press.

Kuttler, S., Myles, B. S., & Carlson, J. K. (1998). The use of Social Stories to reduce precursors to tantrum behavior in a student with autism. *Focus on Autism and Other Developmental Disabilities, 13,* 176–182.

La Greca, A. M. (1999). *Social Anxiety Scales for Children and Adolescents.* Miami, FL: University of Miami.

La Greca, A. M., & Stone, W. L. (1993). Social Anxiety Scale for Children—Revised: Factor structure and concurrent validity. *Journal of Clinical Child Psychology, 22,* 117–127.

Landa, R. (2000). Social language use in Asperger syndrome. In A. Klin, F. R. Volkmar, & S. S. Sparrow (Eds.), *Asperger syndrome* (pp. 125–155). New York: Guilford Press.

Lane, K. L., Wehby, J. H., & Cooley, C. (2006). Teacher expectations of student classroom behavior across the grade span: Which social skills are necessary for success? *Exceptional Children, 72,* 153–167.

Lantz, J. F., Nelson, J. M., & Loftin, R. L. (2004). Guiding children with autism in play: Applying the integrated play group model in school settings. *Teaching Exceptional Children, 37,* 8–14.

Lee, H. J., & Park, H. R. (2007). An integrated literature review on the adaptive behavior of individuals with Asperger syndrome. *Remedial and Special Education, 28,* 132–139.

Lee-Tarver, A. (2006). Are individualized education plans a good thing? A survey of teachers' perceptions of the utility of IEPs in regular education settings. *Journal of Instructional Psychology, 33,* 263–273.

Lickona, T. (1991). *Education for character: How our schools can teach respect and responsibility.* New York: Bantam Books.

Lickona, T., Schaps, E., & Lewis, C. (2007). *CEP's eleven principles of effective character education.* Washington, DC: Character Education Partnership.

Liss, M., Fien, D., Allen, D., Dunn, M., Feinstein, C., Morris, R., et al. (2001). Executive functioning in high-functioning children with autism. *Journal of Child Psychology and Psychiatry, 42,* 261–270.

Lorimer, P. A., Simpson, R. L., Myles, B. S., & Ganz, J. B. (2002). The use of Social Stories as a preventative behavioral intervention in a home setting with a child with autism. *Journal of Positive Behavior Interventions, 4,* 53–60.

Lotter, V. (1967). Epidemiology of autistic conditions in young children: Prevalence. *Social Psychiatry, 1,* 134–137.

Loukusa, S., Leinonen, E., Kuusikko, S., Jussila, K., Mattila, M., Ryder, N., et al. (2007a). Use of context in pragmatic language comprehension by children with Asperger syndrome or high-functioning austism. *Journal of Autism and Developmental Disorders, 37,* 1049–1059.

Loukusa, S., Leinonen, E., Jussila, K., Mattila, M., Ryder, N., Ebeling, H., et al. (2007b). Answering contextually demanding questions: Pragmatic errors produced by children with Asperger syndrome or high-functioning autism. *Journal of Communication Disorders, 40,* 357–381.

Lynn, G. (2007). *The Asperger plus child: How to identify and help children with Asperger syndrome and seven common co-existing conditions.* Shawnee Mission, KS: Autism Asperger Publishing.

MacDonald, R., Clark, M., Garrigan, M., & Vangala, M. (2005). Using video modeling to teach pretend play to children with autism. *Behavioral Interventions, 20,* 225–238.

Macintosh, K., & Dissanayake, C. (2006a). A comparative study of the spontaneous social interactions and social skills of children with high-functioning autism and children with Asperger's disorder. *Autism, 10,* 199–220.

Macintosh, K., & Dissanayake, C. (2006b). Social skills and problem behaviours in school-aged children with high-functioning autism and Asperger's disorder. *Journal of Autism and Developmental Disorders, 36,* 1065–1076.

Maher, C. A., Illback, R. J., & Zins, J. E. (1984). *Organizational psychology in the schools: A handbook for professionals.* Springfield, IL: Thomas.

Maione, L., & Mirenda, P. (2006). Effects of video modeling and video feedback on peer-directed social language skills of a child with autism. *Journal of Positive Behavior Interventions, 8,* 106–118.

Manjiviona, J., & Prior, M. (1995). Comparison of Asperger syndrome and high-functioning autistic children on a test of motor impairment. *Journal of Autism and Developmental Disorders, 25,* 23–29.

March, J. S. (1998). *Multidimensional Anxiety Scale for Children* (MASC). Toronto, Ontario, Canada: Multi-Health Systems.

McAfee, J. (2002). *Navigating the social world: A curriculum for individuals with Asperger's syndrome, high-functioning autism, and related disorders.* Arlington, TX: Future Horizons.

McConaughy, S. H., & Ritter, D. R. (2002) Best practices in multidimensional assessment of emotional or behavioral disorders. In A. Thomas & J. Grimes (Eds.), *Best practices in school psychology: IV* (pp. 1303–1320). Washington, DC: National Association of School Psychologists.

McMahon, S. D., & Washburn, J. (2003). Violence prevention: An evaluation of program effects with urban African-American students. *Journal of Primary Prevention, 24,* 43–62.

McMahon, S. D., Washburn, J., Felix, E. D., Yakin, J., & Childrey, G. (2000). Violence prevention: Program effects on urban preschool and kindergarten children. *Applied and Preventive Psychology, 9,* 271–281.

Meier, C. R., DiPerna, J. C., & Oster, M. M. (2006). Importance of social skills in the elementary grades. *Education and Treatment of Children, 29,* 409–419.

Merrell, K. W. (2007a). *Strong kids—grades 3–5: A social and emotional learning curriculum.* Baltimore: Brookes.

Merrell, K. W. (2007b). *Strong kids—grades 6–8: A social and emotional learning curriculum.* Baltimore: Brookes.

Merrell, K. W., & Gimpel, G. A. (1998). *Social skills of children and adolescents: Conceptualization, assessment, treatment.* Mahwah, NJ: Erlbaum.

Miller, M. C., Cooke, N. L., Test, D. W., & White, R. (2003). Effects of friendship circles on the social interaction of elementary age students with mild disabilities. *Journal of Behavioral Education, 12,* 167–184.

Miltenberger, R. G. (2007). *Behavior modification: Principles and procedures* (4th ed). Belmont, CA: Wadsworth.

Minshew, N. J., & Goldstein, G. (2001). The pattern of intact and impaired memory functions in autism. *Journal of Child Psychology and Psychiatry, 42,* 1095–1101.

Mitchell, P., Parsons, S., & Leonard, A. (2007). Using virtual environments for teaching social understanding to six adolescents with autism spectrum disorders. *Journal of Autism and Developmental Disorders, 37,* 589–600.

Moes, D. R., (1998). Integrating choice-making opportunities within teacher-assigned academic tasks to facilitate the performance of children with autism. *Journal of the Association for the Severely Handicapped, 23,* 319–328.

Moore, D. J. (1998, Autumn). Computers and people with autism/Asperger syndrome. *Communication,* pp. 20–21.

Moore, D., Cheng, Y., McGrath, P., & Powell, N. J. (2005). Collaborative virtual environment technology for people with autism. *Focus on Autism and Other Developmental Disabilities, 20,* 231–243.

Moore, S. T. (2002). *Asperger syndrome and the elementary school experience: Practical solutions for academic and social difficulties.* Shawnee Mission, KS: Autism Asperger Publishing.

Morrison, M. (2008). How to write SMART objectives and SMARTER objectives. Retrieved September 27, 2008, from *www. rapidbi.com/created/WriteSMARTobjectives. html#usesofSMARTERObjectives.*

Mruzek, D. W., Cohen, C., & Smith, T. (2007). Contingency contracting with students with autism spectrum disorders in a public school setting. *Journal of Developmental and Physical Disabilities, 19,* 103–114.

Murray, D., Lesser, M., & Lawson, W. (2005). Attention, monotropism, and the diagnostic criteria for autism. *Autism, 9,* 139–156.

Musarra, N. L. (2006). Information-processing skills related to working memory in individuals with Asperger's disorder. *Dissertation Abstracts International, 66*(8–B), 4494.

Musser, E. H., Bray, M. A., Kehle, T. J., & Jenson, W. R. (2001). Reducing disruptive behavior in students with social and emotional disorders. *School Psychology Review, 30*, 294–304.

Myles, B. S. (2005). *Children and youth with Asperger syndrome: Strategies for success in inclusive settings.* Thousand Oaks, CA: Corwin Press.

Myles, B. S., & Adreon, D. (2001). *Asperger syndrome and adolescence: Practical solutions for school success.* Shawnee Mission, KS: Autism Asperger Publishing.

Myles, B. S., Huggins, A., Rome-Lake, M., Hagiwara, T., Barnhill, G., & Griswold, D. (2003). Written language profile of children and youth with Asperger syndrome: Research to practice. *Education and Training in Developmental Disabilities, 38*, 362–369.

Myles, B. S., Jones-Bock, S., & Simpson, R. (2000). *Asperger Syndrome Diagnostic Scale (ASDS).* Los Angeles: Western Psychological Services.

Myles, B. S., Keeling, K., & Van Horn, C. (2001). Studies using the Power Card strategy. In E. Gagnon (Ed.), *The Power Card strategy: Using special interests to motivate children and youth with Asperger syndrome and autism* (pp. 51–57). Shawnee Mission, KS: Autism Asperger Publishing.

Myles, B. S., Lee, H. J., Smith, S. M., Tien, K., Chou, Y., Swanson, T. C., et al. (2007). A large-scale study of the characteristics of Asperger syndrome. *Education and Training in Developmental Disabilities, 42*, 448–459.

Myles, B. S., & Simpson, R. L. (2001). Understanding the hidden curriculum: An essential social skill for children and youth with Asperger syndrome. *Intervention in School and Clinic, 36*, 279–286.

Myles, B. S., & Simpson, R. L. (2003). *Asperger syndrome: A guide for educators and parents.* Austin, TX: PRO-ED.

Myles, B. S., & Southwick, J. (2005). *Asperger syndrome and difficult moments: Practical solutions for tantrums, rage, and meltdowns.* Shawnee Mission, KS: Autism Asperger Publishing.

Myles, B. S., Trautman, M. L., & Schelvan, M. L. (2004). *The hidden curriculum: Practical solutions for understanding unstated rules in social situations.* Shawnee Mission, KS: Autism Asperger Publishing.

Nation, K., Clarke, P., Wright, B. J., & Williams, C. (2006). Patterns of reading ability in children with autism spectrum disorders. *Journal of Autism and Developmental Disorders, 36*, 911–919.

National Research Council. (2001). *Educating children with autism.* Washington, DC: ational Academy Press.

Nelson, R. O., & Hayes, S. C. (Eds.). (1986). *Conceptual foundations of behavioral assessment.* New York: Guilford Press.

Neumann, L. (2004). *Video modeling: A visual teaching method for children with autism.* Brandon, FL: Willerik.

Nikopoulos, C. K., & Keenan, M. (2004). Effects of video modeling on social initiations by children with autism. *Journal of Applied Behavior Analysis, 37*, 93–96.

No Child Left Behind Act of 2001, 20 U.S.C. § 6301 *et seq.*

Norbury, C. F., & Bishop, D. V. M. (2002). Inferential processing and story recall in children with communication problems: A comparison of specific language impairment, pragmatic language impairment, and high-functioning autism. *International Journal of Language and Communication Disorders, 37*, 227–251.

Norris, C., & Dattilo, J. (1999). Evaluating effects of a Social Story intervention on a young girl with autism. *Focus on Autism and Other Developmental Disabilities, 14*, 180–186.

Nutter, R. E., Algozzine, B., & Lue, M. S. (1982). An evaluation of the implementation of individualized education programs. *Planning and Changing, 13*, 172–180.

Odom, S. L., & Strain, P. S. (1984). Peer-mediated approaches to promoting children's social interaction: A review. *American Journal of Orthopsychiatry, 54*, 544–557.

Office of Special Education Programs. (2004). *Table B4A: Percentage of children served in the 50 states and D.C. (including BIA schools) under IDEA, part B, ages 6–21 by educational environments and disability, 1989–2004.* Retrieved November 20, 2005, from *www.ideadata.org/docs/PartBTrendData/B4A.html.*

O'Connor, I. M., & Klein, P. D. (2004). Exploration of strategies for facilitating the reading comprehension of high-functioning students with autism spectrum disorders. *Journal of*

Autism and Developmental Disorders, 34(2), 115–127.

O'Neill, R. E., Horner, R. H., Albin, R. W., Sprague, J. R., Storey, K., & Newton, J. S. (1997). *Functional assessment and program development for problem behavior: A practical handbook.* Pacific Grove, CA: Brooks/Cole.

Ozonoff, S., Dawson, G., & McPartland, J. (2002). *A parents' guide to Asperger syndrome and high-functioning autism.* New York: Guilford Press.

Ozonoff, S., & Jenson, J. (1999). Brief report: Specific executive function profiles in three neurodevelopmental disorders. *Journal of Autism and Developmental Disorders, 29,* 171–177.

Ozonoff, S., Pennington, B. F., & Rogers, S. J. (1991). Executive function deficits in high-functioning autistic individuals: Relationship to theory of mind. *Journal of Child Psychology and Psychiatry, 32,* 1081–1105.

Ozonoff, S., South, M., & Miller, J. N. (2000). DSM-IV-defined Asperger syndrome: Cognitive, behavioral and early history differentiation from high-functioning autism. *Autism, 4,* 29–46.

Paavonen, E. J., Almqvist, F., Tamminen, T., Moilanen, J., Piha, J., Rasanen, E., et al. (2002). Poor sleep and psychiatric symptoms at school: An epidemiological study. *European Child and Adolescent Psychiatry, 11,* 10–17.

Paine, S. C., Radicchi, J., Rosellini, L. C., Deutchman, L., & Darch, C. B. (1983). *Structuring your classroom for academic success.* Champaign, IL: Research Press.

Patzold, L. M., Richdale, A. L., & Tonge, B. J. (1998). An investigation into sleep characteristics of children with autism and Asperger's disorder. *Journal of Pediatrics and Child Health, 34,* 528–533.

Pelphrey, K. A., Sasson, N. J., Reznick, J. S., Paul, G., Goldman, B. D., & Piven, J. (2002). Visual scanning of faces in autism. *Journal of Autism and Developmental Disorders, 32,* 249–261.

Peterson, S. M., Caniglia, C., & Royster, A. J. (2001). Application of choice-making intervention for a student with multiple maintained problem behavior. *Focus on Autism and Other Developmental Disabilities, 16,* 240–246.

Pierangelo, R., & Giuliani, G. (2008). *Teaching students with autism spectrum disorders.* Thousand Oaks, CA: Corwin Press.

Polimeni, M. A., Richdale, A. L., & Francis, A. J. P. (2005). A survey of sleep problems in autism, Asperger's disorder, and typically developing children. *Journal of Intellectual Disability Research, 49,* 260–268.

Powell-Smith, K. A. (1996). Curriculum-based assessment/curriculum-based measurement. In T. K. Fagan & P. G. Warden (Eds.), *Historical encyclopedia of school psychology* (pp. 100–101). Westport, CT: Greenwood.

Powell-Smith, K. A., & Bradley-Klug, K. L. (2001). Another look at the "C" in CBM: Does it really matter if curriculum-based measurement reading probes are "curriculum-based"? *Psychology in the Schools, 38*(4), 299–312.

Powell-Smith, K. A., & Shinn, M. R. (2004). *AIMSweb training workbook: Administration and scoring of Written Expression Curriculum-Based Measurement (WE-CBM) for use in general outcome measurement.* Eden Prairie, MN: Edformation.

President's Commission on Excellence in Special Education. (2002). *A new era: Revitalizing special education for children and their families.* Washington, DC: U.S. Department of Education.

Prior, M. (2003). *Learning and behavior problems in Asperger syndrome.* New York: Guilford Press.

Quill, K. A. (1997). Instructional consideration for young children with autism. *Journal of Autism and Developmental Disorders, 27,* 607–714.

Quinn, M. M., Kavale, K. A., Mathur, S. R., Rutherford R. B., Jr., & Forness, S. R. (1999). A meta-analysis of social skills interventions for students with emotional and behavioral disorders. *Journal of Emotional and Behavioral Disorders, 7,* 54–64.

Rathvon, N. (2003). *Effective school interventions: Strategies for enhancing academic achievement and social competence.* New York: Guilford Press.

Reschly, D. J. (2008). School psychology paradigm shift and beyond. In A. Thomas & J. Grimes (Eds.), *Best practices in school psychology* (5th ed., pp. 3–15). Bethesda, MD: National Association of School Psychologists.

Redcay, E., & Courchesne, E. (2005). When is

the brain enlarged in autism? A meta-analysis of all brain size reports. *Biological Psychiatry, 58*, 1–9.

Reynhout, G., & Carter, M. (2007). Social Story efficacy with a child with autism spectrum disorder and moderate intellectual disability. *Focus on Autism and Other Developmental Disabilities, 22*, 173–182.

Reynolds, C. R., & Kamphaus, R. W. (2004). *Behavior Assessment System for Children* (2nd ed.). Circle Pines, MN: American Guidance Service.

Reynolds, C. R., & Richmond, B. O. (2008). *Revised Children's Manifest Anxiety Scale* (2nd ed.). Los Angeles: Western Psychological Services.

Reynolds, W. M. (2004). *Reynolds Adolescent Depression Scale* (2nd ed.). Lutz, FL: Psychological Assessment Resources.

Rhode, G., Jenson, W. R., & Reavis, H. K. (1993). *The tough kid book*. Longmont, CO: Sopris West.

Robinson, L. K., & Howell, K. W. (2008). Best practices in curriculum-based evaluation and written expression. In A. Thomas & J. Grimes (Eds.), *Best practices in school psychology: V* (pp. 439–452). Bethesda, MD: National Association of School Psychologists.

Roeyers, H. (1996). The influence of nonhandicapped peers on the social interactions of children with a pervasive developmental disorder. *Journal of Autism and Developmental Disorders, 26*, 303–320.

Roid, G. H. (2003). *Stanford–Binet Intelligence Scale—Fifth Edition*. Itasca, IL: Riverside.

Roid, G. H., & Miller, L. J. (1997). *Leiter International Performance Scale—Revised* (Leiter). Wood Dale, IL: Stoeling.

Rosas, C., Winterman, K. G., Kroeger, S., & Jones, M. M. (2009). Using a rubric to assess individualized education programs. *International Journal of Applied Educational Studies, 4*(1), 47–57.

Rosenberg, M. S., Wilson, R., Maheady, L., & Sindelar, P. T. (2004). *Educating students with behavior disorders*. Boston: Allyn & Bacon.

Rosenfield, S. (1992). Developing school-based consultation teams: A design for organizational change. *School Psychology Quarterly, 7*, 27–46.

Ruth, W. J. (1996). Goal setting and behavior contracting for students with emotional and behavioral difficulties: Analysis of daily, weekly and total goal attainment. *Psychology in the Schools, 33*, 153–158.

Rutter, M., Bailey, A., & Lord, C. (2003). *Social Communication Questionnaire* (SCQ). Los Angeles: Western Psychological Services.

Rutter, M., Le Couteur, A., & Lord, C. (2003). *Autism Diagnostic Interview—Revised* (ADI-R). Los Angeles: Western Psychological Services.

Safran, S. P. (2001). Asperger syndrome: The emerging challenge to special education. *Exceptional Children, 67*, 151–160.

Safran, S. P. (2008). Why youngsters with autistic spectrum disorders remain underrepresented in special education. *Remedial and Special Education, 29*, 90–95.

Sansosti, F. J. (2003). *Effectiveness of Social Story interventions for children with Asperger's syndrome*. Unpublished education specialist thesis, University of South Florida, Tampa, FL.

Sansosti, F. J. (2008). Teaching social behavior to children with autism spectrum disorders using Social Stories: Implications for school-based practice. *Journal of Speech Language Pathology and Applied Behavior Analysis, 2*(4)–*3*(1), 36–45.

Sansosti, F. J., & Powell-Smith, K. A. (2006). High-functioning autism/Asperger's syndrome. In G. Bear & K. Minke (Eds.), *Children's Needs: III. Understanding and addressing the developmental needs of children* (pp. 949–963). Bethesda, MD: National Association of School Psychologists.

Sansosti, F. J., & Powell-Smith, K. A. (2008). Using computer-presented Social Stories and video models to increase the social communication skills of children with high-functioning autism spectrum disorders. *Journal of Positive Behavior Interventions, 10*, 162–178.

Sansosti, F. J., Powell-Smith, K. A., & Kincaid, D. (2004). A research synthesis of Social Story interventions for children with autism spectrum disorders. *Focus on Autism and Other Developmental Disabilities, 19*, 194–204.

Sansosti, J. M. (2008). *The meaning and means of inclusion for students with autism spectrum disorders: A qualitative study of educators' and parents' attitudes, beliefs, and decision-making strategies.* Unpublished doctoral dissertation, University of South Florida.

Satter, D. B. (2007). *Conditions occurring in autism: Other complications in autism spectrum disorder individuals.* Retrieved July 1, 2008, from *autism.suite101.com/article.cfm/conditions_occurring_in_autism.*

Sattler, J. M., & Hoge, R. D. (2006). *Assessment of children: Behavioral and clinical applications* (5th ed.). La Mesa, CA: Sattler.

Scattone, D., Tingstrom, D. H., & Wilczynski, S. M. (2006). Increasing appropriate social interactions of children with autism spectrum disorders using Social Stories. *Focus on Autism and Other Developmental Disabilities, 21,* 211–222.

Scattone, D., Wilczynksi, S. M., Edwards, R. P., & Rabian, B. (2002). Decreasing disruptive behaviors of children with autism using Social Stories. *Journal of Autism and Developmental Disorders, 32,* 535–543.

Seigel, L. M. (2001). *The complete IEP guide: How to advocate for your special ed child* (2nd ed.). Berkeley, CA: Nolo.

Shapiro, E. S. (2004). *Academic skills problems: Direct assessment and intervention* (3rd ed.). New York: Guilford Press.

Sheridan, S. M. (1997). Conceptual and empirical bases of conjoint behavioral consultation. *School Psychology Quarterly, 12,* 119–133.

Sheridan, S. M., Marti, D. C., Burt, J. D., Rohlk, A. M., Garbacz, S. A., Olson, S. C., et al. (2005, April). *Is conjoint behavioral consultation partnership centered?* Paper presented at the annual meeting of the National Association of School Psychologists, Atlanta, GA.

Sheridan, S. M., & Cowan, R. J. (2004). Consultation with school personnel. In R. T. Brown (Ed.), *Handbook of pediatric psychology in school settings* (pp. 599–616). New York: Erlbaum.

Sheridan, S. M., Cowan, R. J., & Eagle, J. W. (2001). Facilitating parental involvement in home–school partnerships for students with disabilities. In C. Telzrow & M. Tankersley (Eds.), *IDEA Amendments of 1997: Practice guidelines for school-based teams* (pp. 307–

350). Bethesda, MD: National Association of School Psychologists.

Sheridan, S. M., Eagle, J. W., Cowan, R. J., & Mickelson, W. (2001). The effects of conjoint behavioral consultation: Results of a four-year investigation. *Journal of School Psychology, 39,* 361–385.

Sheridan, S. M., & Kratochwill, T. R. (1992). Behavioral parent–teacher consultation: Conceptual and research considerations. *Journal of School Psychology, 30,* 117–139.

Sheridan, S. M., & Kratochwill, T. R. (2008). *Conjoint behavioral consultation: Promoting family–school connections and interventions.* New York: Springer.

Sheridan, S. M., Kratochwill, T. R., & Bergan, J. R. (1996). *Conjoint behavioral consultation: A procedural manual.* New York: Plenum.

Sheridan, S. M., Welch, M., & Orme, S. (1996). Is consultation effective? A review of outcome research. *Remedial and Special Education, 17,* 341–354.

Shinn, M. R. (Ed.). (1989). *Curriculum-based measurement: Assessing special children.* New York: Guilford Press.

Shinn, M. R. (Ed.). (1998). *Advanced applications of curriculum-based measurement.* New York: Guilford Press.

Shinn, M. R. (2008). Best practices in curriculum-based measurement and its use in a problem-solving model. In A. Thomas & J. Grimes (Eds.), *Best practices in school psychology: V* (pp. 243–262). Bethesda, MD: National Association of School Psychologists.

Shinn, M. R., & Bamonto, S. (1998). Advanced application of curriculum-based measurement: "big ideas" and avoiding confusion. In M. R. Shinn (Ed.), *Advanced applications of curriculum-based measurement* (pp. 1–31). New York: Guilford Press.

Shinn, M. R., Rosenfield, S., & Knutson, N. (1989). Curriculum-based assessment: A comparison of models. *School Psychology Review, 18,* 299–316.

Sidman, M. (1960). *Tactics of scientific research.* New York: Basic Books.

Siegel, B. (2003). *Helping children with autism learn: A guide to treatment approaches for parents and professionals.* New York: Oxford University Press.

Silverman, S. M., & Weinfeld, R. (2007). *School success for kids with Asperger's syndrome.* Waco, TX: Prufrock Press.

Simonsen, B., Sugai, G., & Negron, M. (2008). Schoolwide positive behavior supports: Primary systems and practices. *Teaching Exceptional Children, 40,* 16–22.

Simpson, R. L., & Myles, B. S. (1998). *Educating children and youth with autism: Strategies for effective practice.* Austin, TX: PRO-ED.

Siperstein, G. N., & Rickards, E. P. (2004). *Promoting social success: A curriculum for children with special needs.* Baltimore: Brookes.

Skiba, R., & Peterson, R. (2003). Teaching the social curriculum: School discipline as instruction. *Preventing School Failure, 47,* 66–73.

Smeeth, L., Cook, C., Fombonne, E., Heavey, O. L., Rodrigues, L. C., Smith, P. G., et al. (2004). MMR vaccination and pervasive developmental disorders: A case–control study. *Lancet, 364,* 963–969.

Smith, B. W., & Sugai, G. (2000). A self-management functional assessment based behavior support plan for a middle school student with EBD. *Journal of Positive Behavior Interventions, 2,* 208–217.

Snell, M. E., & Brown, F. (2005). *Instruction of students with severe disabilities* (6th ed.). Upper Saddle River, NJ: Pearson.

Songlee, D., Miller, S. P., Tincani, M., Sileo, N. M., & Perkins, P. G. (2008). Effects of test-taking strategy instruction in high-functioning adolescents with autism spectrum disorders. *Focus on Autism and Other Developmental Disorders, 23*(4), 217–228.

South, M., Ozonoff, S., & McMahon, W. M. (2005). Repetitive behavior profiles in Asperger syndrome and high-functioning autism. *Journal of Autism and Developmental Disorders, 35,* 145–158.

Sparrow, S. S., Cicchetti, D. V., & Balla, D. A. (2005). *Vineland Adaptive Behavior Scales—Second Edition* (VABS-II). Circle Pines, MN: American Guidance Service.

Steege, M. W., & Watson, T. S. (2008). Best practices in functional behavioral assessment. In A. Thomas & J. Grimes (Eds.), *Best practices in school psychology: V* (pp. 337–348). Bethesda, MD: National Association of School Psychologists.

Steele, S. D., Minshew, N. J., Luna, B., & Sweeney, J. A. (2007). Spatial working memory deficits in autism. *Journal of Autism and Developmental Disorders, 37,* 605–612.

Stoiber, K. C., & Kratochwill, T. R. (2000). Empirically supported interventions and school psychology: Rationale and methodological issues: Part I. *School Psychology Quarterly, 15,* 75–105.

Stokes, T. F., & Baer, D. (1977). An implicit technology of generalization. *Journal of Applied Behavior Analysis, 10,* 349–367.

Sugai, G., & Horner, R. H. (2002). The evolution of discipline practices: School-wide positive behavior supports. *Child and Family Behavior Therapy, 24,* 23–50.

Sugai, G., Horner, R. H., Dunlap, G., Hieneman, M., Lewis, T. J., Nelson, C. M., et al. (2000). Applying positive behavioral support and functional behavioral assessment in schools. *Journal of Positive Behavior Interventions, 2,* 131–143.

Sugai, G., & Lewis, T. J. (1996). Preferred and promising practices for social skills instruction. *Focus on Exceptional Children, 29,* 11–27.

Sundbye, N. (1998). *Goal structure mapping.* Lawrence, KS: Curriculum Solutions.

Swanger-Gagne, M. S., Garbacz, S. A., Witte, A. L., Kunz, G. M., Gill-Hraban, K. A., & Sheridan, S. M. (2007, March/April). *Group-based conjoint behavioral consultation: Responsive support for students' needs.* Paper presented at the annual meeting of the National Association of School Psychologists, New York.

Thede, L. L., & Coolidge, F. L. (2007). Psychological and neurobehavioral comparisons of children with Asperger's disorder versus high-functioning autism. *Journal of Autism and Developmental Disorders, 37,* 847–854.

Thiemann, K. S., & Goldstein, H. (2001). Social Stories, written text cues, and video feedback: Effects on social communication of children with autism. *Journal of Applied Behavior Analysis, 34,* 425–446.

Tiger, J. S., Fisher, W. W., & Bouxsein, K. J. (2009). Therapist- and self-monitored DRO contingencies as a treatment for the self-injurious skin picking of a young man with Asperger syndrome. *Journal of Applied Behavior Analysis, 42,* 315–319.

Tilly, W. D., III. (2008). The evolution of school psychology to science-based practice: Problem solving and the three-tiered model. In A. Thomas & J. Grimes (Eds.), *Best practices in school psychology: V* (Vol. 1, pp. 17–36). Washington, DC: National Association of School Psychologists.

Tonge, B. J., Brereton, A. V., Gray, K. M., & Einfeld, S. L. (1999). Behavioural and emotional disturbance in high functioning autism and Asperger syndrome. *Autism, 3,* 117–130.

Turnbull, A., Edmundson, H., Griggs, P., Wickman, D., Sailor, W., Freeman, R., et al. (2002). A blueprint for schoolwide positive behavior support: Implementation of three components. *Exceptional Children, 68,* 377–402.

Turner, M. (1997). Towards an executive dysfunction account of repetitive behaviour in autism. In J. Russell (Ed.), *Autism as an executive disorder* (pp. 57–100). Oxford, UK: Oxford University Press.

Turner, M. A. (1999). Annotation: Repetitive behavior in autism: A review of psychological research. *Journal of Child Psychology and Psychiatry, 40,* 839–849.

Twachtman-Cullen, D., & Twachtman-Reilly, J. (2002). *How well does your IEP measure up?: Quality indicators for effective service delivery.* Higganum, CT: Starfish Specialty Press.

U.S. Department of Education Office of Special Education and Rehabilitation Services. (2000). A guide to the individualized education program. Retrieved May 1, 2009, from *www.ed.gov/parents/needs/speced/iepguide/index.html.*

VanDerHeyden, A. (2008). Best practices in can't do/won't do assessments. In A. Thomas & J. Grimes (Eds.), *Best practices in school psychology: V* (Vol. 2, pp. 131–140). Washington, DC: National Association of School Psychologists.

Vaughn, B. J., & Horner, R. H. (1997). Identifying instructional tasks that occasion problem behaviors and assessing the effects of student versus teacher choice making among these tasks. *Journal of Applied Behavior Analysis, 30,* 299–312.

Volkmar, F. R., & Klin, A. (2000). Diagnostic issues in Asperger syndrome. In A. Klin, F. R. Volkmar, & S. S. Sparrow (Eds.), *Asperger syndrome* (pp. 25–71). New York: Guilford Press.

Von Brock, M., & Elliott, S. N. (1987). Influence and treatment effectiveness information on the acceptability of classroom interventions. *Journal of School Psychology, 25,* 131–144.

Wahler, R. G., & Fox, J. J. (1981). Setting events in applied behavior analysis: Toward a conceptual and methodological expansion. *Journal of Applied Behavior Analysis, 14,* 327–338.

Wakefield, A. J. (1999). MMR vaccination and autism. *Lancet, 354,* 949–950.

Walker, H. M., Colvin, G., & Ramsey, E. (1995). *Antisocial behavior in schools: Strategies and best practices.* Pacific Grove, CA: Brooks/Cole.

Watkins, M. W. (2000). Cognitive profile analysis: A shared professional myth. *School Psychology Quarterly, 15,* 465–479.

Watkins, M. W. (2003). IQ subtest analysis: Clinical acumen or clinical illusion? *Scientific Review of Mental Health Practice, 2,* 118–141.

Watkins, M. W., & Guttling, J. J. (2000). Incremental validity of WISC-III profile evaluation, scatter, and shape information for predicting reading and math achievement. *Psychological Assessment, 12,* 402–408.

Wechsler, D. (1992). *Wechsler Individual Achievement Test* (WIAT). San Antonio, TX: Psychological Corporation.

Wechsler, D. (2001). *Wechsler Individual Achievement Test—Second Edition* (WIAT-II). San Antonio, TX: Psychological Corporation.

Wechsler, D. (2003). *Wechsler Intelligence Scale for Children—Fourth Edition* (WISC-IV). San Antonio, TX: Psychological Corporation.

Westby, C. (2004, March). *Reading between the lines for social and academic success.* Paper presented at the ninth annual autism spectrum disorders symposium, "Social and Academic Success for Students with ASD," Providence, RI.

Westling, D. L., & Fox, L. (2000). *Teaching students with severe disabilities* (2nd ed.). Englewood Cliffs, NJ: Prentice Hall.

White, O., & Liberty, K. (1976). Evaluation and measurement. In N. G. Haring & R. L. Schielfelbusch (Eds.), *Teaching special children* (pp. 31–69). New York: McGraw-Hill.

Wiederholt, J. C., & Bryant, B. R. (2001). *Gray Oral Reading Test—Fourth Edition* (GORT-4). Austin, TX: PRO-ED.

Wilczynski, S. M., Menousek, K., Hunter, M., & Mudgal, D. (2007). Individualized education programs for youth with autism spectrum disorders. *Psychology in the Schools, 44,* 653–666.

Wilkinson, L. A. (2005). Supporting the inclusion of a student with Asperger Syndrome: A case study of using conjoint behavioural consultation and self-management. *Educational Psychology in Practice, 21*(4), 307–326.

Wilkinson, L. A. (2008). Self-management for children with high-functioning autism spectrum disorders. *Intervention in School and Clinic, 43,* 150–157.

Williams, D., Goldstein, G., & Minshew, N. J. (2006). The profile of memory function in children with autism. *Neuropsychology, 20,* 21–29.

Wimmer, H., & Perner, J. (1983). Beliefs about beliefs: Representation and constraining function of wrong beliefs in young children's understanding of deception. *Cognition, 13,* 103–128.

Wing, L. (2000). Past and future of research on Asperger syndrome. In A. Klin, F. R. Volkmar, & S. S. Sparrow (Eds.), *Asperger syndrome* (pp. 418–432). New York: Guilford Press.

Wing, L., & Gould, J. (1979). Severe impairments of social interaction and associated abnormalities in children: Epidemiology and classification. *Journal of Autism and Developmental Disorders, 9,* 11–29.

Witt, J. C., & Elliott, S. N. (1985). Acceptability of classroom management strategies. In T. R. Kratochwill (Ed.), *Advances in school psychology* (Vol. 4, pp. 251–288). Hillsdale, NJ: Erlbaum.

Witt, J. C., Elliott, S. N., Daly, E. J., III, Gresham, F. M., & Kramer, J. J. (1998). *Assessment of at-risk and special needs children* (2nd ed.). Boston: McGraw Hill.

Wolf, M. M. (1978). Social validity: The case for subjective measurement or how applied behavior analysis is finding its heart. *Journal of Applied Behavior Analysis, 11,* 203–214.

Wolfberg, P. (2003). *Peer play and the autism spectrum: The art of guiding children's socialization and imagination.* Shawnee Mission, KS: Autism Asperger Publishing.

Wolfberg, P., & Schuler, A. L. (1993). Integrated play groups: A model for promoting the social and cognitive dimensions of play in children with autism. *Journal of Autism and Developmental Disorders, 23,* 467–489.

Wolfberg, P., & Schuler, A. L. (1999). Fostering peer interaction, imaginative play and spontaneous language in children with autism. *Child Language Teaching and Therapy, 15,* 41–52.

Womack, R. R. (2002). Autism and the Individuals with Disabilities Education Act: Are autistic children receiving appropriate treatment in our schools? *Texas Tech Law Review, 34,* 189–235.

Woodcock, R. W., McGrew, K. S., & Mather, N. (2001). *Woodcock–Johnson III* (WJ-III). Itasca, IL: Riverside.

Wright, P., & Wright, P. (2006). *Wrightslaw: From emotions to advocacy* (2nd ed.). Hartfield, VA: Harbor House Law Press.

Yang, T., Wolfberg, P., Wu, S., & Hwu, P. (2003). Supporting children on the autism spectrum in peer play at home and school. *Autism: The International Journal of Research and Practice, 7,* 437–453.

Yeargin-Allsopp, M., Rice, C., Karapurkan, T., Doernberg, N., Boyle, C., & Murphy, C. (2003). Prevalence of autism in a U.S. metropolitan area. *Journal of the American Medical Association, 289,* 49–55.

Yell, M. L., Meadows, N. B., Drasgow, E., & Shriner, J. G. (2009). *Evidence-based practice for educating students with emotional and behavioral disorders.* Upper Saddle River, NJ: Merrill.

Yell, M. L., Katsiyannis, A., Drasgow, E., & Herbst, M. (2003). Developing legally correct and educationally appropriate programs for students with autism spectrum disorders. *Focus on Autism and Other Developmental Disabilities, 18,* 182–191.

Zimmerman, S., & C. Hutchins. (2003). *Seven keys to comprehension: How to help your kids read it and get it!* New York: Three Rivers Press.

Index

Note. "f " following a page number indicates a figure; "t" following a page number indicates a table.

A–B–C recording, 191–192, 195f, 196f, 227–228
Abstraction, 8
Academic performance. *see also* Academic performance
    interventions
    assessment of, 51, 53–61, 55t, 58t
    central coherence and, 29
    overview, 21–23, 22f
    present level of performance (PLOP) in the IEP and,
        160–161
Academic performance interventions. *see also* Academic
    performance
    general strategies, 81–86, 83f
    overview, 80–81, 101
    specific strategies, 87–101, 88f, 90f, 91f, 92f–93f, 94t,
        97f, 99f, 100t
Achievement, 160–161. *see also* Academic performance
Adaptive behavior, 61–62
Adaptive Behavior Assessment System—Second Edition
    (ABAS-II), 62
All-Stars Character Education program, 130–131
Anaphoric cuing, 89–90, 90f
Anecdotal reports
    assessing social skills and, 73
    forms for, 227
    overview, 192
Antecedent–Behavior–Consequence (A–B–C) Checklist,
    228
Anxiety, 9, 24–25, 77–78
Applied behavior analysis (ABA) perspective, 40, 114–115
Asperger syndrome, 2–9
Asperger Syndrome Diagnostic Scale (ASDS), 63t, 75
Assessment. *see also* Data collection
    of academic skills, 53–61, 55t, 58t
    of behavioral skills, 61–62, 64–71, 66t
    conjoint behavioral consultation (CBC) and, 41–42
    of diagnostic characteristics, 62–64, 63t

    of emotional difficulties, 77–78
    forms for, 211–216
    goals and objectives on the IEP and, 164
    IEP goals and, 177
    of intellectual functioning, 48–51, 52t
    overview, 46, 78–79
    present level of performance (PLOP) in the IEP and, 158
    reinforcement and, 115
    school-based, 46–47
    social skills and, 71–77, 74t, 76t, 134–135
    task lists and, 83f, 85
    tools for, 50–51, 52t
Assignments. *see also* Homework; Task presentation
    assignment notebooks and, 86
    improving academic performance and, 84–85
    in mathematics, 98, 99f
    reinforcement and, 116
Attentional functioning
    academic performance and, 21–22, 22f, 81
    assessment of intellectual functioning and, 49
    executive functioning and, 27
    seating arrangements and, 82–84
Attention-deficit/hyperactivity disorder (ADHD), 9
Autism Diagnostic Interview—Revised (ADI-R), 63t
Autism Social Skills Profile (ASSP), 76t, 77
Autism spectrum disorders (ASD), 2, 9–11
Average-duration recording, 189–190

B

Background knowledge, 87–89, 88f
Behavior Assessment System for Children—Second
    Edition (BASC-2), 78
Behavior inhibition, 27, 28
Behavior intervention plan (BIP), 129

Behavioral concerns
    assessment of, 64–71, 65*f*, 66*t*
    assessment of adaptive behavior, 61–62
    core impairments and, 15*t*, 17–19
    data collection and, 183–197, 184*f*, 186*f*, 187*f*, 188*f*, 189*f*,
      191*f*, 192*f*, 193*f*–194*f*, 195*f*, 196*f*, 197*f*
    elementary school years, 5–6
    executive functioning and, 27
    middle/high school years and, 7–8
    overview, 102–103
Behavioral consultation, 38–39. *see also* Conjoint
    behavioral consultation (CBC); Consultation
Behavioral contracts, 118–120. *see also* Reinforcement
Behavioral supports
    direct intervention strategies, 113–125, 124*t*
    effective, 103
    overview, 102–103, 125
    preventative approaches, 104–112, 105*t*, 107*f*, 108*f*, 109*f*,
      110*f*–111*f*, 112*f*, 113*f*
Bias in data collection, 199–200
Brain growth, 27

C

CBA for instructional design (CBA-ID), 54. *see also*
    Curriculum-based assessment (CBA)
Central coherence, 28–29
Character education (CE), 130–131
Character Education Partnership (CEP), 130–131
Checklists
    data collection and, 195, 197*f*
    reinforcement and, 115–116
    visual supports and, 108–109, 109*f*, 110*f*
    writing support and, 96, 97*f*
Child Interview of Social Functioning form, 215–216
Children's Depression Inventory (CDI), 78
Children's Intervention Rating Profile (CIRP), 204–205
Choice, 106
Chronosystem, 33*f*, 34, 40
Circle of Friends network, 138
Clarifying strategy, 89
Classroom environment, 82–84, 104–105, 105*t*
Cognitive ability
    assessment of, 48–51, 52*t*
    central coherence and, 28–29
    definitions and issues and, 2–3
    executive functioning and, 27–28
    overview, 21–23, 22*f*
Collaboration. *see* Collaborative consultation
Collaborative consultation, 31–32, 36–37, 45. *see also*
    Conjoint behavioral consultation (CBC)
Collaborative problem solving, 35–36, 37–39
Communication, teacher, 82–84
Communication skills
    assessing social skills and, 74*t*
    assessment of adaptive behavior and, 61–62
    core impairments in, 15*t*, 19–20
    theory of mind and, 26
Community-based providers, 36–37

Comprehension
    academic performance and, 22*f*
    central coherence and, 29
    DIBELS and, 59
    reading support and, 89–90, 90*f*
Computer-based strategies, 151
Conflict resolution, 8
Conjoint behavioral consultation (CBC), 31–32, 38–39,
    40–43, 43–45. *see also* Behavioral consultation;
    Collaborative consultation; Consultation
Consequences, 67–68
Consultation, 37–38, 45. *see also* Collaborative
    consultation
Contingency agreements, 118–120. *see also* Reinforcement
Contingent positive reinforcement, 114–118
Contracts, behavioral, 118–120. *see also* Reinforcement
Criterion-referenced CBA (CR-CBA), 54, 58*t*. *see also*
    Curriculum-based assessment (CBA)
Curriculum-based assessment (CBA), 54, 56–61, 58*t*
Curriculum-based assessment for instructional design
    (CBA-ID), 58*t*
Curriculum-based evaluation (CBE), 54, 56, 58*t*, 60–61.
    see also Curriculum-based assessment (CBA)
Curriculum-based measurement (CBM), 54, 56–57, 58*t*,
    60. *see also* Curriculum-based assessment (CBA)

D

Daily living skills, 61–62
Data collection. *see also* Assessment; Data evaluation
    action plan for, 195, 197
    factors that influence, 199–200
    forms for, 221–229
    graphing of data, 200–201
    how much data to collect, 198–199, 198*f*
    importance of, 182–183
    overview, 181, 207
    process of, 183–197, 184*f*, 186*f*, 187*f*, 188*f*, 189*f*, 191*f*,
      192*f*, 193*f*–194*f*, 195*f*, 196*f*, 197*f*
Data evaluation. *see also* Data collection
    forms for, 221–229
    graphing of data, 200–201
    methods for, 201–205, 202*f*, 203*f*, 204*f*
    overview, 181, 207
Data-based decision making, 181, 207. *see also* Data
    collection; Data evaluation
Decision making, 130. *see also* Problem-solving skills
Depression
    assessment and, 77–78
    middle/high school years and, 7
    overview, 9, 24–25
Developmental course
    behavioral concerns, 18
    brain growth and, 27
    language development, 19
    overview, 4–9
Diagnosis
    core impairments and, 14–20, 15*t*
    definitions and issues regarding, 2–3

developmental course of HFA/AS and, 6
present level of performance (PLOP) in the IEP and, 158
Diagnostic and Statistical Manual of Mental Disorders (DSM-IV-TR), 2–3, 14
Diagnostic characteristics of HFA/AS, 62–64, 63*t*
Differential Ability Scales—Second Edition (DAS-II), 52*t*
Differential reinforcement strategies, 117–118. *see also* Reinforcement
Direct instruction, 94–95
Do2Learn program, 132
Duration recording, 189–190, 191*f*, 193*f*, 223, 225
Dynamic Indicators of Basic Early Literacy Skills (DIBELS), 54, 56, 57–60, 58*t*, 162–163

E

Ecobehavioral consultation, 38–39. *see also* Consultation
Ecological model
    conjoint behavioral consultation (CBC) and, 40
    intervention-based assessment and, 47
    overview, 32–34, 33*f*
    stakeholders and, 34–37
Educational placement, 10–11, 163–175, 170*t*
Effect size, 203–204, 204*f*
Efficacious interventions, 42
Elementary school, 5–6
Emotion regulation, 8, 28
Emotions, 17–18, 26, 77–78
Environmental modifications, 70–71, 104–105, 105*t*, 206
Evaluation
    conjoint behavioral consultation (CBC) and, 42–43
    example of, 44–45
    individualized education program and, 155–157, 156*f*
    social skills training and, 134–135
Evaluation of data. *see* Data evaluation
Evidence-based interventions, 42
Executive functioning, 27–28, 48–49
Exosystem in the ecological model, 32, 33*f*, 40. *see also* Ecological model
Expectancy in data collection, 199–200
Expectations, 109, 111*f*
Experimental analyses, 70–71
Extended school year (ESY) services, 176–177

F

Facial expressions, 16, 26
Fine-motor skills, 24
First…, Then… boards, 112, 113*f*
Five-step problem-solving consultation model, 38–39. *see also* Problem-solving consultation model
Flexible thinking, 49
Free, appropriate public education (FAPE)
    individualized education program and, 154–155, 156–157
    progress monitoring and, 178
    service delivery and, 169, 171–172
Frequency recording, 185, 186*f*, 221

Friendships, 16–17. *see also* Peer relationships
Functional analysis, 70–71
Functional behavioral assessment (FBA)
    behavioral supports and, 113–114
    overview, 64–71, 65*f*, 66*t*
    replacement behaviors and, 113–114
    schoolwide positive behavior support (SWPBS), 128–129
    Social Stories and, 144, 145
Functional performance, 161–162

G

Generalization, 205–207
Gestures, 16
Gilliam Asperger's Disorder Scale (GADS), 63*t*, 75
Gilliam Autism Rating Scale—Second Edition (GARS), 63*t*
Goal setting, 123, 125
Goal structure mapping, 89
Goals, IEP, 164–169, 170*t*, 176–177
Graphic organizers, 88–89, 88*f*, 91–94, 92*f*–93*f*
Gray Center for Social Learning, 144–145, 144*t*
Gray Oral Reading Test—Fourth Edition (GORT-4), 54, 55*t*
Gross-motor skills, 24
Group interventions, 133–143, 134*t*, 136*t*, 139*t*, 142*t*

H

Handwriting skills, 95–96
Health professionals, 36–37
High school, 7–8
High-functioning autism, 2–11
Home Base, 105, 105*t*
Homework, 85–86. *see also* Assignments

I

Idioms, 26
IEP Program Planning Matrix, 220
"IFEED rules", 114–115. *see also* Reinforcement
Impairment. *see also specific areas of impairment*
    associated areas of, 20–25, 22*f*
    core areas of, 14–20, 15*t*
    overview, 14, 29–30
    theoretical perspectives regarding, 25–29
Impulsive behavior, 27
Inattentiveness. *see* Attentional functioning
Independent functioning, 61–62
Individual interventions
    schoolwide positive behavior support (SWPBS), 128–129, 129*f*
    social skills training and, 143–149, 144*t*, 147*t*
Individualized education program (IEP)
    forms for, 218–220
    goals and objectives on, 164–169, 170*t*
    intervention/instructional planning and, 163–175, 170*t*
    overview, 153–155, 180

Individualized education program (IEP) *(cont.)*
  problem analysis and, 162–163
  problem identification, 157–162, 159*t*
  as a problem-solving vehicle, 155–157, 156*f*
  progress monitoring and, 176–178
  tools for enhancing, 178–180, 179*f*
Individuals with Disabilities Education Act (IDEA)
  assessment and, 47
  individualized education program and, 154–155, 180
  present level of performance (PLOP) in the IEP and, 160
  prevalence of HFA/AS and, 10–11
  service delivery and, 169, 171–172
Information processing, 28–29, 49
Instruction, 94–95, 131–133. *see also* Interventions
Instructional consultation, 38–39. *see also* Consultation
Instructional planning, 163–175, 170*t*
Integrated play groups (IPG), 138–140, 139*t*
Intellectual functioning, 48–51, 52*t*. *see also* Cognitive ability
Interests
  academic performance and, 21–22
  assignments and, 85
  central coherence and, 29
  core impairments and, 17–19
  core impairments in, 15*t*
Interval recording
  forms for, 222
  overview, 185, 187–189, 187*f*, 188*f*, 189*f*
Intervention Rating Profile (IRP-15), 204–205
Intervention-based assessment, 47
Interventions. *see also* Academic performance interventions; Behavioral supports; Social skills interventions
  behavioral support and, 113–125, 124*t*
  conjoint behavioral consultation (CBC) and, 42
  data collection and, 198–199, 198*f*
  to improve academic performance, 80–101, 83*f*
  individualized education program and, 163–175, 170*t*
  preventative approaches, 104–112, 105*t*, 107*f*, 108*f*, 109*f*, 110*f*–111*f*, 112*f*, 113*f*
  reading support, 87–95, 88*f*, 90*f*, 91*f*, 92*f*–93*f*, 94*t*
  self-management and, 122–125, 124*f*
  writing support, 95–97, 97*f*
Interviews, 68–69, 72
IQ measures, 48–50, 51, 53
Irony, theory of mind and, 26
Isolation, 7

J

Jackpot Online Reinforcement Survey tool, 116
Job cards, 85
Jokes, theory of mind and, 26

K

Kaufman Assessment Battery for Children—Second Edition (KABC-II), 52*t*

Kaufman Tests of Educational Achievement—Second Edition (KTEA-II), 53–54, 55*t*
Key Math Diagnostic Arithmetic Test—Third Edition (KeyMath-3), 54, 55*t*
Keystone method of analysis, 162–163
Krug Asperger's Disorder Index (KADI), 63*t*

L

Language functioning, 15*t*, 19–20
Large-group instruction, 131–133
Latency recording, 190–191, 192*f*, 194*f*, 224, 226
Least restrictive environment (LRE), 173
Leiter International Performance Scale—Revised (Leiter-R), 52*t*
LifeStories for Kids series, 130–131
Literal interpretations, 20

M

Macrosystem in the ecological model, 32, 33*f*, 40. *see also* Ecological model
Maintenance, 205
Math skills, 57, 97–101, 99*f*, 100*t*
Mean level, 201, 202*f*
Mental flexibility, 27
Mental health needs, 9, 36–37, 77–78. *see also* Anxiety; Attention-deficit/hyperactivity disorder (ADHD); Depression
Mental health professionals/consultation, 37, 38–39. *see also* Consultation
Mesosystem in the ecological model, 32, 33, 33*f*, 40. *see also* Ecological model
Microsystem in the ecological model, 32–33, 33*f*, 40. *see also* Ecological model
Middle school, 7–8
Mindblindness, 16, 26
Mnemonic strategies, 96
Modeling, 89, 145–148, 147*t*, 148–149
Model–lead–test teaching procedure, 94–95
Monotropism, 28–29
Motivators, 115–116. *see also* Reinforcement
Motor abilities, 24
Motor mannerisms, 15*t*, 17–19, 49
Motor skills, 61–62
Multidimensional Anxiety Scale for Children (MASC), 76*t*
Multi-tiered approach to prevention, 38. *see also* Prevention

N

Narrative Antecedent–Behavior–Consequence (A–B–C) Form, 227
National Autism Center, 42
Needs identification and analysis, 41–42, 44, 162–163. *see also* Problem analysis; Problem identification
Negative reinforcement, 114–115. *see also* Reinforcement
No Child Left Behind Act, 160, 171

Nonliterary language, 26
Nonverbal communication, 16, 48–49
Note taking, 85–86

O

Objectives, IEP, 164–169, 170*t*
Observation of Appropriate Social Interaction Skills
    (OASIS), 195, 197*f*, 229
Observational assessment
    assessing social skills and, 72–74, 74*t*
    functional behavioral assessment (FBA) and, 64–71, 65*f*,
        66*t*
    reinforcement and, 115
Observer drift in data collection, 199–200
Obsessive interests. *see* Interests
Occupational therapists, 36. *see also* School personnel
Oral reading fluency, 57
Organizational consultation, 38–39. *see also* Consultation
Organizational skills, 21–22, 22*f*, 59–60
Outcomes of individuals with HFA/AS, 9, 176–178

P

Parent Interview of Social Functioning form, 211–212
Parents, 34–35
PDD Behavior Inventory (PDDBI), 63*t*
Peer Buddies Sociometric form, 217
Peer buddy systems, 140–143, 142*t*
Peer relationships, 6, 15*t*. *see also* Relationships with peers
Peer-mediated approaches, 137–143, 139*t*, 142*t*
Percentage of nonoverlapping data (PND), 202–203, 203*f*
Performance, 27, 135. *see also* Academic performance
Personal space, 16–17
Perspective taking, 74*t*
Physical therapists, 36. *see also* School personnel
Picture Exchange Communication System (PECS), 171
Picture walk strategy, 88–89
Placement, educational, 10–11, 163–175, 170*t*
Plan implementation, 42, 44–45, 155–157, 156*f*
Planning skills, 21–22, 22*f*, 27
Play groups, 138–140, 139*t*
PLEP in the IEP. *see* Present level of educational
    performance (PLEP) in the IEP
PLOP in the IEP. *see* Present level of performance (PLOP)
    in the IEP
Power Cards, 148–149, 150*f*
Praise, 114–115. *see also* Reinforcement
Preconsultation step, 39. *see also* Problem-solving
    consultation model
Predicting strategy, 89
Preference, 106
Preschool years, 4–5
Present level of educational performance (PLEP) in the
    IEP, 157
Present level of performance (PLOP) in the IEP, 157–162,
    159*t*, 177–178
President's Commission on Excellence in Special
    Education, 154

Prevalence of HFA/AS, 9–11
Prevention, 37–38, 59, 104–112, 105*t*, 107*f*, 108*f*, 109*f*,
    110*f*–111*f*, 112*f*, 113*f*
Primary interventions, 128–133, 129*f*
Priming, 84, 87–89, 88*f*, 148–149
Problem analysis. *see also* Needs identification and
    analysis
    conjoint behavioral consultation (CBC) and, 41–42
    individualized education program and, 155–157, 156*f*,
        162–163
Problem identification. *see also* Needs identification and
    analysis
    data collection and, 183–184
    individualized education program and, 155–157, 156*f*,
        157–162, 159*t*
    overview, 39
Problem-solving consultation model. *see also* Collaborative
    consultation
    collaborative problem solving and, 37–39
    individualized education program and, 155–157, 156*f*
    overview, 31–32
    stakeholders and, 35–36
Problem-solving skills
    academic performance and, 21–22, 22*f*, 23
    Character Education Partnership (CEP) and, 130
    executive functioning and, 27
    middle/high school years and, 8
Program planning, 178–180, 179*f*, 220
Progress monitoring
    curriculum-based evaluation (CBE) and, 60–61
    goals and objectives on the IEP and, 166–168
    individualized education program and, 176–178
    social skills training and, 137
Prosody, 20

Q

Questioning strategy, 89
Questioning students in assessment, 68–69

R

Rating scales, 74–77, 76*t*
Reactivity in data collection, 199–200
Reading skills
    academic performance and, 22*f*
    central coherence and, 29
    DIBELS and, 59
    improving, 87–95, 88*f*, 90*f*, 91*f*, 92*f*–93*f*, 94*t*
Reasoning skills, 8
Reciprocity, 16
Reinforcement, 114–118, 136
Rejection. *see* Social rejection
Relationships with peers, 6, 15*t*
Remediation goal, 37–38
Repetitive movements, 15*t*, 17–19
Replacement behaviors, 113–114, 167
Research-based treatments, 42
Responses to sensory stimuli, 20–21

Responsiveness, 74*t*
Retelling, 59–60
Revised Children's Manifest Anxiety Scale—Second
    Edition (RCMAS-2), 78
Rewards, 115–116, 136. *see also* Reinforcement
Reynolds Adolescent Depression Scale—Second Edition
    (RADS-2), 78
Rigidity, 15*t*, 17–19
Rituals, 4, 15*t*, 24–25. *see also* Routines
Routines. *see also* Schedules
    anxiety and, 24–25
    core impairments and, 15*t*
    Home Base and, 105, 105*t*
    preschool years and, 4
    visual supports and, 106–112, 107*f*, 108*f*, 109*f*,
        110*f*–111*f*, 112*f*, 113*f*
Rubrics, 195, 218–219
Rules, 109, 111*f*

S

Sarcasm, 26
Scaffolding, 140
Scales of Independent Behavior—Revised (SIB-R), 62
Schedules. *see also* Routines
    behavioral support and, 104–105
    visual supports and, 106–112, 107*f*, 108*f*, 109*f*,
        110*f*–111*f*, 112*f*, 113*f*
School personnel, 35–36
School-based assessment, 46–47. *see also* Assessment
School-based services, 32–34, 33*f*, 127–128, 128–133,
    129*f*
Schoolwide positive behavior support (SWPBS), 128–130,
    129*f*
Second Step program, 132
Secondary interventions
    schoolwide positive behavior support (SWPBS),
        128–129, 129*f*
    social skills training and, 133–143, 134*t*, 136*t*, 139*t*, 142*t*
Self-awareness, 130
Self-control skills, 8
Self-evaluation, 123, 125
Self-management strategies
    Character Education Partnership (CEP) and, 130
    reinforcement and, 119–120, 122–125, 124*f*
    writing support and, 96
Self-monitoring, 105
Self-regulated strategy development (SRSD) instruction,
    96–97
Self-regulation, 27, 28
Self-reinforcement, 123, 125
Self-Report of Personality Interview (SRP-I), 78
Self-Report of Personality (SRP), 78
Self-stimulatory behaviors, 17–19, 28
Semantic maps, 91–94, 92*f*–93*f*, 96
Sensory stimuli, 20–21
Service delivery
    conjoint behavioral consultation (CBC) and, 40–41
    individualized education program and, 169, 171–172

stakeholders and, 34–37
trends in, 10–11
Setting event, 33
Shifting attention, 49. *see also* Attentional functioning
Simplicity in data collection, 199–200
Sleep disturbances, 23–24
Small-group interventions
    schoolwide positive behavior support (SWPBS),
        128–129, 129*f*
    social skills training and, 133–143, 134*t*, 136*t*, 139*t*, 142*t*
SMART IEP goals, 165–169, 170*t*
Social Anxiety Scale for Children—Revised (SASC-R), 76*t*
Social Anxiety Scale—Adolescent (SAS-A), 76*t*
Social Communication Questionnaire (SCQ), 76*t*
Social interactions, 74*t*
Social learning theory, 145–146
Social play, 74*t*
Social rejection, 4–5, 17
Social responsiveness, 74*t*
Social Responsiveness Scale (SRS), 75, 76*t*
Social skills. *see also* Social skills interventions
    anxiety and, 25
    assessment and, 49, 61–62, 71–77, 74*t*, 76*t*
    core impairments in, 15–17, 15*t*
    elementary school years, 6
    mental health needs and, 77
    middle/high school years and, 7
    theory of mind and, 26
Social Skills Improvement System (SSIS), 75–77, 76*t*
Social skills interventions. *see also* Social skills
    forms for, 217
    future of, 149, 151
    individual interventions and, 143–149, 144*t*, 147*t*
    overview, 126–127, 151–152
    school-based programs for, 127–128
    schoolwide (primary) approaches, 128–133, 129*f*
    small-group (secondary) approaches, 133–143, 134*t*,
        136*t*, 139*t*, 142*t*
Social Skills Rating Scales (SSRS), 75–77
Social skills training (SST) programs, 131–133, 135–137,
    136*t*. *see also* Social skills interventions
Social Stories, 143–145, 144*t*, 182
Social validity, 204–205
Special education services
    educational placement and, 172–175
    free, appropriate public education (FAPE) and, 154–155
    prevalence of HFA/AS and, 10–11
    referrals for, 5–6
    service delivery and, 169, 171–172
Speech features, 20. *see also* Communication skills;
    Language functioning
Speech pathologists, 35–36. *see also* School personnel
Spelling, 96
Stakeholders, 34–37
Stimulus generalization, 206
Strengths, 159–160
Stress cards, 109, 112, 112*f*
Strong Kids program, 132
Student support services personnel, 35–36. *see also* School
    personnel

Study skills, 85–86
Summarizing strategy, 89
Surveys, 115–116
Systematic environmental manipulations, 70–71
Systematic experimental analyses, 70–71
Systematic interventions, 134, 135–137, 136*t*
Systematic observations, 73–74, 74*t*. *see also* Observational assessment

T

Tantrums, 109, 112, 112*f*, 143–144
Task initiation, 27
Task lists, 83*f*, 85
Task presentation. *see also* Assignments
  improving academic performance and, 81–82, 83*f*
  in mathematics, 98, 99*f*
  visual supports and, 106–112, 107*f*, 108*f*, 109*f*, 110*f*–111*f*, 112*f*, 113*f*
Teacher communication, 82–84
Teacher Interview of Social Functioning form, 213–214
Team Social Stories, 144–145, 144*t*
Technology, 151, 200–201
Temper tantrums, 109, 112, 112*f*, 143–144
Tertiary supports, 128–129, 129*f*
Test of Written Language—Fourth Edition (TOWL-4), 54, 55*t*
Test taking, 86, 101
Text structure, 94, 94*t*
Theory of mind, 25–27
Think-aloud strategy, 89
Timed tasks, 101
Token economies, 120–122, 136. *see also* Reinforcement
Tone of voice, 16, 20
Total-duration recording, 189–190
Transition planning, 175
Treatment, 42
Treatment Evaluation Inventory (TEI), 204–205

Treatment planning, 40–41, 42
Trends, 201, 202*f*

U

Universal Nonverbal Intelligence Test (UNIT), 52*t*

V

Validity, social, 204–205
Verbal skills, 48–49
Video modeling, 145–148, 147*t*
Vineland Adaptive Behavior Scales—Second Edition (VABS-II), 62
Visual analysis of data, 201–205, 202*f*, 203*f*, 204*f*
Visual supports
  as a preventative behavioral support, 106–112, 107*f*, 108*f*, 109*f*, 110*f*–111*f*, 112*f*, 113*f*
  self-management and, 123, 125
Vocabulary, 82, 83*f*

W

Weaknesses, 159–160
Wechsler Individual Achievement Test (WIAT), 53, 54, 55*t*
Whole-class instruction, 131–133
Wings for Kids program, 132
Woodcock–Johnson Tests of Academic Achievement—Third Edition (WJ-III), 53–54, 55*t*
Woodcock–Johnson Tests of Cognitive Abilities—Third Edition (WJ-III COG), 52*t*
Word problems in mathematics, 98–99, 100*t*
Word use fluency, 59
Working memory, 27, 49
Writing support, 95–97, 97*f*
Written expression, 57